Download Your Included Ebook Today!

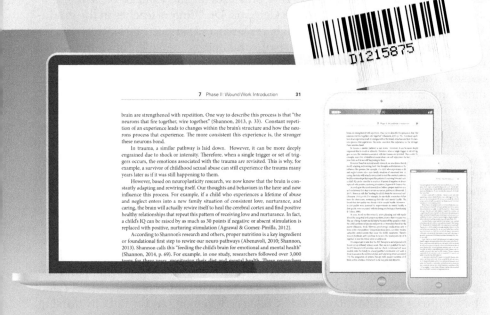

Your print purchase of *Rural Nursing: Concepts, Theory, and Practice*, 5e, **includes an ebook download** to the device of your choice—increasing accessibility, portability, and searchability!

Download your ebook today at:
http://spubonline.com/ruralnurs
and enter the access code below:

14X6KN5DG

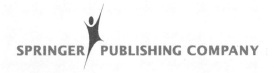

SPRINGER PUBLISHING COMPANY

SPC

springerpub.com

Charlene A. Winters, PhD, RN, is a professor in the College of Nursing at Montana State University, Missoula Campus. Dr. Winters teaches in the graduate program and is actively engaged in research and service. She teaches courses on evidence-based practice and care of rural and vulnerable populations. Her research focuses on the health of rural populations—rural nursing practice, rural nursing theory development, adaptation to and self-management of chronic illness by rural dwellers, and response to environmental exposures in rural communities. She is an active member of the Rural Nurse Organization, the Western Institute of Nursing, Sigma Theta Tau International, the Council for the Advancement of Nursing Science, and is a charter member of the International Council of Nursing—Rural and Remote Nurses Network. She holds a PhD in nursing from Rush University, College of Nursing, Chicago, Illinois, and BSN and MSN degrees in nursing from California State University, Long Beach.

Helen J. Lee, PhD, RN, is professor emerita in the College of Nursing, Montana State University, Missoula Campus. She continues her research interests in rural nursing theory and end-of-life issues. Her professional memberships include the Rural Nurse Organization, the National Rural Health Association, and the Zeta Upsilon Chapter of Sigma Theta Tau International. She holds BSN and MSN degrees from Montana State College, Bozeman, and a PhD in nursing from the University of Texas at Austin.

Rural Nursing
Concepts, Theory, and Practice

FIFTH EDITION

Charlene A. Winters, PhD, RN

Helen J. Lee, PhD, RN

Editors

SPRINGER PUBLISHING COMPANY

Springer Publishing Company, LLC
11 West 42nd Street
New York, NY 10036
www.springerpub.com

Acquisitions Editor: Elizabeth Nieginski
Associate Managing Editor: Kris Parrish
Compositor: diacriTech, Chennai

ISBN: 978-0-8261-6167-3
ebook ISBN: 978-0-8261-6161-0
Instructor's PowerPoints ISBN: 978-0-8261-6181-9

Instructor's Materials: Qualified instructors may request supplements by emailing
textbook@springerpub.com

18 19 20 21 22 / 5 4 3 2 1

The author and the publisher of this Work have made every effort to use sources believed to be reliable to provide information that is accurate and compatible with the standards generally accepted at the time of publication. Because medical science is continually advancing, our knowledge base continues to expand. Therefore, as new information becomes available, changes in procedures become necessary. We recommend that the reader always consult current research and specific institutional policies before performing any clinical procedure. The author and publisher shall not be liable for any special, consequential, or exemplary damages resulting, in whole or in part, from the readers' use of, or reliance on, the information contained in this book. The publisher has no responsibility for the persistence or accuracy of URLs for external or third-party Internet websites referred to in this publication and does not guarantee that any content on such websites is, or will remain, accurate or appropriate.

Library of Congress Cataloging-in-Publication Data
Names: Winters, Charlene A., editor. | Lee, Helen J. (Helen Jacobsen), 1935-
    editor,
Title: Rural nursing: concepts, theory, and practice / [edited by] Charlene
    A. Winters, Helen J. Lee.
Other titles: Rural nursing (Lee)
Description: Fifth edition. | New York, NY: Springer Publishing Company,
    LLC, [2018] | Includes bibliographical references and index.
Identifiers: LCCN 2017056806| ISBN 9780826161673 | ISBN 9780826161710 (ebook)
    | ISBN 9780826161819 (Instructor's PowerPoints)
Subjects: | MESH: Community Health Nursing | Rural Health Services | Rural
    Population | Rural Health
Classification: LCC RT120.R87 | NLM WY 106 | DDC 610.73/43—dc23 LC record available at
    https://lccn.loc.gov/2017056806

Printed in the United States of America.

Contents

---

*Deceased

Contributors

Robin L. Boland, MN, RN, FNP-C Nurse Practitioner, Primary Care Associates, Great Falls, Montana

Victoria Britson, PhD, APRN, CNP, FNP-BC, CNE Assistant Professor/Site Coordinator, College of Nursing, South Dakota State University, Terrance Sullivan Health Science Center, University Center, Sioux Falls, South Dakota

Janice A. Buehler, PhD, RN Associate Professor (retired), Montana State University College of Nursing, Billings, Montana

Ekaterina Burduli, PhD, MS Postdoctoral Research Associate, Washington State University Elson S. Floyd College of Medicine Program of Excellence in Addictions Research, Spokane, Washington

Christy Buttler-Nelson, MN, RN Assistant Clinical Professor, Montana State University College of Nursing, Great Falls, Montana

Renae Christensen, BSN, RN Charge Nurse, Coeducation Coordinator and Pharmacy Technician, Sanford Hospital; Paramedic, Christensen Ambulance Service, Inc., Webster, South Dakota

Jo Ann Walsh Dotson, PhD, MSN, RN Associate Professor and Assistant Dean of Assessment and Evaluation, Washington State University College of Nursing, Program of Excellence in Addictions Research, Spokane, Washington

Becka Foerster, MS, RN Instructor, South Dakota State University College of Nursing, Brookings, South Dakota

Rayn Ginnaty, BSN, MBA, RN Benefis Hospitals, Vice President of Nursing, Great Falls, Montana

Ruiling Guo, DHA, MPH, MLIS, AHIP Associate Professor, Health Care Administration Program, Kasiska School of Health Professions, Division of Health Sciences, Idaho State University, Pocatello, Idaho

Lori Hendrickx, EdD, RN, CCRN, CNL   Professor, South Dakota State University College of Nursing, Brookings, South Dakota

Tanis Hernandez, MSW, LCSW   Formerly Administrative Director, Center for Asbestos Related Disease, Libby, Montana

Barbara B. Hobbs, PhD, RN   Assistant Dean and Associate Professor, West River Nursing Department, South Dakota State University, Rapid City, South Dakota

Laurie J. Johansen, PhD, MS, RN   Chair/Director of Nursing and Associate Professor, Southwest Minnesota State University, Marshall, Minnesota

Elizabeth Kinion, EdD, MSN, RN, FAAN   Professor, Montana State University College of Nursing, Bozeman, Montana

Sandra W. Kuntz, PhD, RN   Associate Professor and Campus Director, Montana State University College of Nursing, Kalispell, Montana

Helen J. Lee, PhD, RN   Professor Emerita, Montana State University College of Nursing, Missoula, Montana

Kathleen A. Long, PhD, APRN, FAAN   Dean and Professor (retired), University of Florida, College of Nursing, Gainesville, Florida

D. "Dale" M. Mayer, PhD, RN   Assistant Professor, Montana State University College of Nursing, Missoula, Montana

Meg K. McDonagh, MN, RN, GNP   Senior Lecturer (Emerita), University of Calgary Faculty of Nursing, Calgary, Alberta, Canada

Sterling McPherson, PhD, MS   Associate Professor and Director for Biostatistics and Clinical Trial Design, Washington State University, Elson S. Floyd College of Medicine, Program of Excellence in Addictions Research, Spokane, Washington

Heidi A. Mennenga, PhD, RN   Associate Professor, South Dakota State University College of Nursing, Brookings, South Dakota

Deana L. Molinari, PhD, RN   Professor (retired), Idaho State University School of Nursing, Pocatello, Idaho

Sheila Ray Montgomery, EdD, MSN, RN   Adjunct Faculty, Becker College, Worcester, Massachusetts

Elizabeth Nichols, PhD, RN Dean and Professor (retired), Montana State University College of Nursing, Bozeman, Montana

Mary Kay Nissen, DNP, APRN, CNP, FNP-BC, COHN-S Clinical Associate Professor, College of Nursing, South Dakota State University, Terrance Sullivan Health Science Center, Sioux Falls, South Dakota

Chad O'Lynn, PhD, RN, CNE, ANEF Director of Evaluation and Innovation, Chamberlain College of Nursing, Downers Grove, Illinois

Judith M. Paré, PhD, RN Director of Education, Workforce Quality and Safety, Massachusetts Nurses Association, Canton, Massachusetts

Polly Petersen, PhD, RN Assistant Professor, Montana State University College of Nursing, Billings, Montana

Susan Wallace Raph, DNP, RN, NEA-BC Campus Director and Associate Clinical Professor, Montana State University College of Nursing, Great Falls, Montana

Andrea Rasmussen, MN, APRN, PMHNP CPG Psychiatry, Missoula, Montana

K. M. Reeder, PhD, RN, FAHA Professor/Associate Dean for Research, College of Nursing, South Dakota State University, Brookings, South Dakota

Marlene Reimer, PhD, RN, CNN(C) [Deceased] Professor, University of Calgary, Faculty of Nursing, Calgary, Alberta, Canada

Jane A. Schantz, MS, FNP-BC, ACHPN Clinical Instructor, Decker School of Nursing, Binghamton University, Binghamton, New York

Jane Ellis Scharff, MN, RN Associate Clinical Professor and Campus Director, Montana State University College of Nursing, Bozeman, Montana

Dayle Boynton Sharp, PhD, DNP, MPH, APRN, FNP-BC Clinical Associate Professor, Director of Family Practitioner Program, Department of Nursing, University of New Hampshire, Durham, New Hampshire

Jenifer Show, DNP, RN, CFNP, Fort Belknap Tribal Health 669, Fort Belknap, Montana

Jean Shreffler-Grant, PhD, RN Professor, Montana State University College of Nursing, Missoula, Montana

Jane Smilie, MPH   Owner, Population Health Partners, LLC, Helena, Montana

Marilyn A. Swan, PhD, RN   Assistant Professor, Minnesota State University School of Nursing, Mankato, Minnesota

Tamara L. Tasseff, MA, RN   Jonas Veterans Healthcare Scholar, Idaho State University School of Nursing, Pocatello, Idaho

Susan S. Tavernier, PhD, APRN-CNS, AOCN   Assistant Professor, Idaho State University School of Nursing, Pocatello, Idaho

Linda M. Torma, PhD, APRN, GCNS-BC   Assistant Professor (retired), Montana State University College of Nursing, Missoula, Montana

Gail M. Wagnild, PhD, RN   Principal, The Resilience Center, Billings, Montana

Clarann Weinert, SC, PhD, RN, FAAN   Professor Emerita, Montana State University College of Nursing, Bozeman, Montana

Charlene A. Winters, PhD, RN   Professor, Montana State University College of Nursing, Missoula, Montana

Jana G. Zwilling, MS, APRN, FNP-C   Clinical Assistant Professor, Director, FNP Program, University of North Dakota College of Nursing and Professional Disciplines, Grand Forks, North Dakota

Foreword

Winters and Lee continue to be the first-line resource toward understanding rural nursing and the interface with culture, health, health beliefs, and healthcare in rural populations. Whether you are developing and disseminating knowledge about rural health and nursing, or learning about rural dwellers or practicing rural nursing, there is much to gain from reading this latest edition of *Rural Nursing: Concepts, Theory, and Practice* (5th ed.). Multiple new chapters are presented in each section. This book highlights the realities of rural nursing from bedside to advanced practice. Community and acute care settings for rural healthcare are examined. Theoretical perspectives, as well as new models of practice and research, are found in this edition. Winters and Lee support rural nurses not only by identifying the challenges, but also by highlighting opportunities in rural healthcare and innovative practice.

The relevance of this text on the development of rural nursing over the past few decades is apparent from the perspective of a nursing educator, researcher, and editor of a journal focusing on rural nursing and healthcare. This text is a staple in graduate nursing education in the rural nursing PhD program at Binghamton University. As an editor, I feel confident that this book and the chapters within are some of the most often cited in the rural nursing literature. Winters and Lee have been, and I am sure will continue to be, in the lexicon of rural nursing.

Pamela Stewart Fahs, PhD, RN
Associate Dean
Professor and Dr. G. Clifford and Florence B. Decker Chair in Rural Nursing
Decker School of Nursing, Binghamton University
Binghamton, New York
Editor-in-Chief, Online Journal of Rural Nursing and Health Care

Preface

The fifth edition of *Rural Nursing: Concepts, Theory, and Practice*, like the editions before it, focuses on the health of rural dwellers, the provision of healthcare in rural settings, and the skills and knowledge required for effective nursing practice, education, and research required within this context.

The genesis of the rural text originated from a vision of Dr. Anna Shannon, dean of the College of Nursing at Montana State University. She was well aware of the early work on nursing theories and noted that little emphasis was placed on environment, and when examining the literature, she found an absence of rural nursing articles. Shortly thereafter, a master's degree program focused on rural nursing was established at Montana State University College of Nursing with a strong emphasis on rural nursing theory. The theory development process grew through the efforts of College of Nursing graduate students, faculty, administrators, and help from consultants. Interviews of rural persons throughout the state of Montana were examined for concepts that frequently emerged from the data. This qualitative material, linked with quantitative studies, led to the theory article published in 1989 by Dr. Kathleen Long and Dr. Clarann Weinert (see Chapter 2). The first edition of the rural text was titled *Conceptual Basis for Rural Nursing* and consisted of chapters written by faculty and students of Montana State University College of Nursing. Subsequent editions were retitled, *Rural Nursing: Concepts, Theory, and Practice*. Each new edition continued to include material written by faculty and students, and then expanded to include authors from across the United States, Canada, and Australia. More than four decades have passed since the College of Nursing developed a master's program that focused on the care of individuals living in a rural/remote environment. Since that time, a doctor of nursing practice (DNP) program with family nurse practitioner and psychiatric/mental health nurse practitioner options has been added to the curriculum at Montana State University College of Nursing to prepare nurses to care for rural and frontier populations.

The four published editions have recorded the progress of our work and the expansion of content beyond Montana to the United States and beyond our borders. The extension of the content areas and the countries represented demonstrate the book's importance to nurse educators, researchers, clinicians, and policymakers. The fifth edition of *Rural Nursing: Concepts, Theory, and Practice* expands our understanding of the rural healthcare environment. As with the first four editions, the quest continues to provide an evidence base and theory structure to help nurses and other providers address the health needs of persons living in rural communities. New chapters have been added on topics important to rural providers, educators, and researchers including a chapter on the history of rural nursing theory development; lack of anonymity; a program of research in rural communities; the lived experience of rural nurses; the rural nurse practitioner; the synergy model for rural nursing; telehealth nursing; trauma care; palliative care; bereavement; workforce issues; public health issues; care for American Indians; complementary therapy; development of a Rural Knowledge Scale; collaborative education models; substance abuse; and community-based participatory research. The fifth edition continues the tradition of including seminal chapters and updated chapters retained from the previous edition.

The text is divided into five sections. Each section includes new chapters as well as updated chapters from previous editions. The first focuses on rural nursing theory and includes the seminal work by Long and Weinert. The focus of Section II is rural nursing practice. In this section is Jane Scharff's chapter on the nature and scope of rural nursing practice that has been so widely quoted since its publication nearly 20 years ago. Section III focuses on healthcare delivery in rural settings. Section IV addresses nursing education for rural populations and Section V focuses on public health. **Qualified instructors may obtain access to ancillary instructor's PowerPoints by emailing textbook@springerpub.com.**

We hope readers will find the latest edition thought provoking and useful in their clinical practice, teaching efforts, and research activities. We look forward to the comments and critiques of our rural colleagues.

Charlene A. Winters
Helen J. Lee

Acknowledgment

We wish to acknowledge the work of our many colleagues, students, consultants, and research participants whose contributions made this text possible.

Rural Nursing Theory

This section opens with a new chapter that features the history of the development of the rural nursing theory (RNT). The beginning work at the College of Nursing at Montana State University is featured and followed by a summary of the ongoing work and proposes what is planned for the future. Chapter 2 is the sentinel chapter, "Rural Nursing: Developing Theory Base" (Long and Weinert), which first appeared in the nursing literature in 1989 and has been a part of the previous four editions of this book. Chapter 3 contains the analyzed concepts included in the RNT chapter; it is updated with the recent work on lack of anonymity. An updated Chapter 4 examines the rural nursing research for the latest findings about concepts contained in the theoretical statements; this activity leads to recommending changes for two of the three theoretical statements in the original RNT.

Chapter 5 provides updated information about a thorough review of the literature that the authors conducted to find specific research studies using the RNT as a theoretical framework. The concept, lack of anonymity, is the topic of Chapter 6; the authors consider the effect of modern technology on the concept and its related concepts of privacy, familiarity, and confidentially. Chapter 7 provides a blueprint for developing a focused research project in rural settings. The research addresses the use of complementary therapy by rural individuals. It considers multiple researchers, distance between the researchers involved, funding from multiple agencies, and the development of an instrument to measure health literacy.

CHAPTER 1

Rural Nursing Theory: Past, Present, and Future

Helen J. Lee and Charlene A. Winters

DISCUSSION TOPICS

- Discuss strategies you might use to initiate and sustain theory development with your colleagues.
- Identify areas within rural nursing theory (RNT) that need further development. Identify specific strategies to address those needs.
- Identify real-world learning experiences for students that allow them to explore health needs and perceptions of rural persons from numerous rural groups.

For this fifth edition of *Rural Nursing: Concepts, Theory, and Practice,* we believe it is important to take a step back and detail the history that led to the development of the theory. We also believe it is critical to provide direction to further its development. Therefore, the purpose of this chapter is to provide the (a) history, context, and assumptions, (b) current status and studies, and (c) future directions and needed research of the RNT. The historical content is divided into three phases.

HISTORY, CONTEXT, AND ASSUMPTIONS

Within the United States, the average population density is 90 persons per square mile (U.S. Census Bureau, 2016) and most persons live in cities. Most states contain rural areas, even New Jersey, where the population density is the highest in the United States at 1,210 individuals per square mile. In contrast,

TABLE 1.1 Least Densely Populated States in the United States

Rank	State	Persons/Square Mile
1	Alaska	1.3
2	Wyoming	6.0
3	Montana	7.1
4	North Dakota	11.0
5	South Dakota	11.3
6	New Mexico	17.2

Source: Worldatlas. (2016). Least densely populated U.S. states. Retrieved from http://www
.worldatlas.com/articles/least-densely-populated-u-s-states.html

based on 2017 U.S. Census Bureau estimates (Worldatlas, 2016), six states have fewer than 20 persons per square mile (Table 1.1). Montana ranks third from the bottom in the population density list.

In 1975, Montana State University (MSU) recruited Anna M. Shannon, a native Montanan, to be dean of the College of Nursing. Dr. Shannon was convinced that nursing practice in a rural environment was different from that in an urban place. Dr. Shannon also noted that there was a paucity in numbers of articles pertaining to *rural* nursing in the literature base. The only articles available were from sociology; the content examined the characteristics of young women entering the nursing profession.

Phase 1 (1977–1998)

Dean Shannon and two faculty members, Drs. Jacqueline Taylor (anthropologist) and Ruth Ludemann (sociologist) wrote federal grant applications to fund the rural generalist master's program beginning in 1977. MSU is a land grant university. The College of Nursing is a state-wide program; the main campus is located in Bozeman and at that time the extended campuses were located in Great Falls, Billings, Butte, and Missoula. Undergraduate students started their nursing courses in Bozeman and then transferred to the extended campuses for clinical courses. A four-quarter master's program was available at the Bozeman campus; students could enroll in adult, family–child, and psychiatric nursing.

Initially, the new graduate rural nursing program rotated around the College of Nursing's campus sites. The length of the program was five quarters. A thesis was required. For two of the rural core nursing courses, students were assigned to select a rural or remote community; in the first course, the community was to be described visually and structurally (population, governance, occupations, healthcare availability). In the second course, titled "Rural Nursing," the students interviewed 10 to 12 persons in the chosen community about their perceptions of their health and their healthcare. Course paperwork for both classes was reports of the findings of both activities. Participants were engaged primarily in the extractive industries—farming, ranching, and logging. Procedures for protection of human subjects were followed.[1]

In the spring of 1982, a podium presentation titled "Sparsely Populated Areas: Towards Nursing Theory" was given to the Western Council on Higher Education, a regional nursing research organization now called the Western Institute of Nursing (WIN), introduced by College of Nursing Dean Shannon. The presentation's purpose was to demonstrate how a nursing school could "maximize its resources, provide opportunities for faculty and student research, and contribute . . . to the development of an empirically based theory of nursing" (pp. 70–71). Dr. Taylor (1982) organized the presentation that included faculty and graduate students' studies about the (a) role of distance in home dialysis, (b) sodium in drinking water and adolescent blood pressure, and (c) beliefs and practices of Crow Indian women, Hmong refugees, and Hutterite colony members. Her concluding remarks included a plan for theory construction and testing using retroduction, a process that includes both inductive and deductive reasoning.

Using the procedures described above, the faculty and student groups continued gathering data for the theory base using the student interviews, the community data they collected, and the student papers describing the health beliefs, values, and practices of the rural participants interviewed. Concepts emerging from the data included *health status, health beliefs, isolation, distance, self-reliance, lack of anonymity, familiarity, insider/outsider, old timer/newcomer,* and *informal healthcare systems.*

In 1983, Dr. Clarann Weinert developed a survey to validate the emerging concepts. Instruments used in the quantitative study and the constructs measured are listed in Table 1.2.

TABLE 1.2 Survey Instruments and Constructs

General Health Perception Scale	Physical health status and health beliefs (Davies & Ware, 1981)
Personal Resource Questionnaire	Informal systems for support and healthcare (Brandt & Weinert, 1981)
Trait Anxiety Scale	Mental health status (Spielberger, Gorsuch, & Lushene, 1970)
Beck Depression Inventory	Mental health status (Beck, 1967)

1. Community and interview data collection were supported in part by U.S. Department of Health and Services, Division of Nursing, Advanced Training Grant to Montana State University Grant (#1816001649AI).

A convenience sample of 62 persons (40 women, 22 men) from 13 sparsely populated counties in Montana responded to the survey. The mean age of the sample was 61.3 years of age; the mean education year was 13.5 years. The survey data were analyzed to inform the qualitative data through the emerging concepts.

"Rural Nursing: Developing the Theory Base," by Drs. Kathleen A. Long and Clarann Weinert, was published in 1989. The following assumptions of the theory guided the process: (a) "Rural" was defined as sparsely populated; the entire state of Montana was considered as sparsely populated despite the population centers that existed within the state; (b) Healthcare needs of rural environments are different from healthcare needs in urban settings; (c) All rural areas have common needs; (d) Urban models of healthcare are not appropriate or adequate for rural areas.

Three theoretical statements were proposed. The first two statements pertain to rural persons. The first states that rural persons "define health primarily as the ability to work, to be productive and do usual tasks" (Long & Weinert, 1989, p. 120). The second statement indicates that "rural persons are self-reliant and resist seeking help from those seen as 'outsiders' or from agencies seen as national or regional 'welfare' programs" (p. 120). A corollary to the second statement was that healthcare is usually sought through the informal rather than the formal system. The third statement applies to rural healthcare providers (HCPs): they "must deal with a lack of anonymity and much greater role diffusion than providers in urban or suburban settings." (p. 119)

Concepts related to the first statement include *health beliefs, work beliefs,* and *health-seeking behavior. Isolation* and *distance* were two concepts that assisted in understanding health-seeking behavior of rural individuals. Despite living long distances from healthcare facilities, rural individuals did not view themselves as isolated.

Related to the second theoretical statement are the concepts of *self-reliance* and *independence.* The desire to care for oneself was common among the interviewed rural individuals.

Lack of anonymity is a major concept for the providers of nursing and healthcare in a rural environment. Closely associated with practice in a rural area are the related concepts of *old-timer/newcomer* and *insider/outsider.* These interrelated concepts guide rural individuals' interactions and relationships with nurses and other HCPs.

Following the publication of Long and Weinert's (1989) article about the RNT base (see a reprint of this paper in Chapter 2 in this text), several MSU faculty members committed to continue work on the theory. Enrolled graduate nursing students continued choosing and describing rural communities and interviewing their residents regarding their health perceptions. A concurrent activity began during this time; interested graduate students and nursing faculty began analyzing the concepts that emerged during the RNT process. Several students developed their community interviews into theses. These along with concept analyses papers became chapters in *Conceptual Basis for Rural Nursing*, a publication edited by Dr. Helen Lee (1998).[2] The text ultimately became the first of the subsequent editions of *Rural Nursing: Concepts, Theory, and Practice*.

Phase 2 (1999–2006)

MSU College of Nursing faculty, Drs. Helen J. Lee and Charlene A. Winters, continued the theory work through the teaching of the rural nursing course in the graduate nursing curriculum. Presentations about the theory, the concepts, and the faculty–student collaboration were accepted at several Communicating Nursing Research Conferences sponsored by WIN, the Western regional nursing research organization (2001, 2002, 2004).

During this time, three events led to the formation of a collaborative effort with nurse researchers in Canada. The first was an independent activity project and visit by Meg K. McDonagh from the University of Calgary to explore the emerging RNT work at MSU. The second and third events were the attendance of the core MSU faculty at two conferences, a Canadian Rural Conference in Saskatoon, Saskatchewan, and the Rural Nursing Research Conference in Binghamton, NY. The collaboration occurred with nurse researchers of the Faculty of Nursing, University of Calgary (Elizabeth H. Tomlinson, Meg K. McDonagh, Dana S. Edge, and Marlene A Reimer). Chad O'Lynn joined the MSU group of researchers. The work, titled North American Study Group (NAS), led to the appointment of Dr. Winters as a visiting scholar at the University of Calgary Faculty of Nursing and a comparison study conducted across international borders about rural/remote health beliefs between participants in Montana and the Canadian provinces of Alberta and Manitoba. The purposes of NAS were to (a) validate existing RNT concepts, (b) explore new emerging concepts, and (c) determine areas for further theoretical development and research.

Following the activity of the comparison study group (Winters et al., 2016), the NAS group made these recommendations regarding RNT:

1. Concepts:
   a. Add identified new concepts to RNT: *health-seeking behavior* and *choices* (residence, HCP).
   b. Most concepts analyses were incomplete and the new concepts identified needed to be developed.
   c. It was noted that validation of all the concepts was needed.

---

2. Funding sources for the publication of *Conceptual* Basis *for* Rrural Nursing was a monetary grant received from the Montana Consortium for Excellence in Healthcare. The Consortium also funded, in part, the content of two chapters within the text. The grant award was facilitated by Jane E. Scharff.

2. These issues arose during the analysis of the data and require further exploration as to their fit with RNT:
   a. Economic
   b. Aging communities
   c. Environmental exposure to chemicals, injury from animals, and safety with regard to driving and farm/ranch work injuries.

Dr. Helen Lee and Ms. McDonagh conducted an extensive review of literature that supported or refuted the RNT theoretical statements and concepts. They found that

> The rural residents' definition of health in the first descriptive statement is changing from that of a functional nature to a more holistic view that includes physical, mental, social, and spiritual aspects. The self-reliance of rural residents in the second relational statement is broadly supported; however, the resistance to seeking help from those seen as 'outsiders' is changing. The third relational statement pertaining to HCPs and their lack of anonymity and role diffusion is supported. The findings for the concept of distance in the original rural theory development work are not supported. This literature appraisal of the rural nursing theory base structure supports a need for change. (Lee & Winters, 2006, pp. 24)

At the end of this phase, Drs. Lee and Winters published the textbook, *Rural Nursing: Concepts, Theory, and Practice* (2006). The Springer Publishers considered it the second edition of *Conceptual Basis for Rural Nursing*. The change in title more accurately reflected the direction of the changing content of the book.

Phase 3 (2007–2012)

The NAS researchers determined that the third relational statement about rural nursing practice would be the next focus of the RNT research group. A study was designed to explore the degree to which nurses and health professionals working in rural and remote settings access and use health research in practice; it was called the Rural Nurse Research Access (RRA) study. The study was initiated with a pilot study in Montana to develop a questionnaire and was conducted in collaboration with graduate nursing students enrolled in the rural nursing course. The qualitative work consisted of a windshield survey of nine rural communities with populations of 3,000 or less and located 50 miles or more from an urban setting. The semi-structured interviews were conducted by 29 rural nurses (age range 31–72; years in nursing 3–50; 11 were baccalaureate prepared and 8 were associate degree graduates; 21 were employed in critical access hospitals [CAHs]). Verbatim transcripts and field notes were analyzed for common themes. The RRA qualitative findings from the pilot study showed that participants (a) equated the word "research" with gathering information, an activity that was done two to three times a day to two to three times a month, (b) considered "research" a work-place activity, (c) stated that their primary sources for health research information were colleagues (managers, staff nurses, physicians), and (d) used the Internet if available.

Following the pilot study initial questionnaire findings, a comparative analysis was done with the literature and revisions were made. Subsequently, the finalized survey instrument was used in Canada to explore practices and attitudes with a mix of healthcare workers including nurses, physicians, and social workers.

Since the U.S. members of the RRA group wanted to focus their study on nurses, the survey was sent to registered nurses working in rural areas in three states—Montana, Oregon, and South Dakota. Human subject procedures were completed for the institutions involved in all three states. The names of participants were obtained through state boards of nursing files. Nurses working in rural counties (Rural–Urban Continuum Codes 6–9, U.S. Department of Agriculture, 2007) were the targeted recipients of the survey questionnaire. There was a 61% response rate (Koessl, Winters, Lee, & Hendrickx, 2010).

The demographics of the RRA quantitative study participants were as follows:

- Their ages ranged from 41 to 60 years.
- Sixty percent had a university degree.
- Sixty percent were employed full time.
- Forty percent were employed in a hospital-based practice.
- More than 50% had been practicing for more than 20 years.
- Less than 50% were practicing in a rural/remote setting.
- Sixty percent did not practice in the same community in which they lived.

The RRA study survey participants indicated that the evidence most frequently used was "a personal experience of caring for patients/clients over time" and "information that I learn about each patient/client as an individual," actions that are consistent with evidence-based practice (EBP; Melnyk, Fineout-Overholt, Stillwell, & Williamson, 2010). They ranked low-level evidence sources as most commonly used, and were least likely to use a research journal. When compared to Olade (2004), the survey participants were (a) more likely to have used research in the last year, (b) less likely to use more research if they could, and (c) unlikely to use research if it contradicted institutional policy or common sense. Their ability to evaluate research quality was lacking. The perception of practice as evidence based was higher in younger nurses (71.5% in nurses less than 30 years of age as compared to 22.2% in those 60 years of age and older).

Members of the research team for this study were Helen Lee, Jean Shreffler-Grant, Charlene Winters, and Susan Luparell from MSU, Dana S. Edge, Meg McDonagh, Lianna Barnieh, and Elizabeth "Betty" Tomlinson from University of Calgary, Chad O'Lynn from the University of Portland, and Lori Hendrickx from South Dakota State University[3]

During this phase, Dr. Lee retired from teaching. The *Rural Nursing: Concepts, Theory, and Practice*, the third edition (2010) by Drs. Winters and Lee was published. This edition contained an update of the RNT from Dr. Lee and Ms. McDonagh to include clearly revised theoretical statements.

1. Rural residents define health as being able to do what they want to do; it is a way of life and a state of mind; there is a goal of maintaining balance in all aspects of their lives.
   Older rural residents and those with ties to extractive industries are more likely to define health in a functional manner—to work, to be productive, and to do usual tasks.
2. Rural residents are self-reliant and make decisions to seek care for illness, sickness, or injury depending on their self-assessment of the severity of their present health condition and of the resources needed and available. Rural residents with infants and children who experience illness, sickness, or injury will seek care more quickly than for themselves. (Lee & McDonagh, 2010, p. 27)

Present Activity (2013–Present)

Dr. Winters continued to teach the rural nursing course as previously described through 2013. After that time, the rural course was broadened to "vulnerable populations"; however, rural remained a significant focus within the course. The fourth edition of *Rural Nursing: Concepts, Theory, and Practice* was published in 2013 with an increased number of international authors and authors from across the United States. As with the previous editions, the focus was on explicating the concepts and propositions that guide nursing practice, rural healthcare delivery issues, and understanding the characteristics and behaviors of rural persons. Winters stated at a Community Forum for Nursing at South Dakota State University and Sanford USD Medical Center (2012) that

> What Drs. Long, Weinert, and Shannon knew is that research data, an understanding of context and resources, as well as rural perceptions of health and healthcare were critical to the provision of EBP. Together, these items constitute the available evidence that should drive rural clinical practice. The rural evidence base is in line with the American Nurses Association (ANA) and other nursing organizations mandate for our EBP interventions.

---

3. Funding sources for the phases of the RRA study included: MSU College of Nursing grant, Sigma Theta Tau International, Zeta Upsilon Chapter (Montana statewide chapter), Sigma Theta Tau, Omicron Chapter (University of Portland), South Dakota State University College of Nursing Intramural Funding.

The American Nurses Association (ANA) standards of nursing practice and professional performance mandate the use of evidence-based interventions and the integration of research findings into practice (2004). EBP is a problem-solving approach to the delivery of healthcare that integrates the best evidence from well-designed studies and patient care data, and combines it with patient preferences and values, combined with clinical expertise (Melnyk et al., 2010). The Institute of Medicine maintained that EBP is a core competency that every healthcare clinician should have to meet the needs of the 21st century healthcare system (Greiner & Knebel, 2003). To achieve EBP as a core competency requires improved communication and collaboration, shared responsibility, synchrony of efforts, drawing close clinical research and practice, and an engaged public.

To facilitate rural research and practice there must be an integration of rural experiences in nursing education, nursing students must be recruited from rural settings, and nursing education must be delivered from rural settings (Bushy & Leipert, 2005). Strategies to integrate research and EBP projects require course assignments, collaboration with clinical partners on research applicable to clinical practice, and provision of networking and educational opportunities–academic/ clinical partnerships (Miller, Bryant MacLean, Coward, & Broeeling, 2009).

Dr. Winters and her faculty colleagues are working to increase collaboration efforts in western Montana. Groups, students (high school, undergraduate, and graduate), and faculty collaboration include the following examples:

- *High school students and faculty collaboration*: MSU researchers collaborated with a Libby MT high school science teacher and students enrolled in a research elective on a community-based participatory research study conducted in Libby, MT (Kuntz et al., 2009; Winters, Kuntz, Weinert, & Rowse, 2008). The faculty presented a class on research process. Human subjects and research protocol training were provided. In the class, there was discussion and approval of a research proposal. A survey was developed and community-based data collection took place. Students were provided a report of the survey findings. Drs. Winters and Kuntz were the faculty mentors.
- *Undergraduate nursing students and faculty collaboration*: To explore community members' understanding of and interest in research, undergraduate MSU nursing students interviewed residents of Libby, MT as part of a community-based participatory research project (CBPR; Winters et al., 2008). The interviews informed the research study and also served as an assignment in the students' senior level community health nursing course. Dr. Kuntz was the faculty mentor.
- *Undergraduate nursing students and faculty collaboration in a clinical course*: To compare BMI of school children (in Missoula, MT), student teams used the compiled data in support of the Coordinated Approach to the Child Health program. Dr. Sandy Kuntz was the faculty mentor.
- *Undergraduate nursing students and faculty collaboration in a research course*: Students in Missoula, MT collaborated with hospital nurses and a faculty

mentor to test whether hospital procedures for nasogastric tube placement and chest tube dressing changes were evidence based. Dr. Dorothy (Dale) Mayer was the faculty mentor.

- *Graduate nursing students and faculty collaboration*: Students conducted a secondary analysis of previously collected qualitative data to explore the rural context and women's self-management of chronic health conditions. Dr. Winters was the faculty mentor.
- *Graduate nursing students and faculty collaboration*: Students enrolled in a vulnerable populations course select a rural community, vulnerable sub-population, and health-related issue to explore throughout the semester from the individual, provider, and health system perspective. Students search and appraise the literature, conduct community and systems assessments, and interview individuals as part of the learning experience. Dr. Winters in the faculty mentor.

From each of these experiences, students and faculty learn valuable information about rural communities and rural persons that inform RNT, practice, and research.[4]

FUTURE DIRECTIONS

The collaborative work of MSU faculty in the above EBP activities represents brief examples of the total number of activities occurring in the MSU College of Nursing. The examples with undergraduate students originated from one College of Nursing campus in western Montana. Collaboration with faculty members from other campuses in the MSU College of Nursing system would be ideal. Reinstating the RNT work group that existed in earlier years to conduct secondary analyses of qualitative data collected by graduate nursing students enrolled in the vulnerable populations course would provide valuable insight into current rural health issues. MSU is collecting funds to support an endowed research chair within the College of Nursing. When that goal is finally realized, may the rich heritage of this work on RNT be a stepping-stone for future work!

As indicated earlier, toward the conclusion of the comparative analysis across borders study, the NAS investigators identified a blueprint of work that was needed related to RNT development:

- Develop and test instruments to measure the concepts
- Test the theoretical and relational statements

4. Funding sources to partially support evidenced-based rural practice activities: HRSA Office of Rural Health Policy [RO4RH07544-01], NIH/NINR P20 Research Center Grant [IP20NR 07790-0], NIH/NNR Partners in Research Grant [1R03NR011242-01], NR/NNR Women to women [1R03NR011242-01]

- Compare and contrast the health perceptions and needs of persons living in differing rural cultures and environments:
  - American Indians and Aboriginal peoples
  - Rural and remote persons in other areas in the United States, Canada, and else where
  - Urban, former urban, and other rural subpopulations
- Compare and contrast the health perceptions and needs of persons of differing circumstances:
  - Ill and well populations
  - Old-timers and newcomers
  - Young and old
  - The urban poor
- Target research on the third relational statement:
  - Effect of technology on generalist role, role diffusion, and professional isolation
  - Explore gender differences

The NAS group generated the following research questions:

1. Are the health-seeking behaviors identified unique to rural residents?
2. How do health-seeking behaviors differ from those of health promotion?
3. How do illness variables affect rural persons' health seeking behaviors? Choice of HCP?
4. What variables affect rural persons' acceptance of "outside" services/HCP?
5. Do various rural groups define health differently?

The above needs and questions are still relevant for the RNT work that needs to be done today.

CONCLUSION

Forty years have passed since the initial work on RNT began. The RNT base as published is in need of revision. Advances in health service and communication technologies, healthcare practices, along with changes in the perceptions and behaviors of rural residents over the past four decades may account for the emerging concepts identified. The work identified and the generation of additional theoretical statements will increase the potential of generating a middle range theory pertaining to the healthcare of rural persons. Relevance of rural nursing will likely be measured by the ability to evolve and change as new knowledge shapes it.

REFERENCES

American Nurses Association. (2004). *Scope and standards of practice*. Washington, DC: Author.

Beck, A. (1967). *Depression: Causes and treatment*. Philadelphia: University of Pennsylvania Press.

Brandt, P., & Weinert, C. (1981). The PRQ: A social support measure. *Nursing Research, 30*, 277–280.

Bushy, A., & Leipert, B. (2005). Factors that influence students in choosing rural nursing practice: A pilot study. *Rural and Remote Health, 5*(387). Retrieved from http://rrh.deakin.edu.au

Davies, A., & Ware, J. (1981). *Measuring health perceptions in the health insurance experiment*. Santa Monica, CA: RAND.

Greiner, A. C., & Knebel, E. (Eds.) (2003). *Health professions education: A bridge to quality*. Washington, DC: National Academies Press. Retrieved from http://www.nap.edu/catalog/10681.html

Koessl, B. D., Winters, C. A., Lee, H. J., & Hendrickx, L. (2010). Rural nurses' attitudes and beliefs toward evidence-based practice. In C. A. Winters & H. J. Lee (Eds.), *Rural nursing: Concepts, theory, and practice* (3th ed., pp. 327–344). New York, NY: Springer Publishing.

Kuntz, S. W., Winters, C. A., Hill, W., Weinert, C., Rowse, K., Hernandez, T., & Black, B. (2009). Rural public health policy models to address an evolving environmental asbestos disaster. *Public Health Nursing, 26*(1), 70–78. doi:10.1111/j.1525-1446.2008.00755.x

Lee, H. J. (Ed.). (1998). *Conceptual basis for rural nursing*. New York, NY: Springer Publishing.

Lee, H. J., & McDonagh, M. K. (2010). Updating the rural nursing theory base. In Winters, C. A. & Lee, H. J. (Eds.). *Rural nursing: Concepts, theory, and practice* (3rd ed., pp. 19–39). New York, NY: Springer Publishing.

Lee, H. J., & Winters, C. A. (Eds.). (2006). *Rural nursing: Concepts, theory, and practice* (2nd ed.). New York, NY: Springer Publishing.

Long, K. A., & Weinert, C. (1989). Rural nursing: Developing the theory base. *Scholarly Inquiry for Nursing Practice: An International Journal, 3*, 113–127.

Melnyk, B. M., Fineout-Overholt, E., Stillwell, S. B., & Williamson, K. M. (2010). The seven steps of evidence-based practice. *American Journal of Nursing, 110*(1), 51–53.

Miller, J., Bryant MacLean, L., Coward, P., & Broemeling, A. M. (2009). Developing strategies to enhance health capacity in a predominantly rural Canadian health authority. *Rural and Remote Health, 9*(1266).

Olade, P. (2004). Evidence-based practice and research utilization activities among rural nurses. *Journal of Nursing Scholarship, 36*(3), 220–225.

Olsen, L. et al. (2007). *The learning healthcare system: Workshop summary*. Washington, DC: National Academies Press. Retrieved from http://www.nap.edu/catalog.php?record_id=11903

Shannon, A. (1982). Introduction: Nursing in sparsely populated areas. In J. Taylor, Sparsely populated areas: Toward nursing theory. *Western Journal of Nursing Research, 4*(Suppl. 3), 70–71.

Spielberger, C., Gorsuch, R., & Lushene, R. (1970). *STAI manual for the State-Trait Anxiety Questionnaire*. Palo Alto, CA: Consulting Psychologist.

Taylor, J. (1982). Sparsely populated areas: Toward nursing theory. *Western Journal of Nursing Research*, 4(3), 69–77.

U.S. Census Bureau. (2016). Quick facts: Montana. Retrieved from https://www.census .gov/quickfacts/table/PST045216/30,00

U.S. Department of Agriculture Economic Research Service (2007). Rural-urban continuum codes. Retrieved from https://www.ers.usda.gov/data-products/rural -urban-continuum-codes

Winters, C. A. (2012, April). *Rural nursing theory & nursing research: Developing evidence-based care for rural dwellers*. Presentation at a Community Forum for Nursing, South Dakota State University & Sanford USD Medical Center, Sioux Falls, SD.

Winters, C. A. (Ed.). (2014). *Rural nursing: Concepts, theory, and practice* (4th ed.). New York, NY: Springer Publishing.

Winters, C. A., Kuntz, S. W., Weinert, C., & Rowse, K. (2008). *Exploring research communication & engagement in a rural community: The Libby Partnership Initiative*. National Institutes of Health/National Institute of Nursing Research.

Winters, C. A., & Lee, H. J. (Eds.). (2010). *Rural nursing: Concepts, theory, and practice* (3th ed.). New York, NY: Springer Publishing.

Winters, C. A., Thomlinson, E. H., O'Lynn, C., Lee, H. L., McDonagh, M. K., Edge, D. S., & Reimer, M. A. (2006). Exploring rural nursing across borders. In H. J. Lee & C. A. Winters (Eds.), *Rural nursing: Concepts, theory and practice* (2nd ed., pp. 27–39). New York, NY: Springer Publishing.

Worldatlas. (2016). Least densely populated U.S. states. Retrieved from http://www .worldatlas.com/articles/least-densely-populated-u-s-states.html

CHAPTER 2

Rural Nursing: Developing the Theory Base[*]

Kathleen A. Long and Clarann Weinert

DISCUSSION TOPICS

- Select a rural or frontier community to explore. Conduct a windshield survey of the community, gather epidemiographic data about the community, and interview residents to further define both the common and the locale-specific conditions and characteristics of the rural populations. Compare and contrast findings with concepts identified by Long and Weinert.
- Design strategies to tailor the formal healthcare system to suit the preferences of rural persons for family and community help during times of illness and injury.
- Identify opportunities to reduce professional isolation and increase professional networking for advanced practice nurses working in rural and frontier settings.

A logger suffering from "heart lock" does not have a cardiovascular abnormality. He is suffering from a work-related anxiety disorder and can be assisted by an emergency department nurse who accurately assesses his needs and responds with effective communication and a supportive interpersonal relationship. A farmer who has lost his finger in a grain thresher several hours earlier does not have time during the harvesting season for a discussion of occupational safety. He will cope with his injury assisted by a clinic nurse who can adjust the timing of his antibiotic doses to fit with his work schedule in the fields.

Many healthcare needs of rural dwellers cannot be adequately addressed by the application of nursing models developed in urban or suburban areas, but require unique approaches emphasizing the special needs of this population. Although nurses are significant, and frequently the sole healthcare providers for people living in rural areas, little has been written to guide the practice of rural nursing. The literature provides vignettes and individual descriptions, but there is a need for an integrated, theoretical approach to rural nursing.

Rural nursing is defined as the provision of healthcare by professional nurses to persons living in sparsely populated areas. Over the last 8 years, graduate students and faculty members at the Montana State University College of Nursing have worked toward developing a theory base for rural nursing. Theory development has used primarily a retroductive approach, and data have been collected and refined using a combination of qualitative and quantitative methods. The experiences of rural residents and rural nurses have guided the identification of key concepts relevant to rural nursing. The goal of the theory-building process has been to identify commonalities and differences in nursing practice across all rural areas and the common and unique elements of rural nursing in relation to nursing overall. The implications of developing a theory of rural nursing for practice have been examined as a part of the ongoing process.

The theory-building process was initiated in the late 1970s. At that time, literature and research related to rural healthcare were limited and focused primarily on the problem of retaining physicians in rural areas and providing assessments of rural healthcare needs and prescriptions for rural healthcare services based on models and experiences from urban and suburban areas (Coward, 1977; Flax, Wagenfeld, Ivens, & Weiss, 1979). The unique health problems and healthcare needs of extremely sparsely populated states, such as Montana, had not been addressed from the perspective of the rural consumer. No organized theoretical base for guiding rural healthcare practice in general, or rural nursing in particular, existed.

QUALITATIVE DATA

The target population for qualitative data collection was the people of Montana. Montana, the fourth largest state in the United States, is an extremely sparsely populated state, with nearly 800,000 people and an average population density of approximately five persons per square mile. One-half of the counties in Montana have three or fewer persons per square mile, with six of those counties having less than one person per square mile. There is only one metropolitan center in the state; it is a city of nearly 70,000 people, with a surrounding area that constitutes a center of approximately 100,000 (Montana State University Center for Data Systems and Analysis, 1985).

Qualitative data were collected through ethnographic study by Montana State University College of Nursing graduate students. These data provided the initial ideas about health and healthcare in Montana. Since general propositions about rural health and rural healthcare did not exist, gathering of concrete data was the first step toward subsequent development of more general theoretical propositions.

Graduate students used ethnographic techniques as described by Spradley (1979) to gather information from individuals, families, and healthcare providers. Interview sites were selected by students on the basis of specific interest and convenience. During a 6-year period, data were gathered from approximately 25 locations. In general, each student worked in depth in one community, collecting data from 10 to 20 informants over a period of at least 1 year. Data were gathered primarily from persons in ranching and farming areas and from towns of less than 2,500 persons. In some instances, student interest led to extensive interviews with specific rural subgroups, such as men in the logging industry or older residents in a rural town (Weinert & Long, 1987). Open-ended interview questions were developed using Spradley's guidelines. The questions emphasized seeking the informants' views without superimposing the cultural biases of the interviewer. The opening question in the interview was, "What is health to you . . . from your viewpoint? . . . your definition?" Interviewers used standard probes and a standard format of questions regarding health beliefs and healthcare preferences.

Spradley (1979) indicated that the goal of ethnographic study is to "build a systematic understanding of all human cultures from the perspective of those who have learned them" (p. 10). The goal of data collection in Montana was to learn about the culture of rural Montanans from rural Montanans. Emphasis in the cultural learning process was on understanding health beliefs, values, and practices. Rigdon, Clayton, and Diamond (1987) have noted that understanding the meaning that persons attach to subjective experiences is an important aspect of nursing knowledge. The ethnographic approach captured the meanings that rural dwellers ascribe to the subjective states of health and illness and facilitated the development of a rich database.

As the database developed, the following definitions and assumptions were accepted as a foundation for theory development. "Rural" was defined as meaning sparsely populated. Within this context, states such as Montana, which are sparsely populated overall, are viewed as rural throughout, despite the existence of some population centers within them. Further, based on this definition, rural regions or areas can be identified within otherwise heavily populated states. An assumption is made that, to some degree, healthcare needs are different in rural areas from those of urban areas. Also, all rural areas are viewed as having some common healthcare needs. Finally, another assumption is made that urban models are not appropriate to, or adequate for, meeting healthcare needs in rural areas.

Retroductive Theory Generation

Faculty work groups were developed to examine and organize the qualitative data. The work groups involved three to five nursing faculty members, each with rural nursing experience, but with varied backgrounds and expertise. Thus, a work group included experts from various clinical areas, as well as persons with direct experience either in small rural hospitals or in larger metropolitan centers within rural states. Standard ethnographic content analysis (Spradley, 1979) was used to sort and categorize the ethnographic data. Groups worked toward consensus about the meaning and organization of specific data. Recurring themes were identified and viewed as having relevance and importance for the rural informants in relation to their views of health.

A retroductive approach, as originally described by Hanson (1958), was used for examining the initial ethnographic data and to build the theory base. Specific concepts and relational statements were derived from the data, and more general propositions were induced from these statements. The new propositions were then used for developing additional specific statements that could be supported by existing data or were categorized for later testing. The retroductive approach was literally a "back and forth" process that permitted persons familiar with the data to move between the data and beginning-level theoretical propositions. The process was orderly and consistent, and required group consensus about data interpretation and the relevance of derived propositions. The retroductive process continued in work groups over several years as additional ethnographic data were gathered. Consultants participated at key points in the process, to raise questions, add insights, and critically evaluate the group's theory-building approach. Walker and Avant (1983) have noted that the retroductive process "adds considerably to the body of theoretical knowledge. It is, in fact, the way theory develops in the 'real world'" (p. 176).

QUANTITATIVE DATA

Following several years of ethnographic study, the faculty members involved in theory development wished to enrich the qualitative database by collecting relevant quantitative data. Kleinman (1983) stated, "Qualitative description, taken together with various quantitative measures, can be a standardized research method for assessing validity. It is especially valuable in studying social and cultural significance, for example, illness beliefs interaction norms, social gain, ethnic help seeking, and treatment responses" (p. 543). Hinds and Young (1987) noted, "The combination of different methodologies within a single study promotes the likelihood of uncovering multiple dimensions of a phenomenon's empirical reality" (p. 195).

A survey developed by Weinert in 1983 attempted to validate some of the rural health concepts that had emerged from the ethnographic data.

These concepts were health status and health beliefs, isolation and distance, self-reliance, and informal healthcare systems. Survey instruments with established psychometric properties were selected to measure the specific concepts of interest. A mail questionnaire completed by the respondents included the Beck Depression Inventory (Beck, 1967) and the Trait Anxiety Scale (Spielberger, Gorsuch, & Lushene, 1970) to tap mental health status, and the General Health Perception Scale (Davies & Ware, 1981) to measure physical health status and health beliefs. A background information form assessed demographic variables, including the period of residence and geographic locale. The Personal Resource Questionnaire (Brandt & Weinert, 1981) assessed the use of informal systems for support and healthcare.

The convenience sample of survey participants was located through the agricultural extension service, social groups, and informal networks. All the participants lived in Montana, completed the questionnaires in their homes, and returned them by mail to the researcher. The 62 survey participants were middle-class Whites, with an average of 13.5 years of education and a mean age of 61.3 years, who had lived in Montana for an average period of 45.6 years. The survey sample consisted of 40 women and 22 men residing in one of the 13 sparsely populated Montana counties. The most populated county has a population density of 5.9 persons per square mile, and one town of nearly 6,000 people. In the most sparsely populated county, there is one town with 600 people and an average population density of 0.5 persons per square mile.

Findings from the quantitative study were used throughout the theory development process to support or refute concept descriptions and relational statements derived from the ethnographic data. Survey findings are discussed in the following section as they relate to key concepts and relational statements.

REFINING THE BUILDING BLOCKS OF THEORY

To order the data and foster the formation of relational statements, an organizational scheme for theory development was adopted. Using the paradigm first described by Yura and Torres (1975) and later by Fawcett (1984), ethnographic data were categorized under the four major dimensions of nursing theory: person, health, environment, and nursing. The data were then ordered from the more general to the more specific. This process led to the identification of constructs, concepts, variables, and indicators.

An example helps in illustrating this process. Ethnographic data had been gathered from "gypo" loggers. These men are independent logging contractors from northwestern Montana who work in rugged isolated areas, usually living in trailers or tents while working. Examples of quotes from these loggers and their associates as found in the data: A logger states, "We worry about the here and now"; a local physician says, "Loggers enter the healthcare system during

TABLE 2.1 Data Ordering Scheme

Dimension	Psychological/sociocultural
Concept	"Present time" orientation
	Crisis orientation to health
Variable	Definitions of time
	Definitions of crisis
Indicator	Hours, minutes, days
	Seasons, work seasons
	Number of injuries
	Number of illnesses

times of crisis only"; and the public health nurse in the area says, "Loggers don't want to hear about healthcare problems; they don't return until the next accident." Table 2.1 shows the scheme used for organizing these data. The concepts "present time" orientation and crisis orientation to health are identified. These are placed under the person dimension. In this example, the constructs are not fully developed, but are viewed as either psychological or sociocultural, or both. The important variables identified thus far are definitions of time and of crisis. Possible indicators are measures of time, such as hours or seasons, and measures of crisis, such as numbers of illnesses or injuries.

Key Concepts

In the process of data organization, it was noted that some concepts appeared repeatedly in ethnographic data collected in several different areas of the state. In addition, aspects of several of these concepts were supported by the quantitative survey data (Weinert, 1983). Using Walker and Avant's (1983) model of concept synthesis, these concepts were identified as key concepts in relation to understanding rural health needs and rural nursing practice. These key concepts are as follows: work beliefs and health beliefs, isolation and distance, self-reliance, lack of anonymity, outsider/insider, and old-timer/newcomer.

As key concepts in this theory, work beliefs and health beliefs are viewed differently in rural dwellers as contrasted with urban or suburban residents. These two sets of beliefs appear to be closely interrelated among rural persons. Work or fulfilling one's usual functions is of primary importance. Health is assessed by rural people in relation to work role and work activities, and health needs are usually secondary to work needs.

The related concepts of isolation and distance are identified as important in understanding rural health and nursing. Specifically, they help in understanding healthcare-seeking behavior. Quantitative survey data indicated that rural informants who lived outside towns traveled a distance of almost 23 miles, on an average, for emergency healthcare, and over 50 miles for routine healthcare. Despite these distances, ethnographic data indicated that rural dwellers tended to see health services as accessible and did not view themselves as isolated.

Self-reliance and independence of rural persons are also seen as key concepts. The desire to do for oneself and care for oneself was strong among the rural persons interviewed; this has important ramifications in relation to the provision of healthcare.

Two key concept areas, lack of anonymity and outsider/insider, have particular relevance to the practice of rural nursing. Lack of anonymity, a hallmark of small towns and surrounding sparsely populated areas, implies a limited ability for rural persons to have private areas of their lives. Rural nurses almost always reported being known to their patients as neighbors, as part of a given family, as members of a certain church, and so on. Similarly, these nurses usually know their patients in several different social and personal relationships beyond the nurse–patient relationship. The old-timer/newcomer concept, or the related concept of outsider/insider, is relevant in terms of the acceptance of nurses and of all healthcare providers in rural communities. The ethnographic data indicated that these concepts were used by rural dwellers in organizing their view of the social environment and in guiding their interactions and relationships. Survey data revealed that those who had lived in Montana for over 10 years, but less than 20 years, still considered themselves to be "newcomers" and expected to be viewed as such by those in their community (Weinert & Long, 1987).

Relational Statements

In an effort to move from a purely descriptive theory to a beginning-level explanatory one, some initial relational statements were generated from the qualitative data and were supported by the quantitative data that had been collected thus far. The statements are in the early stages of testing.

The first statement is that rural dwellers define health primarily as the ability to work, to be productive, and to do usual tasks. The ethnographic data indicate that rural persons place little emphasis on the comfort, cosmetic, and life-prolonging aspects of health. One is viewed as healthy when he or she is able to function and is productive in one's work role. Specifically, rural residents indicated that pain was tolerated, often for extended periods, so long as it did not interfere with the ability to function. The General Health Perception Scale indicated that rural survey participants reported experiencing less pain than an age-comparable urban sample (Weinert & Long, 1987). Further, scores on the Beck Depression Inventory and the Trait Anxiety Scale (Weinert, 1983) revealed that they experienced less anxiety and less depression.

The second statement is that rural dwellers are self-reliant and resist accepting help or services from those seen as "outsiders" or from agencies seen as national or regional "welfare" programs. A corollary to this statement is that help, including needed healthcare, is usually sought through an informal rather than a formal system. Ethnographic data supported both the second statement and its corollary. Numerous references were found to show, for example, a preference for "the 'old doc' who knows us" over the new specialist who was unfamiliar. Data from the Personal Resource Questionnaire (Weinert, 1983) indicated that rural dwellers relied primarily on family, relatives, and close friends for help and support. Further, the rural survey respondents reported using healthcare professionals and formal human service agencies much less frequently than did comparable urban respondents in previous studies.

A third statement is that healthcare providers in rural areas must deal with a lack of anonymity and a much greater role diffusion than providers in urban or suburban settings. This statement has a marked significance for rural nursing practice. Although limited ethnographic and survey data have been collected from rural nurses thus far, some emerging themes have been identified. In addition to identifying a sense of isolation from professional peers, rural nurses emphasize their lack of anonymity and a sense of role diffusion. There is an inability to keep separate the activities and the behaviors of the individual nurse's various roles. In a small town, for example, the nurse's behavior as a wife, a mother, and a church attendee are all significantly related to her effectiveness as a healthcare professional in that community. Further, in their professional role, nurses reported experiencing role diffusion. Nurses are expected to perform a variety of diverse and unrelated tasks. During a single shift, a nurse may work in obstetrics delivering a baby, care for a dying patient on the medical–surgical unit, and initiate care of a trauma patient in the emergency department. Likewise, during an evening shift or on weekends, a nurse may be required to carry out tasks reserved for the pharmacist or dietitian on the day shift.

RELATIONSHIP OF CONCEPTS AND STATEMENTS TO THE LARGER BODY OF NURSING KNOWLEDGE

How people define health and illness has a direct impact on how they seek and use healthcare services and is a key concept in understanding client behavior and in planning intervention.

Definition of Health

The rural Montana dwellers defined health primarily as the ability to work and to be productive. The work of other researchers supports the finding that residents of sparsely populated areas view health in terms of ability to work and to remain productive. Ross (1982), a nurse anthropologist, studied the health perceptions of women living in the Lake District along the coast of Nova Scotia. She conducted in-depth interviews with 60 women of both British and French backgrounds in small coastal fishing communities. Similar to the rural dwellers in Montana, these women described good health as being "able to do what you want to do" and to be "able to work." Lee's (1991) recent work in Montana supports earlier findings on which the rural nursing theory was built. She found that work and health practices were closely related among farmers and ranchers; health is viewed as a functional state in relation to work. Scharff's (1987) interviews with nurses practicing in small rural hospitals in eastern Washington, northern Idaho, and western Montana indicated that they viewed the health needs of rural people as overlapping those of people living in urban situations in many instances. The nurse informants, however, noted that rural people equate health with the ability to work or function in their daily activities. Rural people were viewed as delaying healthcare until they were very ill, thus often needing hospitalization at the point of seeking care.

Self-Reliance

The statement derived from the Montana data that "rural dwellers resist accepting help from outsiders or strangers" has been supported by data from research in rural Maryland (Salisbury State College, 1986). People living in the rural eastern shore area were described as highly resistant to care from persons viewed as outsiders, and rural shore residents often refused to go "across the bridge" to Baltimore to seek healthcare, even though this was a trip of less than 100 miles and would allow access to sophisticated, specialized treatment. Like the rural people in Montana, these Maryland residents sought healthcare information and assistance from local, and often informal, sources. The self-reliance of rural persons and their resistance to outside help were also reported by Counts and Boyle (1987) in relation to the residents of the Appalachian area. Self-reliance was noted as a major feature that must be considered in planning nursing care services for this population.

The rural Nova Scotia women studied by Ross (1982) indicated informal personal networks of family, friends, and neighbors as important sources of health information who also provided the physical, financial, emotional, and social support that contributed to well-being. When these women were asked what connection there was between health and the availability of hospitals, doctors, and other medical care, 42% indicated that health knowledge and care was the individual's responsibility; 25% thought professionals were useful to a certain point in providing advice and services such as routine physical exams; 19% indicated that these services were for sick persons, not healthy persons; and 9% felt the formal healthcare system had no relationship to health (Ross, 1982, p. 311). One woman commented, "Health is not a topic to discuss with doctors and nurses" (Ross, 1982, p. 309).

Rural Nursing

The Montana data and the theory derived from it indicate that nurses and other healthcare providers in rural areas must deal with a lack of anonymity. Nurses are known in a variety of roles to their patients, and in turn, know their patients in a variety of roles. Most of the nurses interviewed by Scharff (1987) felt that by knowing their patients personally they could give better care. Other nurses, however, noted that providing professional care for family or friends can be a frightening experience. Nurses indicated that there was no anonymity for them in the rural community, which at times was reassuring and at other times, constricting (Scharff, 1987).

The concept of role diffusion in the rural hospital setting was very apparent in Scharff's (1987) work. She reported that a rural hospital nurse must be a jack-of-all-trades who often practices within the realm of numerous other healthcare disciplines, including respiratory therapy, laboratory technology, dietetics, pharmacy, social work, psychology, and medicine. Examples of the intersections between rural nursing and other disciplines include doing ECGs, performing arterial punctures, running blood gas machines, drawing blood, setting up cultures, going to the pharmacy to pour drugs, going to the local drugstore to get medications for patients, ordering x-rays and medications, delivering babies, directing the actions of physicians, and cooking meals when the cook gets snowed in. As Scharff noted, some of these functions are carried out by urban nurses practicing in particular settings such as a trauma center or an intensive care unit. Rural nurses, however, are usually not circumscribed by assignment to a particular unit or department and are expected to function in multiple roles, even during one work shift.

This generalist work role and the lack of anonymity of rural nurses are substantiated by findings and descriptions from several other rural areas of the United States (Biegel, 1983; St. Clair, Pickard, & Harlow, 1986). A study of nurses in rural Texas noted, "Nurses play roles as nurse, friend, neighbor, citizen, and family member" within a community; further, rural nurses in their work roles were described as needing to be "all things to all people" (St. Clair et al., 1986, p. 28).

Generalizability

The issue of a situation or locale-specific theory and its relationship to the larger body of nursing knowledge needs serious consideration. The work of Scharff (1987) indicated that the core of rural nursing is not different from that of urban nursing. The intersections, however, those "meeting points at which nursing extends its practice into the domains of other professions"; the dimensions, that is, the "philosophy, responsibilities, functions, roles, and skills"; and the boundaries that "respond to new and growing needs and demands from society" (American Nurses Association, 1980), appear to be very distinct for rural nursing practice.

Questions still remain as to how generalizable findings from Montana residents are to other rural populations. Clearly, there is a need for more organized and rigorous data collection in relation to rural nursing before these questions can be answered. A sound theory base for rural practice requires a continued research, conducted across diverse rural settings.

IMPLICATIONS FOR NURSING PRACTICE

The findings from the Montana research about people living in sparsely populated areas have implications for nursing practice in rural areas. Since work is of major importance to rural people, healthcare must fit within work schedules. Healthcare programs or clinics that conflict with the rural economic cycle, such as haying or calving, will not be used. Since health is defined as the ability to work, health promotion must address the work issue. For example, health education related to cardiovascular disease should highlight strategies for preventing conditions that involve long-term disability such as stroke. These aspects will be more meaningful to rural dwellers than preventive aspects that emphasize a longer, more comfortable life.

The self-reliance of rural dwellers has specific nursing implications. Rural people often delay seeking healthcare until they are gravely ill or incapacitated. Nursing approaches need to address two distinct aspects: nonjudgmental intervention for those who undergo a delayed treatment and a strong emphasis on imparting knowledge of preventive health. If the nurse can provide adequate information regarding health, the rural dwellers' desire for self-reliance may lead to health-promotion behaviors. With a good information base, rural people can make appropriate decisions regarding self-care versus the need for professional intervention.

Healthcare services must be tailored to suit the preferences of rural persons for family and community help during periods of illness. Nurses can provide instruction, support, and relief to family members and neighbors, who are often the primary care providers for sick and disabled persons.

The formal healthcare system needs to fit into the informal helping system in rural areas. A long-term community resident, such as the drugstore proprietor, can be assisted in providing accurate advice to residents through the provision of reference materials and a telephone backup system. One can anticipate greater acceptance and use by rural residents of an updated but old and trusted healthcare resource, rather than a new professional but "outsider" service (Weinert & Long, 1987).

Nurses who enter rural communities must allow for extended periods prior to acceptance. Involvement in diverse community activities, such as civic organizations and recreational clubs, may assist the nurse in being known and accepted as a person. In rural communities, acceptance as a healthcare professional is often tied to personal acceptance. Thus, it appears that rural communities are not appropriate practice settings for nurses who prefer to maintain entirely separate professional and personal lives.

The stresses that appear to affect nurses in rural practice settings have particular importance. Rural nurses see themselves as cut off from the professional mainstream. They are often in situations where there is no collegial support to assist in defining an appropriate practice role and its boundaries. The educational preparation of those who wish to practice in rural settings needs to emphasize not only generalist skills, but also a strong base in change theory and leadership techniques. Nurses in rural practice need a sound orientation to techniques for accessing diverse sources of current information. If the closest library is several hundred miles away, for example, can all arrangements for interlibrary loan and access to material via telephone, bus, or mail be arranged? Networks that link together nurses practicing in distant rural sites are particularly useful, both for information exchange and for mutual support.

CONCLUSION

It is becoming increasingly clear that rural dwellers have distinct definitions of health. Their healthcare needs require approaches that differ significantly from urban and suburban populations. Subcultural values, norms, and beliefs play key roles in how rural people define health and from whom they seek advice and care. These values and beliefs, combined with the realities of rural living—such as weather, distance, and isolation—markedly affect the practice of nursing in rural settings. Additional ethnographic and quantitative data are needed to further define both the common and the locale-specific conditions and characteristics of rural populations. Continued research can provide a more solid base for the nursing theory that is required to guide the practice and the delivery of healthcare to rural populations.

ACKNOWLEDGMENTS

Qualitative data collected and analyzed by the Montana State University College of Nursing graduate students and faculty form the basis for a substantial portion of this chapter. Ethnographic data collection and analysis were supported, in part, by a U.S. Department of Health and Human Services, Division of Nursing, and Advanced Training Grant to the Montana State University College of Nursing (#1816001649AI). The project that provided the survey data was funded by a Montana State University Faculty Research/Creativity Grant. This chapter is based partially on a paper presented at the Western Society for Research in Nursing Conference, Tempe, AZ, May 1987.

REFERENCES

American Nurses Association. (1980). *Nursing. A social policy statement (No. NP-6320M 9/82R)*. Kansas City, MO: Author.

Beck, A. (1967). *Depression: Causes and treatment*. Philadelphia: University of Pennsylvania Press.

Biegel, A. (1983). Toward a definition of rural nursing. *Home Health Care Nursing, 1*, 45–46.

Brandt, P., & Weinert, C. (1981). The PRQ: A social support measure. *Nursing Research, 30*, 277–280.

Counts, M., & Boyle, J. (1987). Nursing, health and policy within a community context. *Advances in Nursing Science, 9*, 12–23.

Coward, R. (1977). Delivering social services in small towns and rural communities. In R. Coward (Ed.), *Rural families across the life span: Implications for community programming* (pp. 1–17). West Lafayette: Indiana Cooperative Extension Services.

Davies, A., & Ware, J. (1981). *Measuring health perceptions in the health insurance experiment*. Santa Monica, CA: RAND.

Fawcett, J. (1984). *Analysis and evaluation of conceptual models of nursing*. Philadelphia, PA: F. A. Davis.

Flax, J., Wagenfeld, M., Ivens, R., & Weiss, R. (1979). *Mental health and rural America: An overview, and annotated bibliography*. Rockville, MD: U.S. Government Printing Office.

Hanson, N. (1958). *Patterns of discovery*. Cambridge, UK: Cambridge University Press.

Hinds, P., & Young, K. (1987). A triangulation of methods and paradigms to study nurse-given wellness care. *Nursing Research, 36*, 195–198.

Kleinman, A. (1983). The cultural meanings and social uses of illness: A role for medical anthropology and clinically oriented social science in the development of primary care theory and research. *Journal of Family Practice, 16*, 539–545.

Lee, H. J. (1991). Relationship of hardiness and current life events to perceived health and rural adults. *Research in Nursing and Health, 14*(5), 351–359.

Montana State University Center for Data Systems and Analysis. (1985). *Population profiles of Montana counties: 1980*. Bozeman, MT: Author.

Rigdon, I., Clayton, B., & Diamond, M. (1987). Toward a theory of helpfulness for the elderly bereaved: An invitation to a new life. *Advances in Nursing Science, 9*, 32–43.

Ross, H. (1982). *Women and wellness: Defining, attaining, and maintaining health in Eastern Canada*. Dissertation Abstracts International, 42, DEO 82–12624.

Salisbury State College. (1986, June). *Discussion of Salisbury State College rural health findings*. Presented at the Contemporary Issues in Rural Health Conference, Salisbury, MD.

Scharff, J. (1987). The nature and scope of rural nursing: Distinctive characteristics. Unpublished master's thesis, Montana State University–Bozeman, Montana.

Spielberger, C., Gorsuch, R., & Lushene, R. (1970). *STAI manual for the State-Trait Anxiety Questionnaire*. Palo Alto, CA: Consulting Psychologist.

Spradley, J. (1979). *The ethnographic interview*. New York, NY: Holt, Rinehart, & Winston.

St. Clair, C., Pickard, M., & Harlow, K. (1986). Continuing education for self-actualization: Building a plan for rural nurses. *Journal of Continuing Education in Nursing, 17*, 27–31.

Walker, L., & Avant, K. (1983). *Strategies for theory construction in nursing*. Norwalk, CT: Appleton-Century-Crofts.

Weinert, C. (1983). Social support: Rural people in their new middle years. Unpublished raw data.

Weinert, C., & Long, K. (1987). Understanding the health care needs of rural families. *Journal of Family Relations, 36*, 450–455.

Yura, H., & Torres, G. (1975). *Today's conceptual frameworks with the baccalaureate nursing programs* (NLN Pub. No. 15–1558, pp. 17–75). New York, NY: National League for Nursing.

CHAPTER 3

Concept Analysis

Helen J. Lee, Charlene A. Winters,
Robin L. Boland, Susan Wallace Raph,
and Janice A. Buehler

DISCUSSION TOPICS

- In the Swan and Hobbs (2017) concept analysis of lack of anonymity, the consequences of the concept include familiarity, privacy, and anonymity. Select another concept and determine linkages between it and other identified rural nursing concepts.
- Select a concept, look at the attributes listed, and list potential empirical referents that might be used to measure the concept.
- The concept of work beliefs has yet to be analyzed. What search terms would you select to begin your search?

Long and Weinert (1989) stated that during the initial "process of data organization . . . some concepts appeared repeatedly in the ethnographic data collected in several different areas of the state" (p. 118). Following the initial publication of their article in 1989, faculty in the Rural Nursing Theory Special Committee within the Montana State University (MSU)-Bozeman College of Nursing embarked on a plan to analyze identified concepts. The committee's efforts were enhanced through course work involvement of graduate nursing students enrolled in the MSU College of Nursing's rural generalist program. The purpose of this chapter is to summarize the analyzed concepts contained in *Conceptual Basis of Rural Nursing* (Lee, 1998), other conducted relevant research (Boland & Lee, 2006; Raph & Buehler, 2006), and the concept analysis work on lack of anonymity (Swan & Hobbs, 2017). The summary provides a quick reference of the analyzed concepts and allows for easy identification of areas needing further work.

THE CONCEPTS

The concepts are organized according to the framework provided in the rural nursing theory base. Following each theoretical statement are concept summaries pertinent to that particular statement. Each concept summary is presented using the analysis framework selected by the chapter authors from *Conceptual Basis of Rural Nursing* (Lee, 1998). Elements of the framework, whether explicit or implicit, contained in the chapters are presented; elements not evident are indicated by statements such as "none given" or "not identified."

First Statement: How Rural Dwellers Define Health

The first statement is that "rural dwellers define health primarily as the ability to work, to be productive, to do usual tasks" (Long & Weinert, 1989, p. 120). Work beliefs and health beliefs were key concepts; isolation and distance were identified as related concepts. Health beliefs, isolation, and distance were three of the four concepts analyzed.

HEALTH BELIEFS (LONG, 1993)

Method of analysis: Smith's (1983) four models of health—clinical, role performance, adaptive, and eudaemonistic.

Definition: Rural dwellers often conceptualize health within the role performance model (Long, 1993).

Defining attributes:

- "Ability to work . . . [and] perform one's daily activities" (p. 124).
- "Determine health needs primarily in relation to work activities" (p. 124).
- "As a result of their environment, rural dwellers are more frequently called upon to be independent and self-reliant" (p. 124).

Antecedents: Beliefs held will affect "health-promotion behaviors, healthcare seeking, and acceptance of preventive and treatment interventions" (p. 123).

Consequences: Knowledge of client's concept of health is important for development of relevant and acceptable assessment approaches and intervention strategies (p. 123).

Empirical referents: Not identified.

ISOLATION (LEE, HOLLIS, & McCLAIN, 1998)

Method of analysis: Wilson's method (Walker & Avant, 1995).

Definition: None given.

Essential attributes:

1. Separation—"Being divided from the rest" (Lee et al., 1998, p. 69).

2. Relativeness—"Something dependent on external conditions for its specific nature . . . existing or having its specific nature only by relation to something else; not absolute or independent" (p. 69).

3. Perception—"Consciousness or awareness" (p. 69).

Antecedents: "Presence of an indicator directing attention to the condition of isolation (geographical terrain, distance, changes imposed by weather, economic costs, time, or personal preference)" (p. 69).

Consequences: "Decreased communication or interaction with other individuals that results in social or professional isolation" (p. 70).

Empirical referents: Not identified.

DISTANCE (HENSON, SADLER, & WALTON, 1998)

Method of analysis: Wilson's method (Walker & Avant, 1988).

Definition: "Implies a degree of separation between two or more entities. . . . The nature of separation may be in space, time or behavior" (Henson et al., 1998, p. 51).

Essential attributes:

1. Mileage—"Total number of miles traveled" (p. 56).

2. Time—"Measurement in minutes it takes to travel from one place to another" (p. 56).

3. Perception—"Variation in awareness of data that is different from others' awareness" (p. 56).

Antecedent: "Access to healthcare" (p. 58).

Consequence: "Potential for compromised healthcare" (p. 58).

Empirical referents:

1. Objective:
   a. "Distance" (miles, kilometers) (p. 58).
   b. "Travel time" (p. 58).
   c. MSU Rurality Index (county of residence population, distance to emergency care) (Weinert & Boik, 1995).

2. Subjective:
   a. "Perception" (Henson et al., 1998, p. 58).

Second Statement: Self-Reliance

The second statement states that

> . . . rural dwellers are self-reliant and resist accepting help or services from those seen as "outsiders" or from agencies seen as national or regional "welfare" programs. A corollary to this statement is that help, including needed healthcare, is usually sought through an informal rather than a formal system. (Long & Weinert, 1989, p. 120)

Key concepts analyzed were self-reliance, outsider, insider, old-timer, newcomer, resources, informal networks, and lay care network.

SELF-RELIANCE (CHAFEY, SULLIVAN, & SHANNON, 1998)

Method of analysis: Qualitative research inquiry (Morse, 1995).

Definition:

1. "The capacity to provide for one's own needs" (Agich, 1993, as cited in Chafey et al., 1998, p. 158).
2. "The desire to do for oneself and care for oneself" (Long & Weinert, 1989, p. 119).

Sample: Cohort of nine women between 70 and 85 years of age, living in small rural towns.

Data collection: Interview using structured guide developed to elicit participants' perceptions of self-reliance (Chafey et al., 1998, p. 160).

Characteristics:

1. Primary
   a. Learned—"A skill emanating from previous learning events that started in their youth (family chores and assumption of responsibilities), continued into adulthood, and was reinforced by later life events (retirement, death of a parent or spouse)" (p. 162).
   b. Decisional choice—"Making one's own decisions and choices" (p. 164).
   c. Independence—"Independence or dependence on self, dependence on others, self-assertion or freedom of action, and self-identity" (p. 166).
2. Secondary—Embodied an aspect of their self-reliance experience.
   a. Self-confidence (p. 170).
   b. Self-competence (pp. 170–171).

OUTSIDER (BAILEY, 1998)

Method of analysis: Wilson's method (Walker & Avant, 1988).

Definition: "Being exterior to the group, matter, or boundary in question" (Bailey, 1998, p. 140).

Defining attributes:

1. Differentness—"In terms of cultural orientation, standards, lifestyle, education, religion, occupation, social status, worldview, interests, or experience"; "the quality or state of being different" (pp. 143–144).

2. Unfamiliarity—With the matter in question (p. 144).

3. Unconnectedness—"Having no family or personal ties" (p. 144).

Antecedents: "Lacking understanding or knowledge of the social context, beliefs, rituals, customs, and history of the community" (p. 144).

Consequences: "One may be excluded from access to knowledge and information, not be accepted, not be recognized, be isolated, and be distrusted" (p. 144).

Empirical referents: Not identified.

INSIDER (MYERS, 1998)

Method of analysis: Wilson's method (Walker & Avant, 1995).

Definition: "Someone who is a member of a group and has access to special or privileged information" (Myers, 1998, p. 127).

Defining attributes:

1. "Member of a group" (p. 132).

2. "Having access to privileged information" (p. 132).

3. "An awareness of implicit assumptions and social context" (p. 132).

4. "A long-time occupant" (p. 132).

Antecedents: "Acceptance by the group" (p. 135).

Consequences:

1. "Power . . . because of having information that others lack" (p. 135).

2. "Reserved social position . . . that is unavailable to others" (p. 135).

3. "Lack of objectivity" (p. 135).

4. "Committed to the group" (p. 135).

Empirical referents: Not identified.

OLD-TIMER (CANIPAROLI, 1998)

Method of analysis: Wilson's method (Walker & Avant, 1995).

Definition:

1. "One who is long established in a place or position" (Caniparoli, 1998, p. 103).

2. "A man who has lived in the county a long time" (American slang, 1968, as cited in Caniparoli, 1998, p. 103).

Defining attributes:

1. "Age" (p. 108).

2. "Length of time spent in a community" (p. 108).

3. "Establishment of a relationship within the community" (p. 108).

Antecedents: "Identification as an old-timer" (p. 110).

Consequences: "Establishes a relationship within the community . . . [that] can be viewed as positive or negative depending on the role of the viewer" (p. 110).

Empirical referents: Not identified.

Concept Verification Research

Boland conducted a qualitative study with a convenience sample of nine participants living in small rural communities in central Montana (Boland & Lee, 2006). The study findings confirmed the three defining attributes for old-timer and identified land ownership as the key element of the third attribute. The old-timers spoke of their functions within the community as working together for survival, holding social events to accomplish work and play, to share traditions, and act as historians.

Most participants identified themselves as "old-timers" despite earlier historical literature describing "old-timers" as persons who were "mysterious, unusual and fiercely independent" (Caniparoli, 1998, p. 106). These study participants expressed doubt about their level of influence within the communities, originally attributed to them in the earlier rural nursing theory development. Loss of influence was attributed to changing times (fewer farms and ranches, increased identification with the nearby larger towns and cities) and "the loss of respect for elderly people in today's society" (Boland & Lee, 2006, p. 50).

NEWCOMER (SUTERMASTER, 1998)

Method of analysis: Wilson's method (Walker & Avant, 1995).

Definition: "One that has recently arrived" (Sutermaster, 1998, p. 113).

Defining attributes:

1. "Newly arrived" (p. 120).

2. "Unaware of the history of the area/institution" (p. 120).

3. "Their existence may result in change" (p. 120).

Antecedents: "Individuals or families would have had a need or desire to move" (p. 121).

Consequences: "There is a new individual or family living in the community" (p. 121).

Empirical referents: Not identified.

RESOURCES (BALLANTYNE, 1998)

Method of analysis: Wilson's method (Walker & Avant, 1995).

Definition: "Resources are properties, resorts, or assets that are finite by nature and are made available for use by populations through an allocation process. Resources are accessed and used in response to a population's or individual's motivation for need satisfaction. . . . Furthermore, these three elements can be visualized in a circle with the flow of energy between the allocated resource, accessibility of the resource, and use of the resource" (Ballantyne, 1998, p. 181).

Defining attributes:

1. Property—"Resource is a property or an asset that has value for consumption by populations in need of that property" (p. 181).

2. Expedient—"Continuance or plan for solution of a particular problem" (p. 181).

3. Resort—"Turning inward to one's resources" (p. 181).

Antecedents: Knowledge of "local, regional, and national availability" (p. 187).

Consequences: "Allocation, accessibility, and use" (p. 187).

Empirical referents: Not identified.

INFORMAL NETWORKS (GROSSMAN & MCNERNEY, 1998)

Method of analysis: Wilson's method (Walker & Avant, 1995).

Definition: "Networks are interconnected relationships, durable patterns of interactions, and interpersonal threads that comprise a social fabric" (Grossman & McNerney, 1998, pp. 201–202).

Defining attributes:

1. Volunteer—includes family members, coworkers, and neighbors who offer assistance free of charge (p. 204).

2. Information exchange (p. 204).

3. Support—has two components: Emotional component (being a friend, listening) and physical (assistance with daily living, health promotion, and maintenance activities) (p. 204).

4. Guidance—"May be given as advice, consultation (availability of resources, referral to healthcare providers, sources of alternative treatments), and information" (p. 204).

Antecedents:

1. "A bond . . . the tie that exists among . . . the core of the informal network (family, friends, neighbors, and coworkers)" (p. 206).

2. "Are generated in response to a perceived need" (p. 206).

3. Consequences: "The perceived need is met or not met" (p. 206).

Empirical referents: Not identified.

Lay Care Network (Turnbull, 1998)

Method of analysis: Wilson's method (Walker & Avant, 1988).

Definition: None given.

Defining attributes:

1. Interconnection or net—"An interconnection is the means by which one thing connects with another, whereas a net consists of fibers woven together for catching something" (Turnbull, 1998, p. 195).

2. Of the people—"Belonging to, concerned with, or performed by the 'people' in a nonprofessional capacity" (p. 195).

3. Sense of concern—"The idea that one develops or maintains an interest in the well-being of a person or object, to oversee with the intent to protect" (Oxford, 1989 as cited in Turnbull, 1998, p. 195).

Antecedents: Not identified.

Consequences: Not identified.

Empirical referents: Not identified.

Conclusion: Turnbull (1998) recommended "further refinement of the concept, 'lay care provider,' and suggests a change in the wording of the concept itself"

(p. 198). The literature review clearly delineates between lay providers and informal care providers, whereas the wording "lay care providers" combines two different concepts.

Third Statement: Lack of Anonymity and Role Diffusion

The third statement states that "Health care providers in rural areas must deal with a lack of anonymity and much greater role diffusion than providers in urban or suburban settings" (Long & Weinert, 1989, p. 120). The key concepts are lack of anonymity and role diffusion. Related concepts are familiarity and professional isolation. Analyzed were lack of anonymity, familiarity, and professional isolation.

Lack Of Anonymity (Lee, 1998; Swan & Hobbs, 2017)

In the rural nursing theory literature base, this concept was first analyzed by Lee (1998). Recently, Swan and Hobbs have completed extensive work on the concept of lack of anonymity and one article is blended with this summary. A second article is a chapter in this edition of *Rural Nursing: Concepts, Theory, and Practice* (see Chapter 6).

Method of analysis: Wilson's method (Walker & Avant, 1995, 2011)

Definition: "A condition in which one cannot remain nameless or unknown" (Lee, 1998, p. 77)

Defining attributes: (Lee, 1998)

1. Visible—"That which can be seen, is apparent or obvious" (p. 83).

2. Identifiable—"Being able to recognize or establish the condition or character of a person" (p. 83).

3. "Diminished personal/professional boundaries: Borders or perimeters through which one functions are smaller, more circumscribed" (p. 83).

Swan and Hobbs (2017, p. 1078) derived these defining 3 attributes:

"Identifiable"

"Establishing boundaries for public and private self"

"Interconnectedness in a community"

Antecedents: "Lack of anonymity occurs in an environmental context characterized by a low level of stimulation. It contains fewer numbers of individuals and/or objects (e.g., automobiles, buildings) needing to be considered in the normal deliberation of one's activities" (Lee, 1998, pp. 83–84).

Swan and Hobbs's antecedent update includes "(a) environmental context, (b) opportunities to become visible, (c) developing relationships, and (d) unconscious or limited awareness of public or personal privacy" (p. 1080).

Consequences: "A relationship [in which] one's actions are visible and readily observed" (Lee, 1998, p. 84). Greater difficulty in maintaining personal and professional privacy exists because of the relationship.

Swan and Hobbs consequence update includes "(a) familiarity, (b) visibility, (c) collective responsibility, (d) awareness of privacy, and (e) manage/balance lack of anonymity" (p. 1080).

Empirical referents: None were identified by Lee.

Swan and Hobbs (2017) identified several referents for each of the three attributes:

Identifiable: "accountable for actions, known by others, visible member of the community, awareness of personal and professional reputation" (p. 1081).

Establishing boundaries for public and private self:

> Develop strategies to maintain boundaries, regularly encounter current or former clients outside of professional setting, isolation is used to distance self from social encounters, personal privacy is limited, location of home and how to be reached after hours is known, stopped attending a group activity due to being known, other individuals have crossed personal and professional boundaries, personal and professional boundaries have been crossed by choice. (p. 1081)

Interconnectedness in a community:

> Have numerous personal connections in the community, understand the history and culture of the community, engages in mutually trusting relationships, may have intimate knowledge of others, maintain appropriate and meaningful connections with others, encounters pressure to conform to ideas that run counter to personal beliefs, opportunity to support others. (p. 1081)

Concept Verification Research

Raph conducted a pilot study focusing on the phenomenon "lack of anonymity" with four informants employed in a western rural "frontier" county health department (Raph & Buehler, 2006). Using grounded theory technique, four differing interactive categories emerged through the data analysis: (a) Personally affirming interactions were defined as "friendly encounters that did not place the informant in a professional role" (p. 199); (b) professional affirming interactions were those seeking clarification on "general information about vaccines, appointments, or needed after-hour services . . . usually (taking place in) public places in the community" (pp. 199–200); (c) professionally threatening interactions "placed health care providers in a position of potentially doing harm if not handled correctly" (p. 200); and (d) personally threatening encounters were those that "provoked fear and anger" (p. 201). The four categories, placed in a continuum from positive to negative, extend the second and third defining attributes of the lack of anonymity (Lee, 1998, p. 84) and verify the consequences of the "greater difficulty in maintaining personal and professional privacy."

FAMILIARITY (MCNEELY & SHREFFLER, 1998)

Method of analysis: Wilson's method (Walker & Avant, 1995).

Definition:

> . . . an antithetical concept that includes the positive ideas of thorough knowledge of or an acquaintance with and closeness and intimacy, such as one would find in a family or deep friendship, and the contrasting perspective of offensive, unwarranted, intimate conduct that might include behaviors such as flirting, sexual harassment, domestic violence, abusive relationships, or incest. (McNeely & Shreffler, 1998, p. 91)

Defining attributes:

1. "Friendly relationship or close acquaintance" (p. 98)

2. "Intimacy" (p. 98)

3. "Informality" (p. 98)

4. "The exhibited familiarity is welcome or unwelcome depending on the perceptions of the receiver" (p. 98)

Antecedents: Not identified.

Consequences: Not identified.

Empirical referents: Not identified.

PROFESSIONAL ISOLATION (SHREFFLER, 1998)

Method of analysis: Wilson's method (Walker & Avant, 1988).

Definition: None given.

Defining attributes:

1. "an actual separation from or a deficiency in a resource needed to fulfill one's professional responsibilities or needs (objective component)" (Shreffler, 1998, p. 426)

2. "professional need is perceived as partially or wholly unmet (subjective component)" (p. 426)

3. "the actual separation or deficiency is on a continuum" (p. 426)

4. "the individual is not voluntarily separating herself/himself from an available professional resource" (p. 426)

5. "the objective component is more likely to be present in rural areas" (p. 426)

Antecedents: The individuals

1. experience "separation from or deficiency in resources needed to fulfill professional responsibilities" (p. 429)

2. have "needs for resources to fulfill their professional responsibilities" (p. 429)

3. "can make choices about the use of available resources" (p. 429)

4. "are able to perceive whether professional needs are met" (p. 429)

Consequences: They "are specific to the need that is unmet and the vulnerabilities of the individual in the occupation or job position" (p. 429).

Empirical referents:

1. "The availability of the needed resource is measured and found deficient" (p. 429).

2. "Individuals. . . . express awareness of an unmet need or exhibit signs of the consequence of the unmet need" (pp. 429–430).

CONCLUSION

The concepts contained in *Conceptual Basis of Rural Nursing* (Lee, 1998) and updated content about lack of anonymity published by Swan and Hobbs (2017) have been explicated in this chapter. Most analyses were conducted using the Wilson method (Walker & Avant, 1988, 1995, 2011). However, some of the elements (e.g., definitions, antecedents, consequences, and empirical referents) were not addressed. Furthermore, some key concepts were not analyzed (e.g., work beliefs, role diffusion). Further development of the concepts is needed. Paramount is the need for validation of concepts with rural dwellers.

REFERENCES

Bailey, M. C. (1998). Outsider. In H. J. Lee (Ed.), *Conceptual basis for rural nursing* (pp. 139–148). New York, NY: Springer Publishing.

Ballantyne, J. (1998). Health resources and the rural client. In H. J. Lee (Ed.), *Conceptual basis for rural nursing* (pp. 178–198). New York, NY: Springer Publishing.

Boland, R., & Lee, H. (2006). Old-timers. In H. J. Lee & C. A. Winters (Eds.), *Rural nursing: Concepts, theory, and practice* (2nd ed., pp. 43–52). New York, NY: Springer Publishing.

Caniparoli, C. D. (1998). Old-timer. In H. J. Lee (Ed.), *Conceptual basis for rural nursing* (pp. 102–112). New York, NY: Springer Publishing.

Chafey, K., Sullivan, T., & Shannon, A. (1998). Self-reliance: Characteristics of their own autonomy by elderly rural women. In H. J. Lee (Ed.), *Conceptual basis for rural nursing* (pp. 156–177). New York, NY: Springer Publishing.

Grossman, L. L., & McNerney, S. (1998). Informal networks. In H. J. Lee (Ed.), *Conceptual basis for rural nursing* (pp. 200–208). New York, NY: Springer Publishing.

Henson, D., Sadler, T., & Walton, S. (1998). Distance. In H. J. Lee (Ed.), *Conceptual basis for rural nursing* (pp. 51–60). New York, NY: Springer Publishing.

Lee, H. J. (1998). Lack of anonymity. In H. J. Lee (Ed.), *Conceptual basis for rural nursing* (pp. 76–88). New York, NY: Springer Publishing.

Lee, H. J., Hollis, B. R., & McClain, K. A. (1998). Isolation. In H. J. Lee (Ed.), *Conceptual basis for rural nursing* (pp. 139–148). New York, NY: Springer Publishing.

Long, K. A. (1993). The concept of health: Rural perspectives. *Nursing Clinics of North America, 28,* 123–130.

Long, K. A., & Weinert, C. (1989). Rural nursing: Developing the theory base. *Scholarly Inquiry for Nursing Practice: An International Journal, 3*(2), 113–132.

McNeely, A. G., & Shreffler, M. J. (1998). Familiarity. In H. J. Lee (Ed.), *Conceptual basis for rural nursing* (pp. 89–101). New York, NY: Springer Publishing.

Morse, M. J. (1995). Exploring the theoretical basis of nursing using advanced techniques of concept analysis. *Advances in Nursing Science, 17*(3), 31–46.

Myers, D. D. (1998). Insider. In H. J. Lee (Ed.), *Conceptual basis for rural nursing* (pp. 125–138). New York, NY: Springer Publishing.

Raph, S., & Buehler, J. A. (2006). Rural health professionals' perceptions of lack of anonymity. In H. J. Lee, & C. A. Winters (Eds.), *Rural nursing: Concepts, theory, & practice* (2nd ed., pp. 197–204). New York, NY: Springer Publishing.

Shreffler, M. J. (1998). Professional isolation: A concept analysis. In H. J. Lee (Ed.), *Conceptual basis for rural nursing* (pp. 420–432). New York, NY: Springer Publishing.

Smith, J. A. (1983). *The idea of health: Implications for the nursing profession.* New York, NY: Teachers College Press.

Sutermaster, D. J. (1998). Newcomer. In H. J. Lee (Ed.), *Conceptual basis for rural nursing* (pp. 113–124). New York, NY: Springer Publishing.

Swan, M. A., & Hobbs, B. B. (2017). Concept analysis: Lack of anonymity. *Journal of Advanced Nursing, 73*(5), 1075–1084. doi:10.1111/jan.13236

Turnbull, T. S. (1998). Lay care network. In H. J. Lee (Ed.), *Conceptual basis for rural nursing* (pp. 189–199). New York, NY: Springer Publishing.

Walker, L., & Avant, K. (1988). *Strategies for theory construction in nursing* (2nd ed.). Norwalk, CT: Appleton-Century-Crofts.

Walker, L., & Avant, K. (1995). *Strategies for theory construction in nursing* (3rd ed.). Norwalk, CT: Appleton-Century-Crofts.

Walker, L., & Avant, K. (2011). *Strategies for theory construction in nursing* (5th ed.). Columbus, OH: Prentice Hall.

Weinert, C., & Boik, R. (1995). MSU rurality index: Development and evaluation. *Research in Nursing and Health, 18,* 453–464.

CHAPTER 4

Updating the Rural Nursing Theory Base

Helen J. Lee and Meg K. McDonagh

DISCUSSION TOPICS

- Select one of the relational statements from the rural nursing theory statements and diagram it. Include additional concepts that might be related to the statement.
- Lack of anonymity has changed over the years since it was first identified as a concept in rural nursing theory. Identify if there are other concepts that have changed over time? In what way?
- Identify a concept and select the fields of study from which you could analyze it.

Many disciplines exist to generate, test, and apply theories that will improve the quality of people's lives.

(Fawcett, 1999, p. 1)

"Sparsely Populated Areas: Toward Nursing Theory" was the title of a symposium presented by Montana State University (MSU) College of Nursing at the Western Council on Higher Education for Nursing (now Western Institute of Nursing). It was introduced by Dean Anna Shannon who stated that it would demonstrate how the school could "maximize its resources, provide opportunities for faculty and student research and contribute . . . to the development of an empirically based theory of nursing" (1982, pp. 70–71). This chapter includes a summary of the rural nursing theory structure subsequently published in 1989 by Long and Weinert. It is followed by a review of the literature supporting or refuting the viability of the theoretical statements and concepts. Based on the review, we propose a revised rural nursing theory structure and make suggestions for future work.

THE ORIGINAL RURAL NURSING THEORY STRUCTURE

The quality of the lives of rural persons and the lack of empirical studies about their healthcare was of concern to MSU College of Nursing researchers. A middle-range theory emerged from a recognized need for a framework that acknowledges the unique perceptions of rural persons and the generalist experience of nurses who practice in rural settings. Prior to the development of the theory, it was assumed that nursing care of rural persons was similar to the care of persons living in urban environments.

The resulting descriptive theory is the "most basic type of middle-range theory" (Fawcett, 1999, p. 15). Middle-range theory focuses "on a limited dimension of the reality of nursing" and grows at the "intersection of practice and research to provide guidance for everyday practice and scholarly research rooted in the discipline of nursing" (Smith & Liehr, 2003, p. xi). The theory emerged from observations gathered through qualitative and quantitative descriptive studies conducted in the sparsely populated rural setting of Montana. It describes specific characteristics and observations made of rural persons seeking healthcare and their healthcare providers. The published theory contains three theoretical statements and several key concepts (Long & Weinert, 1989).

The first statement is descriptive and states that "*rural dwellers define health primarily as the ability to work, to be productive, to do usual tasks*" (Long & Weinert, 1989, p. 120). Key concepts associated with this statement are work beliefs and health beliefs. The second statement is relational and proposes that "*rural dwellers are self-reliant and resist accepting help or services from those seen as 'outsiders' or from agencies seen as national or regional 'welfare' programs*" (Long & Weinert, 1989, p. 120). Rural persons preferred to seek healthcare from insiders, persons with whom they were familiar. Additional key concepts pertaining to this statement are "old-timer" and "newcomer." A corollary to the second statement is that "help, including needed medical care, is usually sought through an informal rather than a formal system" (p. 120). The third statement is relational and focuses on healthcare providers; it indicates that *lack of anonymity and role diffusion are experienced more acutely among rural providers than among providers in urban or suburban settings*. Lack of anonymity also applies to the recipients of healthcare in rural areas, as all persons in that environment have a "limited ability . . . to have private areas of their lives" (Long & Weinert, 1989, p. 119).

In addition to the abovementioned three statements, an understanding of the concepts "isolation" and "distance" is important in the healthcare–seeking behavior of rural residents. Isolation refers to separation from or being placed alone (Lee, Hollis, & McClain, 1998). Distance is measurable time, physical space between places, and personal perception of that space (Henson, Sadler, & Walton, 1998). Qualitative data upon which the theoretical work was based indicated that rural residents did not feel isolated, despite the fact that they averaged 23 miles of travel to their nearest emergency department (ED) and over 50 miles to their primary healthcare source (Long & Weinert, 1989, p. 119).

RELATED NURSING LITERATURE

The content of Long and Weinert's (1989) rural nursing theory article was and is widely quoted in nursing literature, including community health and rural nursing texts, and in presentations given about rural nursing. However, periodic rural nursing literature reviews contain few citations specifically focusing on health perceptions and needs of rural persons. We located three qualitative studies through conference proceedings, the contents of which were subsequently published (Bales, Winters, & Lee, 2006; Lee & Winters, 2004; Thomlinson, McDonagh, Reimer, Crooks, & Lees, 2004). Other sources included two nursing master's theses (Bales, 2006; Moran, 2005), a study that focused on the healthcare meanings, values, and practices of Anglo-American male population in the rural American Midwest (Sellers, Poduska, Propp, & White, 1999), a study exploring rurality and health in midlife women (Thurston & Meadows, 2003), and a study examining the health-information-seeking experiences of rural women in Ontario, Canada (Wathen & Harris, 2006, 2007). We also located several journal articles, mostly qualitative rural research, that included rural concepts found in Long and Weinert's article. In the following sections, each theoretical statement is followed by findings from the literature supporting or refuting the statement.

Theoretical Statement 1 (Descriptive)

> . . . [R]ural dwellers define health primarily as the ability to work, to be productive, to do usual tasks. (Long & Weinert, 1989, p. 120)

Four qualitative studies conducted in the United States examined health perceptions; one with rural men aged 25 to 49, one with rural men and women aged 28 to 63, and two with older rural persons aged 60 to 85. Three provided support for the abovementioned descriptive statement that defines health as the ability to carry out important functions (Niemoller, Ide, & Nichols, 2000; Pierce, 2001; Sellers et al., 1999). In the fourth study, Averill (2002) found that definitions of health varied across her southwest United States sample that included older retirees, more recent retirees, and Hispanic elders. The older retirees from mining and ranching communities viewed health in a similar manner to the original qualitative theory development samples, whereas more recent retirees focused on strategies to remain healthy—proper diet, regular exercise, and regular health exams. The Hispanic elders in Averill's sample frequently mentioned incorporating home remedies and herbal preparations into their health maintenance practices.

Participants in the several health perceptions and needs studies (Bales, 2006; Bales et al., 2006; Lee & Winters, 2004; Moran, 2005; Thomlinson et al., 2004; Winters, Thomlinson, et al., 2006) conducted in the United States and Canada were more likely to define health holistically. Lee and Winters (2004) found that for rural persons working in service occupations, being able to function included being physically, mentally, and emotionally fit. Participants in a study conducted by Bales et al. (2006) thought that being healthy meant being mentally and physically active, eating well, and having an overall sense of well-being. Thomlinson et al. (2004) interpreted their participants' responses by saying that health was a "holistic relationship between the physical, mental, social and spiritual aspects of their lives" (p. 261). This same view of health was echoed by Canadian middle-aged women in Thurston and Meadows's (2003) study and by the older adults residing in Appalachia who completed surveys and participated in focus groups (Goins, Spencer, & Williams, 2011).

Australian women in de la Rue and Coulson's (2003) study, aged 73 to 87, equated health with not being ill. They knew maintenance of their health was influenced by their geographical location and their desire to remain living on the land.

SUMMARY

The literature both supports and refutes the first theoretical statement. Support appears in studies of rural male adults and of older persons and retirees from the extractive industries (mining, farming). Lack of support for the functional definition of health emerges from a variety of settings and from differing rural samples. It may be that age, the rural environmental setting, the influence of the work ethic, and the culture are factors in defining health (de la Rue & Coulson, 2003). Potentially, younger rural participants may be influenced by increased media exposure and its emphasis on health promotion and the use of preventive health practices. In addition, healthcare providers may be expanding their view of health beyond the illness care model and may be sharing this with their clients.

Theoretical Statement 2 (Relational)

> . . . [R]ural dwellers are self-reliant and resist accepting help or services from those seen as 'outsiders' or from agencies seen as national or regional welfare programs. (Long & Weinert, 1989, p. 120)

The attribute of self-reliance dominates the literature about rural persons and their health-seeking behaviors (Davis & Magilvy, 2000; Jirojwong & MacLennan, 2002; Lee & Winters, 2004; Niemoller et al., 2000; Sellers et al., 1999; Thomlinson et al., 2004; Wathen & Harris, 2006, 2007; Winters, Thomlinson, et al., 2006). Care was sought by rural residents after first "consulting books" (Jirojwong & MacLennan, 2002, p. 251) and trying "to deal with an illness themselves" (Thomlinson et al., 2004, p. 10). Because of the presence of chronic illnesses, older adults were knowledgeable about nearby medical care resources, including physicians, physician's assistants, and nurse practitioners (Niemoller et al., 2000; Pierce, 2001; Roberto & Reynolds, 2001), and if available, would use them "to achieve their desired level of independence" (Niemoller et al., 2000, p. 39). However, if the desired resources were not available, these same older adults stated they would "manage" (Niemoller et al., 2000, p. 39).

Canadian women (aged 20–82) in the study conducted by Wathen and Harris (2006) shared differing strategies when faced with an urgent health situation. Some would visit a hospital ED while others would self-medicate and wait until the next morning to contact their family doctor. Decision making was influenced by perception of the knowledge and skills of available professional practitioners and, in some situations, by the results of previous interactions about managing their chronic illnesses. In addition, decisions were affected by the distances they needed to travel, particularly in winter.

COROLLARY TO RELATIONAL STATEMENT 2 (DESCRIPTIVE)

. . . [H]elp, including needed healthcare, is usually sought through an informal rather than a formal system. (Long & Weinert, 1989, p. 120)

The literature revealed a variety of findings related to the relational statement corollary. Bales (2006) found that mothers with children living in U.S. frontier settings would seek advice from family, friends, and neighbors and would initiate self-care activities if healthcare situations were not considered serious. However, if the illness or injury was gauged as serious, professional healthcare was immediately accessed no matter the distance involved. Bypassing the informal for the formal system because of the seriousness of the illness or injury also was found in studies conducted by Buehler, Malone, and Majerus (1998) and Thomlinson et al. (2004).

Participants in two Canadian studies (Thomlinson et al., 2004; Wathen & Harris, 2006, 2007) indicated that family, friends, and neighbors were cited as a major source of support, particularly during the information-gathering phase (Wathen & Harris, 2006). Those particularly valued were persons who held a healthcare professional role or had experienced a disease or illness firsthand (Wathen & Harris, 2006). Although older rural women in the U.S. study conducted by Pierce (2001) stated that they were eager to help neighbors and the less fortunate, they also shared their reluctance to tell family and neighbors about their own needs unless really necessary.

Help gained through accessing informal knowledge via the media, popular magazines, books, libraries, and the Internet was cited in three studies (Roberto & Reynolds, 2001; Thomlinson et al., 2004; Wathen & Harris, 2007). A sample of older women living in the United States actively sought information about living with their osteoporosis (Roberto & Reynolds, 2001): Members of a Canadian sample stated that they frequently made use of formal information sources through libraries, books, and computers (Thomlinson et al., 2004; Wathen & Harris, 2007).

Summary

The second theoretical statement and its corollary are both sustained and refuted by the findings in the literature. Self-reliance continues to be a characteristic attribute of rural persons and influences the way they respond to illness or injury and their subsequent care-seeking behaviors. The informal system (family, friends, and neighbors) is still frequently used as a resource. However, the rural cultural barrier to accessing care through formal resources appears to be changing. The increased knowledge and the need to have information about health and the chronic illnesses they are experiencing may be removing the cultural barrier of approaching "outsiders" for health and medical care. In part, this may be occurring because desired health information can now be obtained through use of the Internet while maintaining anonymity. Prior to the current age of information technology, maintaining anonymity while seeking health information was not an option.

Theoretical Statement 3 (Relational)

> . . . [H]ealth care providers in rural areas must deal with a lack of anonymity and much greater role diffusion than providers in urban or suburban settings. (Long & Weinert, 1989, p. 120)

The findings for the two concepts forming this relational statement—lack of anonymity and role diffusion—are sustained in the literature about healthcare providers from Australia, New Zealand, and the United States. In relation to the lack of anonymity, authors stated that "in close knit communities ... news travels fast" (Lau, Kumar, & Thomas, 2002, Results and Discussion, paragraph 7) and that "social life realities in small communities frequently blur professional boundaries" (Blue & Fitzgerald, 2002, pp. 319–320). Social factors pertaining to practice in rural communities include privacy issues for both the professional and the clients for whom they give care (Lau et al., 2002). Healthcare practitioners in rural environments who are known by their clients may find that older women prefer receiving professional care from a familiar person (Courtney, Tong, & Walsh, 2000; Pierce, 2001), whereas middle-aged women prefer to go elsewhere for care because of that familiarity (Brown, Young, & Byles, 1999; Lee & Winters, 2004). Lee and Winters found this is particularly true for women's healthcare and mental health.

According to the work by Swan and Hobbs (2017), the meaning of the concept, "lack of anonymity," has also undergone change since the earlier work of

Long and Weinert (1989). With the advent of widespread access to the Internet and the use of social media, maintaining any sense of anonymity has become increasingly difficult for everyone, including rural nurses. And while Lee (1998) found that personal and professional boundaries may be diminished, Swan and Hobbs and Chipp et al. (2011) found that the issue may be related to how one establishes boundaries for one's personal and professional self. Another key factor related to the current meaning of lack of anonymity is the environmental context of those involved, specifically rural nurses. Previously this was thought to be a physical, geographic, and relational context and now it would seem that "environment" also includes digital and temporal.

Role diffusion was found in studies conducted with psychiatrists and nurses in Australia (Lau et al., 2002) and by Rosenthal (1996) in her study of rural nursing in America. Hegney (1997) described role diffusion in both generalist and extended roles in her study of Australian rural nursing practice. Role diffusion was evident in the practice of hospice nurses in New Zealand (McConigley, Kristjanson, & Morgan, 2000). The reality in sparsely populated areas is that with fewer persons available to perform multiple tasks, more tasks must be undertaken by the individuals who practice in these areas.

SUMMARY

The third theoretical statement about lack of anonymity and role diffusion is well supported in the literature. Familiarity, the opposite of anonymity, can be a facilitator or a barrier to seeking health and illness care from local healthcare practitioners. Familiarity is a distinguishing feature of rural nursing that allows rural nurses a special knowledge of those for whom they provide care within their communities (Hegney, 1997).

The lack of anonymity that healthcare providers experience in rural communities is in itself a paradox. On the one hand, it is often the familiarity and knowing of community members and the lack of anonymity that draws healthcare professionals to rural areas. Yet, it is often these same attributes that can later drive them away.

CONCLUSION

The review of the literature pertaining to the descriptive middle-range rural nursing theory base revealed a variety of findings. The rural residents' definition of health in the first descriptive statement is changing from that of a functional nature to a more holistic view that includes physical, mental, social, and spiritual aspects. The self-reliance of rural residents in the second relational statement is broadly supported; however, the resistance to seeking help from those seen as "outsiders" is changing. The third relational statement pertaining to healthcare providers and their lack of anonymity and role diffusion is supported. The findings for the concept of distance in the original rural theory development work are not supported. This literature appraisal of the rural nursing theory base structure supports a need for change.

THE REVISED RURAL NURSING THEORY

Based on this review of the literature, we recommended the following revisions to the first two theoretical statements originally proposed by Long and Weinert in 1989.

Theoretical Statement 1 (Descriptive)

> Rural residents define health as being able to do what they want to do; it is a way of life and a state of mind; there is a goal of maintaining balance in all aspects of their lives. (Lee & McDonagh, 2006, p. 314)
>
> Older rural residents and those with ties to extractive industries are more likely to define health in a functional manner—to work, to be productive, and to do usual tasks. (Lee & McDonagh, 2006, p. 314)

Essential to understanding rural persons' motivation for illness treatment, health maintenance, and health promotion is knowledge of their health perceptions (Long, 1993). The abovementioned replacement statements provide a broader view of the health perceptions that have been found with more recent research among rural individuals, families, and communities. They reflect both the earlier emphasis on role performance evident among older residents and among those employed in extractive industries and the expanded view of health perception definitions elicited from other individuals living in rural communities.

Theoretical Statement 2 (Relational)

> Rural residents are self-reliant and make decisions to seek care for illness, sickness, or injury depending on their self-assessment of the severity of their present health condition and of the resources needed and available. (Lee & McDonagh, 2006, p. 315)
>
> Rural residents with infants and children experiencing illness, sickness, or injury will seek care more quickly than for themselves. (Lee & McDonagh, 2006, p. 315)

These theoretical statements refer to the health-seeking behaviors of rural residents. Key concepts from the 1989 model included self-reliance, seeking care from insiders, and the use of the informal system. Research findings continue to assert that self-reliance is a key characteristic identified in the management of healthcare situations by rural persons. However, changes were seen in the health-seeking behaviors of these residents as they seek advice and care from insiders and outsiders and also make use of both informal and formal systems of care.

Additional concepts emerged from the comparative research about rural persons' health behaviors: *health-seeking behaviors* and *choice* (Winters, Thomlinson, et al., 2006). *Health-seeking behaviors*, defined as "conscious behaviors designed to promote healthy relationships among physical, mental, social and spiritual aspects of one's life so that life balance is maintained" (Winters, Thomlinson, et al., 2006), include three subthemes: symptom–action–timeline process (SATL; Buehler et al., 1998), resources, and self-reliance.

Conscious *choice* is made in at least two domains of rural persons' lives. The first is the choice to live in a rural environment; the second is in accessing healthcare resources. Choosing to live in a rural environment is closely associated with the concept of place (see discussion later in this chapter).

Theoretical Statement 3 (Relational)

Healthcare providers in rural areas continue to experience lack of anonymity and role diffusion. Although the literature review demonstrates that the meaning of "lack of anonymity" has been expanded, the concept is still well supported. Therefore, the original statement was well supported in the literature review; no changes are recommended.

FUTURE DIRECTIONS

Exploration of the literature regarding rural health perceptions and needs revealed many new avenues for future exploration. Themes of *distance* and *resources* were identified repeatedly in the literature reviewed. Newly proposed concepts emerging from the literature review included *health-seeking behaviors, choice, environmental context,* and *social capital*. Each of these concepts is addressed in the following sections.

Distance

Although *distance* was not part of the three theoretical statements making up the rural nursing theory base, the content of the rural literature we accessed for this review frequently touched on the concept. In the seminal article by Long and Weinert (1989), the participants included in the multiple studies tended to see health services as accessible and did not view themselves as isolated. Canadian authors MacLeod, Browne, and Leipert (1998) stated that distance may not be a problem but said the concept exerts a strong influence in providing healthcare in rural areas. This view affirms Johnson, Ratner, and Bottorff's (1995) assertion that one's geographic location may influence or even determine the form of health-seeking behaviors rural residents demonstrate. Pierce (2001) found that the older women described distance and geographical barriers with concern; yet, they seemed to take problems with accessibility "in stride" (p. 52). In addition, the study participants did express concern about the quality of nearby health services.

The remainder of the research all refuted the initial findings about distance and access to healthcare in Long and Weinert's (1989) theory-based article. Fitzgerald, Pearson, and McCutcheon (2001), Moran (2005), Pieh-Holder, Callahan, and Young (2012), and Racher and Vollman (2002) stated that access to healthcare services is a major concern for rural and remote residents and for the health professionals serving them in Australia, Canada, and the United States. In a quantitative study examining the relationship between distance to the nearest mammography facilities in Kentucky, researchers found a significant relationship between the presence of advanced diagnoses and longer average travel distances (Huang, Digan, Han, & Johnson, 2009).

Australian rural healthcare experts were asked how rural and remote areas are different; Wakerman, Bourke, Humphreys, and Taylor (2017) found "geographic distance" and "access to healthcare" to be the chief characteristics of that difference.

Access to care is particularly a concern for rural individuals with chronic illness; an expressed problem was finding the "best" doctor (Fitzgerald et al., 2001). Distance to emergency care was an expressed concern of service providers in rural areas (Lee & Winters, 2004) and of mothers of children living in frontier areas (Bales, 2006; Pieh-Holder et al., 2012). Wong and Regan's (2009) study participants averaged at least two chronic illnesses each; they made tradeoffs between their safety because of poor winter driving conditions and meeting their health needs. In a survey of middle-aged women, Brown et al. (1999) concluded that experiencing difficulties with accessing healthcare results in greater reliance on self-treatment and self-care, thereby leading to development of "attitudes of independence and self-reliance [sic]" (p. 151).

Resources

In addition to distance, the concept of *resources* directly impacts access to healthcare services. Gulzar (1999) and Racher and Vollman (2002) discuss the complexity of accessing health services. The rurality or remoteness of a given place affects access to health services. Within the rural environment, factors such as geography, politics, and economics, as well as the acceptability and the education of healthcare providers, all influence the residents' access to and choice of health resources. Studying patterns of healthcare use and feedback loops among residents may add to the understanding of the complexity of accessing healthcare services in rural and remote areas (Racher & Vollman, 2002).

Delivery of health services across sparsely populated areas presents unique challenges because of the vast distances involved and the scarcity of health professionals. For example, the greater the nurse-to-patient or physician-to-patient ratio and the more rural or remote the community, the more limited the health resources are for rural and remote community members.

Health-Seeking Behaviors

Health-seeking behaviors were defined as "conscious behaviors designed to promote healthy relationships among physical, mental, social and spiritual aspects of one's life so that life balance in maintained" (Winters, Thomlinson, et al., 2006, p. 34). The authors included three subthemes, SATL process, resources, and self-reliance, as part of health-seeking behaviors. The SATL process (Buehler et al., 1998) is used to describe the social process and to identify symptoms of sickness, illness, or injury and then seek the appropriate level of requisite care. The level of care sought may be self, lay, or professional, depending upon the perceived seriousness and type of symptom. Accessing resources is a part of the SATL process (see Chapter 16). Self-reliance, defined as behaviors to promote or maintain health without seeking assistance from others, was prevalent in the data from Montana and the Canadian provinces of Alberta and Manitoba. Winters, Thomlinson, et al. (2006, p. 35) considered self-reliance a subtheme of health-seeking behavior because of its paramount influence on a person's seeking healthcare in sparsely populated rural areas.

Choice

Choice, the making of conscious decisions to live in a rural environment and access healthcare resources, was a new theme that emerged from the comparison study (Winters, Thomlinson, et al., 2006). Explicitly evident in the Montana data and implicitly identified in the Canadian study through the participants' expressions of the benefits of living in rural environments, the theme of choice is associated with the concept of "place." Although we think of place in a geographical context, it is a broader entity that shapes one's political, economic, spatial, geographic, and cultural views of the world (Kelly, 2003). De la Rue and Colson (2003) found that rural participants' well-being and health were influenced by the "geographical location of living on the land" (p. 5). "Place" provided these rural residents with a kind of emotional or spiritual connectedness that affected the outcomes of their health experiences.

Wathen and Harris (2007) stated that rural living affected the choice of resources that members of their Canadian study would consult about a chronic health concern or an acute medical problem. If the available rural doctor "might not be the best or too up-to date" (p. 643), they preferred their informal system (colleagues, friends, family), medical books, pharmacists, and/or the veterinarian.

Choice in making decisions related to accessing healthcare can be affected by several factors. Questions often asked to aid in determining a course of action are: Where is the closest facility that will provide the healthcare needed? What are the qualifications of the persons who staff that facility? What level of confidence is there in the local facility's healthcare providers? Does familiarity with the professionals who staff the facility make a difference in making the choice of where to go? Is anonymity an important factor in this situation? Does the healthcare facility accept the insurance (true in the U.S. healthcare system) carried by the individual or family seeking care (Moran, 2005)? What hours does the facility stay open? What are the weather conditions? During stormy conditions, what roads are better maintained (freezing rain, snow, and ice; summer rain, wind, and flooding). In an acute emergency, can a fixed-wing aircraft or helicopter land nearby? These represent only a fraction of the factors and questions that play a role in the decision making for accessing healthcare.

Environmental Context

Appearing repeatedly throughout the literature reviewed were terms like *place, geographical location, context,* or *environmental context.* According to Jones and Ross (2003, p. 16), nursing practice is "shaped by its situatedness" (p. 16). Authors speak of the context of a place and the resources needed that are particular to a context or place (Andrews, 2002, 2003; Andrews & Moon, 2005; MacLeod et al., 2008; Poland, Leboux, Holmes, & Andrews, 2005; Thurston & Meadows, 2004; Winters, Cudney, Sullivan, & Thuesen, 2006). According to Lauder, Reel, Farmer, and Griggs (2006), "'Context' is an important unit of analysis . . . A rural heath context is both physical and relational and aspects of rural environments . . . may enhance or impede health" (p. 75). According to Swan and Hobbs's (2017) work on lack of anonymity, with the prevalence of Internet use and social media, "environmental context" should now also include the cyber or digital realm.

Health perceptions, needs, and actions of rural persons are also influenced by the environmental context. This was particularly evident in the research reported by de la Rue and Coulson (2003), Thomlinson et al. (2004), and Winters, Cudney, et al. (2006). In their intervention study of rural women with chronic illnesses, Winters and her colleagues found that four themes emerged through the "overarching theme of distance: (a) physical setting, (b) social/cultural/economic environment, (c) nature of women's work, and (d) accessibility/quality of health care" (pp. 284–285).

Social Capital

Social capital is a concept that comes from sociology and has come into increasing importance over the last 25 years (Shookner, Scott, & Vollman, 2008). Rankin (2002, as cited in Lauder et al., 2006) defines social capital as "forms of association that express trust and norms of reciprocity" (p. 75). The Policy Research

Initiative for the government of Canada (PRI; 2005 as cited in Shookner et al., 2008) further clarifies social capital as the "networks of social relations that may provide individuals and groups with access to resources and supports" (p. 87). "Creating supportive environments is about building social capital" (p. 87) and is similar to the notion of building "rural health services research capacity" (Hartley, 2005, p. 12).

Nurses practicing in rural settings tend to be more actively engaged professionally and personally in the rural communities in which they live and work (Bushy, 2000; Scharff, 1998). However, the present role of nurses in creating supportive healthcare environments is not well understood; recognition, conceptualization, and measurement are needed "to more fully appreciate the impact nurses have on rural health access and services" (Lauder et al., 2006, p. 74).

Three qualitative studies about nurses spoke to the necessity of developing social capital within rural communities (Conger & Plager, 2008; Gibb, Livesey, & Zyle, 2003; MacKinnon, 2008). APRN graduates realized the importance of "rural connectedness" through development of support networks with other healthcare providers, relationships with urban healthcare centers, connections with local communities, and support through electronic means (Conger & Plager, 2008). Nurses providing maternity care realized that they needed to know "their community—who lives in their community, what their skills are, and whether they are available to address local health needs or respond to emergency situations" (MacKinnon, 2008, p. 6). Nurses in solo mental health practice recognized the necessity of assisting rural and remote clients "to achieve a level of social functioning to integrate the person back into their community network" (Gibb, 2003, p. 248). To do this, they found that they needed to work more closely with the potential support structures identified within the clients' community. This was best achieved by fostering a caring home environment, trying to keep people with their families and in their place of employment (Gibb et al., 2003). By having such a support structure, rural mental practitioners can avoid sending the mental health client to a psychiatric institution when a crisis occurs.

SUMMARY

Theories are developed for the purposes of describing, explaining, and predicting phenomena (Fawcett, 2000). The intent of the early theory development work at the College of Nursing at MSU was to use the descriptive research data collected in sparsely populated rural areas to develop a middle-range theory, one that would provide a framework for nurses providing care to rural dwellers (Shannon, 1982). What evolved was a descriptive theory, the most basic type of middle-range theory (Fawcett, 1999).

Although controversy exists about the placement and abstraction level of middle-range theories within the hierarchical structure of nursing theories (Peterson & Bredow, 2004), the basic theory structure, regardless of level, is similar—theoretical statements that describe or link key concepts (Fawcett, 1999). The interweaving of those concepts and statements provides a pattern of ideas, which provide a new perspective on phenomena (Smith & Liehr, 2003). The pattern, once published and subjected to testing, should remain open to scrutiny, debate, and if necessary, to change and the incorporation of new ideas.

By subjecting the middle-range rural nursing theory to testing in several studies (Bales, 2006; Bales et al., 2006; Lee & Winters, 2004; Moran, 2005; Thomlinson et al., 2004; Winters, Thomlinson, et al., 2006) and in the findings from several related studies, it was evident that change had occurred over the past 30 years that had altered the applicability of the original published rural nursing theory base by Weinert and Long (1989). This change is demonstrated by the revisions to theoretical statements and the new emerging concepts

VISION FOR THE FUTURE

Because of the descriptive nature of the middle-range rural nursing theory, additional descriptive research is needed (Fawcett, 1999). Concept analysis methods can take several approaches, including the Wilson method (Walker & Avant, 1995), the evolutionary method (Rogers, 1993), the empirical or inductive approach (Morse, 1995), or a combination thereof. Testing of the proposed changes to the rural nursing theory relational statements through qualitative studies (ethnography, grounded theory, phenomenology, narrative inquiry, historical inquiry, and photovoice) and participatory action research needs to take place in other sparsely populated areas. Development and testing of instruments to measure the concepts are also needed. Conducting surveys to measure attributes, attitudes, knowledge, and opinions using open-ended and semistructured interviews and questionnaires is required (Fawcett, 1999). With a compilation of these focused research efforts can emerge a model, a schema, or a list of logically ordered statements that, when present, will provide guidance for the care of rural dwellers (Smith & Liehr, 2003).

Moving the Work Forward

A core group of nurse researchers from Montana and Alberta periodically met to review and critique theoretical material and models. Members of this North American Study (NAS) group discussed and planned projects to further rural nursing theory development while offering research and educational opportunities to graduate students within their courses or independent studies. A rural nursing and theory listserv group, initiated several years ago, provided a mechanism for online discussion for furthering rural nursing research and theory development. While this listserv is now dormant, a resource is potentially available for reestablishment of communication: The International Council of Nurses (ICN) Rural and Remote Nursing Network, www.icn.ch/rrn_network.htm, and

Improving Health Among Rural and Vulnerable Populations, www.facebook.com/#!/groups/395662340465359.

The NAS and listserv members did identify the following questions for continued exploration of rural healthcare behaviors: (a) Are these health-seeking behaviors unique to rural residents? (b) Will health-seeking behavior activities of the Health-Needs–Action Process (HNAP; Chapter 16) process fit under the same middle-range theory framework as those for health promotion? (c) How do illness variables affect rural persons' health-seeking behaviors? (d) How do illness variables affect rural people's choices of healthcare providers? (e) Are rural dwellers more accepting of "outsiders" if they are healthcare professionals working in partnerships with the rural community and local health professionals?

CONCLUSION

The *revised statements* for the middle-range rural nursing theory as published by Lee and McDonagh (2010) are ready for testing. The emerging concepts identified in the review of the rural nursing literature are also ready for exploration, testing, and tool development. Continued research and theoretical development efforts will increase the potential for a middle-range theory that can provide a structure for acceptable, adaptable, and evidence-based nursing care interventions for rural persons.

REFERENCES

Andrews, G. J. (2002). Towards a more place-sensitive nursing: An invitation to medical and health sensitive health geography. *Nursing Inquiry, 9*(4), 221–238.

Andrews, G. J. (2003). Locating a geography of nursing: Space, place, and the progress of geographical thought. *Nursing Philosophy, 4*, 231–248.

Andrews, G. J., & Moon, G. (2005). Space, place, and the evidence base: Part I—An introduction to health geography. *Worldviews on Evidence Based Nursing, 2*, 55–62.

Averill, J. B. (2002). Voices from the Gila: Health care issues for rural elders in southwestern New Mexico. *Journal of Advanced Nursing, 40*, 654–662.

Bales, R. L. (2006). Health perceptions, needs, and behaviors of remote rural women of childbearing and childrearing age. In H. J. Lee & C. A. Winters (Eds.), *Rural nursing: Concepts, theory and practice* (2nd ed., pp. 66–78). New York, NY: Springer Publishing.

Bales, R. L., Winters, C. A., & Lee, H. J. (2006). Health needs and perceptions of rural persons. In H. J. Lee & C. A. Winters (Eds.), *Rural nursing: Concepts, theory, and practice* (2nd ed., pp. 53–65). New York, NY: Springer Publishing.

Blue, I., & Fitzgerald, M. (2002). Interprofessional relations: Care studies of working relationships between registered nurses and general practitioners in rural Australia. *Journal of Clinical Nursing, 11*, 314–321.

Brown, W. J., Young, A. F., & Byles, J. E. (1999). Tyranny of distance? The health of mid-age women living in five geographical areas of Australia. *Australian Journal of Rural Health, 7*, 148–154.

Buehler, J. A., Malone, M., & Majerus, J. M. (1998). Patterns of responses to symptoms in rural residents: The symptom-action-time-line process. In H. J. Lee (Ed.), *Conceptual basis for rural nursing* (pp. 318–328). New York, NY: Springer Publishing.

Bushy, A. (2000). *Orientation to nursing in the rural community*. Thousand Oaks, CA: Sage.

Chipp, C., Dewane, S., Brems, C., Johnson, M. E., Warnwe, T. D., & Roberts, L. W. (2011). "If only someone had told me ...": Lessons from rural providers. *The Journal of Rural Health, 27*(1), 122–130.

Conger, M. M., & Plager, K. A. (2008). Advanced practice nursing practice in rural areas: Connectedness versus disconnectedness. *Online Journal of Rural Nursing and Health Care, 8*(1), 24–38. Retrieved from http://rnojournal.Binghamton.edu/index.php/RNO/article/view/127

Courtney, M., Tong, S., & Walsh, A. (2000). Older patients in the acute care setting: Rural and metropolitan nurses' knowledge, attitudes and practices. *Australian Journal of Rural Health, 8*, 94–102.

Davis, R., & Magilvy, J. K. (2000). Quiet pride: The experience of chronic illness by rural older adults. *Journal of Nursing Scholarship, 32*, 385–390.

de la Rue, M., & Coulson, I. (2003). The meaning of health and well-being: Voices from older rural women. *Rural and Remote Health, 3*(192), 1–10. Retrieved from htpps://www.rrh.org.au/journal/article/192

Fawcett, J. (1999). *The relationship of theory and research* (3rd ed.). Philadelphia, PA: F. A. Davis.

Fawcett, J. (2000). *Analysis and evaluation of contemporary nursing knowledge: Nursing models and theories*. Philadelphia, PA: F. A. Davis.

Fitzgerald, M., Pearson, A., & McCutcheon, H. (2001). Impact of rural living on the experience of chronic illness. *Australian Journal of Rural Health, 9*, 235–240.

Gibb, H. (2003). Rural community mental health nursing: A grounded theory account of sole practice. *International Journal of Mental Health Nursing, 12*, 243–250.

Gibb, H., Livesey, L., & Zyla, W. (2003). At 3 am who the hell do you call? Case management issues in sole practice as a rural community mental health nurse. *Australasian Psychiatry, 11*(Suppl. 1), S127–S130.

Goins, R. T., Spencer, S. M., & Williams, K. (2011). Lay meanings of health among rural older adults in Appalachia. *The Journal of Rural Health, 27*(1), 13–20.

Gulzar, L. (1999). Access to health care. *Journal of Nursing Scholarship, 31*, 13–19.

Hartley, D. (2005). Rural health research: Building capacity and influencing policy in the United States and Canada. *Canadian Journal of Nursing Research, 37*(1), 7–13.

Hegney, D. (1997). Rural nursing practice. In L. Siegloff (Ed.), *Rural nursing in the Australian context* (pp. 25–43). Deacon Act, Australia: Royal College of Nursing.

Henson, D., Sadler, T. & Walton, D. (1998). Distance. In H. J. Lee (Ed.) *Conceptual basis for rural nursing* (pp. 51–60). New York, NY: Springer Publishing.

Huang, B., Dignan, M., Han, D., & Johnson, O. (2009). Does distance matter? Distance to mammography facilities and stage at diagnosis of breast cancer in Kentucky. *Journal of Rural Health, 25*(4), 366–371.

Jirojwong, S., & MacLennan, R. (2002). Management of episodes of incapacity by families in rural and remote Queensland. *Australian Journal of Rural Health, 10*, 249–255.

Johnson, J. L., Ratner, P. A., & Bottorff, J. L. (1995). Urban–rural differences in the health-promoting behaviors of Albertans. *Canadian Journal of Public Health, 86*, 103–108.

Jones, S., & Ross, J. (2003). *Describing your scope of practice: A resource for rural nurses*. Christchurch, NZ: Centre for Rural Health. Retrieved from http://www.moh.govt.nz

Kelly, S. E. (2003). Bioethics and rural health: Theorizing place, space, and subjects. *Social Science & Medicine, 56*, 2277–2288.

Lau, T., Kumar, S., & Thomas, D. (2002). Practicing psychiatry in New Zealand's rural areas: Incentives, problems and solutions. *Australasian Psychiatry, 10*(1), 33–38.

Lauder, W., Reel, S., Farmer, J., & Griggs, H. (2006). Social capital, rural nursing and rural nursing theory. *Nursing Inquiry, 13*(1), 73–79.

Lee, H. J., Hollis, B. R., & McClain, K. A. (1998). Isolation. In H. J. Lee (Ed.), *Conceptual Basis for Rural Nursing* (pp. 61–75). New York, NY: Springer Publishing.

Lee, H. J. & McDonagh, M. K. (2006). Examining the rural nursing theory base. In H. J. Lee, & C. A. Winters (Eds), *Rural Nursing: Concepts, Theory, and Practice* (2nd ed., pp. 17–26). New York, NY: Springer Publishing.

Lee, H. J., & McDonagh, M. K. (2010). Updating the rural nursing theory base. In C. A. Winters & H. J. Lee (Eds.), *Rural nursing: Concepts, theory, and practice* (3rd ed., pp. 19–39). New York, NY: Springer Publishing.

Lee, H. J., & Winters, C. A. (2004). Testing rural nursing theory: Perceptions and needs of service providers. *Online Journal of Rural Nursing and Health Care, 4*(1), 51–63. Retrieved from http://www.rno.org/journal/issues/vol-4/issue.1/Lee_article.htm

Long, K. A. (1993). The concept of health: Rural perspectives. *The Nursing Clinics of North America, 28*(1), 123–130.

Long, K. A., & Weinert, C. (1989). Rural nursing: Developing the theory base. *Scholarly Inquiry for Nursing Practice: An International Journal, 3*, 113–127.

MacKinnon, K. A. (2008). Labouring to nurse: The work of rural nurses who provide maternity care. *Rural and Remove Health Care, 8*, 1–15. Retrieved from http://www.rrh.org.au

MacLeod, M., Browne, A. J., & Leipert, B. (1998). International perspective: Issues for nurses in rural and remote Canada. *Australian Journal of Rural Health, 6*, 72–78.

MacLeod, M. L. P., Misener, R. M., Banks, K., Morton, A. M., Vogt, C., & Bentham, D. (2008). "I'm a different kind of nurse": Advice from nurses in rural and remote Canada. *Canadian Journal of Nursing Leadership, 21*(3), 40–53.

McConigley, R., Kristjanson, L., & Morgan, A. (2000). Palliative care nursing in rural Western Australia. *International Journal of Palliative Nursing, 6*(2), 80–90.

Moran, C. A. (2005). *Replication study of rural nursing theory: A Missouri perspective* (Unpublished thesis). University of Central Missouri, Warrensburg, MO.

Morse, M. J. (1995). Exploring the theoretical basis of nursing using advanced techniques of concept analysis. *Advances in Nursing Science, 17*(3), 31–46.

Niemoller, J. K., Ide, B. A., & Nichols, E. G. (2000). Issues in studying health-related hardiness and use of services among older rural adults. *Texas Journal of Rural Health, 18*, 35–43.

Peterson, S. J., & Bredow, T. S. (2004). *Middle range theories: Application to nursing research.* Philadelphia, PA: Lippincott Williams & Wilkins.

Pieh-Holder, Callahan, C., & Young, P. (2012). Qualitative needs assessment: Healthcare experiences of underserved populations in Montgomery County, Virginia, USA. *Rural and Remote Health, 12*, 2045. Retrieved from http://www.rrh.org.au

Pierce, C. (2001). The impact of culture of rural women's descriptions of health. *The Journal of Multicultural Nursing and Health, 7*, 50–53, 56.

Poland, B., Lehoux, P., Holmes, D., & Andrews, G. J. (2005). How place matters: Unpacking technology and power in health and social care. *Health & Social Care in the Community, 13*, 170–180.

Racher, F. E., & Vollman, A. R. (2002). Exploring the dimensions of access to health services: Implications for nursing research and practice. *Research and Theory for Nursing Practice: An International Journal, 16*, 77–90.

Roberto, K. A., & Reynolds, S. G. (2001). The meaning of osteoporosis in the lives of rural women. *Health Care for Women International, 22,* 599–611.

Rogers, B. L. (1993). Concept analysis: An evolutionary view. In B. L. Rogers & K. A. Kraft (Eds.), *Concept development in nursing: Foundations, techniques and application* (pp. 73–92). Philadelphia, PA: Saunders.

Rosenthal, K. A. (1996). *Rural nursing: An exploratory narrative description* (Unpublished dissertation). University of Colorado, Denver.

Scharff, J. (1998). The distinctive nature and scope of rural nursing practice: Philosophical bases. In H. Lee (Ed.), *Conceptual basis for rural nursing* (pp. 19–38). New York, NY: Springer Publishing.

Sellers, S. C., Poduska, M. D., Propp, L. H., & White, S. E. (1999). The health care meanings, values, and practices of Anglo-American males in the rural Midwest. *Journal of Transcultural Nursing, 10,* 320–330.

Shannon, A. (1982). Introduction: Nursing in sparsely populated areas. In J. Taylor (Ed.), Sparsely populated areas: Toward nursing theory. *Western Journal of Nursing Research, 4*(3, Suppl.), 70–71,

Shooker, M., Scott, C. M., & Vollman, A. R. (2008). Creating supportive environments for health: Social network analysis. In A. R. Vollman, E. T. Anderson, & J. McFarlane (Eds.), *Canadian community as partner: Theory & multidisciplinary practice* (2nd ed.). Philadelphia, PA: Lippincott Williams & Wilkins.

Smith, M. K., & Liehr, P. R. (Eds.). (2003). *Middle range theory of nursing.* New York, NY: Springer Publishing.

Swan, M. A., & Hobbs, B. B. (2017). Concept analysis: Lack of anonymity. *Journal of Advanced Nursing, 73*(5) 1075–1084. doi:10.1111/jan.13236

Thomlinson, E. H., McDonagh, M. K., Reimer, M., Crooks, K., & Lees, M. (2004). Health beliefs of rural Canadians: Implications for practice. *Australian Journal of Rural Health, 12,* 258–263.

Thurston, W. E., & Meadows, L. M. (2003). Rurality and health: Perspectives from mid-life women. *Rural and Remote Health, 3*(219), 1–12. Retrieved from https://www.rrh.org.au/journal/article/219.

Wakerman, L., Bourke, L., Humphreys, J. S., & Taylor, J. (2017). Is remote health different to rural health? *Rural and Remote Health, 17,* 3832. Retrieved from http://www.rrh.org.au

Walker, L., & Avant, K. (1995). *Strategies for theory construction in nursing* (3rd ed.). Norwalk, CT: Appleton-Century-Crofts.

Wathen, C. N., & Harris, R. M. (2006). An examination of the health information seeking experience of women in rural Ontario, Canada. *Information Research, 11*(4). Retrieved from https://eric.ed.gov/?id=EJ1104643

Wathen, C. N., & Harris, R. M. (2007). "I try to take care of it myself." How rural women search for health information. *Qualitative Health Research, 17*(5), 639–651.

Winters, C. A., Cudney, S. A., Sullivan, T., & Thuesen, A. (2006). The rural context and women's self-management of chronic health conditions. *Chronic Illness, 2,* 273–289.

Winters, C. A., Thomlinson, E. H., O'Lynn, C., Lee, H. J., McDonagh, M. K., Edge, D. S., & Reimer, M. A. (2006). Exploring rural nursing theory across borders. In H. J. Lee & C. A. Winters (Eds.), *Rural nursing: Concepts, theory, and practice* (2nd ed., pp. 27–39). New York, NY: Springer Publishing.

Wong, S., & Regan, S. (2009). Patient perspectives on primary health care in rural communities: Effects of geography on access, continuity, and efficiency. *Rural and Remote Health, 9,* 1142. Retrieved from http://www.rrh.org.au

CHAPTER 5

An Updated Literature Review of the Rural Nursing Theory

Deana L. Molinari and Ruiling Guo

DISCUSSION QUESTIONS

- What are the six core themes of the rural nursing theory (RNT)?
- Why are systematic literature reviews considered a high level of evidence?
- What barriers hinder rural nursing research studies?
- How can researchers test the effectiveness of the RNT?

This qualitative systematic literature review screened publications for the years 2012 to 2017 using the terms "rural nursing" and "rural nursing theory" (RNT). The review updates a previous analysis conducted in 2011. The aim of the review was to examine the state of the science regarding use of the RNT in research. The review focused on the latest uses of the theory, levels of evidence, research purposes, and methodologies.

THE RURAL NURSING THEORY

K. A. Long and Weinert synthesized graduate student and faculty studies conducted in Montana and Canada into a midrange RNT (1989, 1991; K. A. Long, 1999). The conceptual framework provided a formula for examining rural and remote health status and intervention testing. Their desire was to increase research to reduce health disparities (Bushy, 2000; Lee, 1998; Winters et al., 2006). The theory is based on the nursing principles of person, nurse, environment, and health.

Theories help scientists decide what is known and what yet needs to be understood about concepts (Parsons, 1961). Researchers utilize theories to describe, predict, and explain nursing phenomena as well as to guide research design and control potential errors (Chinn & Jacobs, 1978). Theories are created to move scientific thought beyond intuitive opinion (Croyle, 2005). Once created, a theory is tested for performance.

The frequency with which researchers apply a theory often tests the theory's efficacy. The more a theory is employed, the more knowledge expands (Chinn & Jacobs, 1978). Frequency of use enables researchers to discover a theory's limitations. Readers can identify logical trains of thought. For example, Swan and Hobbs (2017) examined the concept of lack of anonymity and Williams (2012) examined feelings of professional isolation. The two studies examined the concepts during nursing interventions allowing the theory to be analyzed at the same time as the intervention was studied.

Another approach to advancing science is to compare the usefulness of theories in one situation. Burdette (2012) stated the RNT concept of self-care is not congruent with Orem's definition of self-care. Comparisons are important in understanding concepts. The Burdette study also reported rural women's definition of health supported both the Orem and RNT definition. More study will clarify a theory's parameters, promoting new ideas and interventions (Ross, 2008).

When interventional studies fail to base research designs on a specific theoretical foundation, logical connections among publications cannot develop. Each study stands alone without a theoretical foundation. The work cannot advance science because connections with previous reason cannot be identified. Bushy stated research studies without theoretical foundations reduce science to the equivalent of inductive vignettes or anecdotes (2000). Generalizability is then impossible and bias is supported.

Reporting theoretical foundations also controls research design error. When a researcher tests an intervention based on incomplete or an unsupported theoretical framework, the findings are negated. For instance, applying a psychosocial stress theory to a physiological intervention is a major design error. Researchers must understand the philosophical differences among theories before using them.

Researchers guard against logical errors throughout the study planning and implementation processes. A method of protecting a project against design errors is to report both conceptual and methodological theories. When scientists show their logical development from philosophical to technological application, readers can then compare research processes. Understanding conceptual and methodological theories is basic to comprehending the state of science.

Theories standardize research and account for sample diversity. Rural populations include diversity of both thought and environment. Theory presents construct definitions and explains logical diversities. Failures to understand a study's conceptual foundation prevents advancing science. Therefore, testing a theory's concepts is foundational to scientific advancement. Theories can be dynamic supporting change based on experiments.

A midrange theory's purpose is to analyze specific situations with a limited number of variables. For example, the environment affects nursing practice.

Therefore, the RNT can be applied to questions like: What are the characteristics of rural health? How do rural care providers/patients define health? What environmental parameters affect self-care? Which nursing intervention produces the best outcome?

During the last decade, the published number of rural studies increased. At the same time, the cultural, political, economic, and environmental alterations prompted qualitative rather than quantitative explorations. Researchers sought to understand the impact of evolutionary shifts in practice and funding. Studies without theoretical designs reduced the value of study outcomes to evidence-based practice. The next generation of readers cannot determine if study outcomes were due to cultural shifts, financial limitations, biology, or the research design until a number of random sample experiments test interventions.

The RNT is needed for understanding rural health according to Long and Weinert (1989) and Lee and Winters (2004). Bushy (2004) stated rural and urban lifestyles differ. Environmental context prevents echoed practice. Patient-care practitioners as well as educational and healthcare administrators must understand population differences in order to provide optimum health services (Jackman, Myrick, & Yonge, 2012; Jackman, Yonge, Myrick, Janke, & Konkin, 2016; Sellers, Poduska, Propp, & White, 1999).

An example of diversity's impact on practice can be seen in the use of professional language. Rural and urban "generalists" function differently. The term "generalist" is not defined the same in rural and urban facilities. Rural generalists are nurses who practice in multiple specialty areas simultaneously using a wide range of advanced clinical knowledge in crisis assessment and management (Long & Weinert, 1991; Scharff, 2006). An urban generalist practices medical–surgical practice only and is often new to the nursing profession receiving orientation and supervision. Rural generalists are experienced nurses who practice independently in a small community caring for patients who suffer a wide range of health issues and with ages ranging from birth to death. Rural hospitals support limited personnel and need specialists as well as generalists. Therefore, rural generalists often specialize in an additional nursing discipline such as maternity or oncology. Rural specialists practice generalist skills until there is need for their advanced specialty knowledge.

Nursing salaries reflect the importance healthcare providers place on the word "generalist" (Barrett, Terry, Quynh, & Ha, 2015; Molinari & Bushy, 2012). Several studies compare the knowledge and salaries of rural and urban generalists (Bratt, Baernholdt, & Pruszynski, 2014). Research indicates rural generalists receive lower salaries although they may have more experience and specialty knowledge than urban generalists.

The RNT's midrange model describes the "provision of healthcare by professional nurses to persons living in sparsely populated areas" (Long & Weinert, 1989, p. 119; Yonge, Myrick, Ferguson, & Grundy, 2013). The theory's core themes include "work and health beliefs, isolation and distance, self-reliance, lack of anonymity, outsider/insider, and old-timers/newcomers" (Long & Weinert, 2013; Bushy & Winters, 2013; Ortiz, Bushy, Zhou, & Hong, 2013). The statement "rural dwellers define health as primarily the ability to work, and to be productive" has been studied over time and demonstrates the dynamic nature of theories (Bushy, 2013; Bushy & Winters, 2013; Hurme, 2009; K. A. Long & Weinert, 1989; Skillman, Palazzo, Hart, & Butterfield, 2007; Winters et al., 2007).

Lee and associates suggest a change in one of the RNT core themes to a concept called "functionality" (Lee, Winters, Boland, Ralph, & Buehler, 2013). The concept is defined as "performing or able to perform a regular function" and "contributes to the development or maintenance of a larger whole" (Bennett, 2009, p. 109). The new concept requires further testing to see if being ambulatory, able to work, feeling good—not just surviving, caring for family, and self-determining—are adequate definitions for the new term. Functionality relies on the interplay between mental, physical, and spiritual well-being and is measured by individual actions. When any one of these measures is lacking, health declines (see Table 5.1).

TABLE 5.1 RNT Concepts

Concept	Rural Dimensions of Nursing Concepts

Person	Genetic and biological variations
	    Diversity
	Human relationships
	    Familiarity among residents
	    Rural culture
	Values/perceptions
	Caregiving support systems
	    Caregiving by known persons
	Spiritual relationships
	    Health and caregiving beliefs
	    Duties and responsibilities (friends, country)
	    Newcomer/old-timer
	    Insider/outsider

Environment	Physical/social/cultural
	    Distance and space
	    Sparse population
	    Geographical terrain
	Values formation and orientation
	Time orientation
	Belief systems and manifestations
	    Lifestyle orientation to natural environment
	    Occupations/recreation

Health	Definitions of health and illness Functionality

(continued)

TABLE 5.1 RNT Concepts (*continued*)

Concept	Rural Dimensions of Nursing Concepts
	Major beliefs
	Spiritual emphasis
	Cultural variations
	Worldview
	Healing practices
	Health and illness behaviors
	Symptom-time-help seeking
	Healthcare systems
	Informal and formal supports
The Professional Nurse	Nursing—definition and roles
	Interprofessional role diffusion
	Interrelationships
	Lack of anonymity
	Client familiarity
	Community expectation and responsibilities
	Generalist role with specialist skills
	Role diffusion
	Multiple community roles
	Nurse–client interactions
	Caring concepts and practices
	Provider culture

RNT, rural nursing theory.

METHODOLOGY

This qualitative study performed a literature search for the terms: "RNT" and "rural nursing." Online databases and rural publications using both manual and computer search strategies were employed. The aim of the study was to find what percentage of rural nursing studies used the RNT or one of its components during the period of 2012 to 2017.

All volumes of the *Online Journal of Rural Nursing and Healthcare* from 2012 to 2017 were searched manually; other journals were not. Eligibility for inclusion in the study required mention of the RNT or one of its components or claimed a rural sample.

The searched databases included PubMed, Web of Science, Cumulative Index to Nursing and Allied Health Literature (CINHAL), Cochrane Library, PsycINFO, Psychology and Behavioral Sciences Collection, Dissertations & Theses Abstracting and Indexing (A&I) Database, Pro Quest, Education Research Complete, and Google Scholar. The search was limited to publication of journals, dissertations and theses, books, and conference proceedings related to rural nursing during the 2012 to 2017 period.

Databases

A brief introduction of each database searched is provided.

PubMed is a comprehensive medical database sponsored by the National Library of Medicine. It comprises more than 27 million citations for biomedical literature including nursing. Publications include case reports, randomized controlled trials, clinical guidelines, and reviews.

Web of Science is an online subscription–based database originally produced but now maintained by Clarivate Analytics. It includes Science Citation Index and Social Sciences Citation Index. So far, it covers over 33,000 journals in the sciences and social sciences. The database also includes nursing-related journal articles for worldwide access.

CINAHL is considered the authoritative and premier resource for nursing and allied health. It contains more than 5.4 million records, including journals, book reviews, and conference proceedings dating back to 1937.

Cochrane Library is an online collection of evidence-based medicine and clinical practice literature. It comprises seven databases. They are Cochrane Database of Systematic Reviews (CDSR), Database of Abstracts of Reviews of Effectiveness (DARE), Cochrane Central Register of Control Trials (CENTRAL), Cochrane Database of Methodology Reviews (CDMR), Cochrane Methodology Register (CMR), Health Technology Assessment Database (HTA), and NHS Economic Evaluation Database (NHS EED). Bringing together seven databases allows users to look at the effectiveness of different healthcare treatments and interventions (Hanan, 2013).

PsycINFO contains about 3 million citations and summaries of scholarly journal articles, book chapters, and dissertations on psychological aspects of topics like bioethics, sociology, education, pharmacology, physiology, and medicine. The journal coverage spans from the 1840s to the present. It includes more than 2,400 journals in about 30 languages.

Psychology and Behavioral Sciences Collection is another comprehensive database covering topics in emotional and behavioral characteristics, psychiatry and psychology, mental processes, anthropology, and observational and experimental methods. This database provides access to hundreds of full-text journals related to psychology.

ProQuest Dissertations and Theses, A&I provides the largest single repository of graduate dissertations and theses that provides access to 4 million works from universities in 88 countries. It covers a variety of disciplines, including nursing.

Education Research Complete is a resource for educational research. Indexing and abstracts from more than 2,400 journals include all levels of education from early childhood to higher education, and all educational specialties, such as multilingual education, health education, and testing. The search engine also includes full text for more than 530 books and monographs and 1,300 educational journals.

Google Scholar is an online search engine for articles, theses, books, abstracts, and court opinions, from academic publishers, professional societies, online repositories, universities, and other websites across many disciplines and sources. Selection criteria included the words "RNT" and "rural health." Articles and book chapters discussing these topics were chosen. Article data were then placed in a matrix with fields listing theories, citation, dates, sample size, research design, outcome concepts, and study location. A synthesis of findings for frequency and diversity was conducted.

RESULTS

Two hundred and fifteen articles met inclusion criteria. Forty articles, 19%, employed the RNT. Six additional studies used the RNT in conjunction with another theory bringing the total number of publications featuring the RNT to 22% (Table 5.2).

Sixty-four publications or 30% of the eligible studies used other models to structure their logic. The following theories were mentioned: Orem's Self-Care, Peplau's Theory of Interpersonal Relations, Active Ageing, Rural Development, Cantor's Social Care, Effect Theory, Rural Health, Theory of Engagement, Virginia Henderson's Need Theory, Risk Management, Ecological Systems, Bandura Social Learning Theory, and Interdisciplinary Cultural Competency and Mutual Respect. Selected studies also used models such as Preceptor, Bright Future Framework, Chronic Care, National Healthcare Agenda, Social Ecological, Vulnerable Population Conceptual Model, Health Promotion, and Corporate Governance. Authors mentioned methodological strategies such as various grounded and phenomenological theories. Although methodological theories are not required to be mentioned before a qualitative study begins, a thorough description of the literature is expected somewhere in the report.

TABLE 5.2 Articles in Databases

Year	Eligible Items	RNT
2012	34	3
2013	73	36
2014	35	2
2015	26	5
2016	39	4
2017	8	3
Total	215	43

Note: 22% of the total eligible articles used the RNT.
RNT, rural nursing theory.

Forty-eight percent of the eligible studies failed to mention any theoretical foundation. While the current statistics represent a slight increase in the use of the RNT since the 2011 literature review, the majority of nursing research publications did not report using a theory.

Authors studied many nursing concepts such as the development of the RNT (Long & Weinert, 1989; Swan & Hobbs, 2017; Williams, 2012); workforce analysis (Baernholdt, Jennings, & Lewis, 2013; Bushy & Winters, 2013; Molinari & Bushy, 2012); patient care (Kitchen et al., 2013; Mallow, Theeke, Barnes, Whetsel, & Mallow, 2014); healthcare administration (Bopp & Fallon, 2013; Rohatinsky & Ferguson, 2013); and nursing education (Molinari, 2011; Molinari, Monserud, & Hudzinski, 2008; Pierce, Thompson, Govoni, & Stiener, 2012; Yonge, Myrick, & Ferguson, 2011; Yonge et al., 2013; Yonge, Myrick, Ferguson, & Grundy, 2015). Several limited scope literature reviews were performed during this period.

The most frequently mentioned research design was the Glaserian Grounded Theory (Seright, 2011). The majority of publications were descriptive research accounts employing systematic literature reviews, interviews, surveys, and focus groups methods for data gathering. Ethnography, phenomenology, and content analysis were also employed (Shookner, Scott, & Vollman, 2008). Few articles reported random samples or experimental interventional designs although several publications were intervention projects using evaluative methods.

More global rural studies were found this year than in the previous study. The 2017 study found a few more international studies in the search engines. Scientists from Australia, Canada, China, Mexico, Africa, India, Haiti, Great Britain, Pakistan, Brazil, Tasmania, Indonesia, and Greenland were included in the search engines. Not enough articles were provided to compare findings among countries. Most articles originated in all regions of the United States. Few articles provided a theoretical foundation in the international studies. Reports of the RNT were found only in English-speaking nation designs. Language translation limitations, diversity in educational values, practice standards, or search engine problems could account for the failure to report nursing research from around the world. Most international articles reviewed did not provide a theoretical foundation.

DISCUSSION

The literature review noted several issues pertaining to search engines, research methodologies, research education, and publication. Search engine limitations inhibited finding and synthesizing rural studies. Many qualitative designs were included with only three random sample clinical trials noted. Few articles provided a theoretical foundation. The scarcity of experimental designs inhibits generalization to diverse rural settings. These limitations affect future practice based on evidence.

PubMed and Web of Science databases identified few articles related to RNT, but the search engines did not provide many results. Reasons cannot be discussed at this time without more evidence. Some of the most influential rural health journals are not included in well-known databases. For instance, the official journal of the Rural Nursing Organization, the *Online Journal of Rural Nursing and Health Care*, focuses exclusively on rural nursing. The PubMed database did not include the journal until 2010 and is still selective about what articles are accepted. *The Journal of Rural Health* covers many rural health topics and is the official publication of the National Rural Health Association, and yet the journal was not selected by the Web of Science for indexing. The journal often provides economic and administrative studies with few rural/urban comparisons. The journals' content restrictions inhibit study synthesis. Few systematic reviews or meta-analyses were found in any database. Other rural and remote health organizations' journals were not included in the databases. In addition, search engines hosted by individual journals were often difficult to use. The inability to access studies is a major problem for both researchers and program developers.

Google Scholar was added to the search strategy to identify articles addressing RNT applications. A database relevance issue was identified. The database produced findings older than 5 years. Google Scholar allows metadata searching on the Internet while most databases use limited searching fields.

Sophisticated search options are needed. For instance, comparison studies require many database search options. The larger the sample, the more useful the study is considered and yet the search engines seem unable to manage a large number of variables. Without search capabilities, many research questions cannot be answered. Researchers wishing to test the RNT need to compare rural and urban disease treatments, behaviors, issues, and characteristics. Policy and funding issues for specific treatments also require sophisticated search strategies. New data analysis methodologies also need sophisticated search methods.

In 2011, 19% of the articles mentioned conceptual components of the RNT compared to the 22% found in 2017. The updated review identified mostly qualitative studies and project reports with few experimental outcomes. The reasons for the lack of experimental studies may relate to basic educational issues, small samples, few rural resources, and the nature of nursing practice. More interventional research is needed if the profession is not to lose ground as a respected profession.

Identification of the reasons for infrequent theory application in publications should be a top priority. Supposition for the infrequent use of RNT cannot be identified since the majority of articles failed to identify any conceptual framework, cannot be narrowed beyond opinions such as researchers' lack of theoretical knowledge, the nature of the publication culture, or a lack of the theory's appropriateness. A lot of analysis is needed. More conceptual analysis of the RNT's themes can be done with small samples and then published in nursing journals.

Although "rural" is defined by a small local context, nurse education varies by country. The lack of articles with a theoretical foundation indicates a poor understanding of the research process and prevents answering questions like, Does the Rural Nurse Theory fit the needs of nurses around the world? Perhaps new research methodologies will fit the specific needs of rural nursing. Gary Donaldson (Nakamura et al., 2017), a nursing researcher, believes technology provides the tools for new research methodologies that will then answer complex questions.

Nursing research in advanced practice requires comparative, random samples. Since most studies are performed by advanced practitioners, analysis of their publications is needed. Educational projects can be experimental, comparative, or descriptive. Evaluation research upgrades the value of projects. Descriptive studies will improve with rigorous evaluation research protocols. The profession demands practitioners understand evidence-based practice that includes the gathering and reporting of data. Educators can hasten improvements by teaching methods of producing higher evidential levels.

The number of interdisciplinary studies will continue to increase as healthcare systems change. Nurses should understand their own discipline's approach to evidence gathering in order to participate in larger interdisciplinary studies. Interdisciplinary researchers continually update their understanding of study designs that support various professions' data gathering. Rural researchers can problem solve and communicate factors that impact rural populations.

Journals can help further science by analyzing the articles they publish. Comparative and experimental methodologies should replace the more frequently published descriptive studies if evidence-based practice is to advance. Educators and administrators will improve their research practices when publishers hold stringent standards for article acceptance. Several universities no longer require the publication of research projects for graduation in part because journals are willing to accept descriptive projects. Such decisions weaken the profession. Students exposed to designing experiments and evaluation studies will recognize opportunities to answer questions in daily practice. No practitioner should believe his or her practice cannot support scientific study. Asking oneself scientific questions is foundational to safe practice.

Currently, rural research characteristics such as "small" sample sizes and limited local research resources restrict the number of experimental studies conducted in small communities. Rural studies are often qualitative due to the small samples available. Nursing knowledge will not advance without answers based on experimental designs. New study tools described by Gary Donaldson (Reblin et al., 2017) suggest new designs, statistical methods, and causal modeling can overcome barriers to experimental research. Qualitative analyses of quantitative results provide new types of outcomes. A focus on comparative intervention effectiveness or the analysis of treatment responses requires fewer participants and more variables per individual in order to understand why some individuals/communities respond to interventions and others do not.

This type of study can be integrated into the initial data gathering or act as a secondary study.

Other strategies can also increase the number of rural studies. Regional research committees including large and small communities can plan to overcome barriers. Sharing technologies becomes possible. Using each unit's strength overcomes perceived barriers. Funding holders can collaborate with rural researchers if they are willing to listen to each other's concerns. Sophisticated analysis strategies can compare samples while limiting costs.

The traditional definition of rural relates to space and distance. "Being rural means being a long way from anywhere and pretty close to nowhere" (Scharff, 2006). Rural populations often invent new ways of addressing old problems using local resources. Rural researchers can apply this rural strength to research designs. Poland, Lehoux, Holmes, and Andrews (2005) suggest making "place" the lens through which research is viewed. They draw upon the literature of many diverse disciplines. Since evidence-based practice research often does not fit the needs of rural investigators, alternative methodologies such as small samples with a large number of variables can meet the needs of rural communities and patient care.

Cloke's (2003) definition of "rurality" as a socially and culturally constructed phenomenon rather than as a location might alter the RNT. Traditionally, a rural nurse is one who cares for people in locations with sparse populations. Place and distance are commonly mentioned in rural and frontier studies but differing rural perceptions are rarely mentioned. Recent studies indicate residents' perceptions of rural are changing as the agrarian population declines and other groups such as retired, aging, and recreational increase. Collaboration with sociologists, anthropologists, and health administration researchers can increase the funding pool while testing theories.

Local researcher collaborations may increase the number of studies conducted in sparsely populated areas. Rural community insiders could gather data and collaborate with urban outsiders on separate data analysis and population comparisons (McNeely & Shreffler, 1998). A simple variable like "community identity" may point out logical reasons for diversity in rural and urban findings.

Research is influenced by national initiatives such as health reform (Hartley, 2005). Accountable care organizations and medical homes and regional healthcare centers may alter rural resident's expectation of healthcare providers. Reforms modify the concept of "place." Telemedicine technologies also alter what constitutes "care." The time for comparative and experimental telemedicine studies has arrived. More comparisons of rural and urban diet, child care, and various primary healthcare practices are needed as regional healthcare centers develop. What are the expectations of rural residents to more computer and less face-to-face care? Who is conducting health education in the newly funded healthcare systems? Is the increase in the number of advanced practice nurses and the decreasing numbers of basic nurses changing the way nurses are perceived, what they do, and how the profession is administered? Comparison studies are mandatory.

Few publications in this study focused on the economics of healthcare except in terms of access, work setting, and resources. Little was presented about the value of nurse generalists. This review indicates most researchers study small community deficiencies rather than strengths. Many cultural and social aspects of "rural" were ignored. The strengths of collaboration, teamwork, cultural diversity, innovations, survival strengths, family, governance, and networking are currently ignored in most studies (Bunce, 2003; Cloke, 2003). Mallow et al. (2014) approached the medication error issue by applying a red light to the medication cart in small hospitals. Experiments measured the effectiveness of communicating the nurses' need not to be disturbed. The experiments required few resources and improved care using the strengths of rural identity. This type of study can be implemented by most student populations. Comparing hospitals and locations can also improve the effectiveness of patient care and nursing research.

CONCLUSION

Testing the RNT appears imperative to understanding the rural person, nurse, environment, and health interventions. The RNT can change nursing research and improve patient care. Using theory enables researchers to provide a logic genealogy for concept development. The literature review of the RNT indicates a pressing need for more theory testing.

Fast-paced healthcare reforms require deeper understanding of how rural perceptions and practices are changing (Molinari, Jaiswal, & Hollinger-Forrest, 2011; Molinari, Jaiswal, & Peterson, 2012). This study found researchers describing basic concepts whereas today's science requires theoretically based treatment outcome studies. There is much for rural researchers to accomplish before local health can improve.

Most midrange theories apply to one population such as rural patients. The RNT discusses nurses' thoughts as well as patients' behaviors that may complicate the theory's use. Grand theories generally pertain to a concept rather than to an environment. The RNT explains a variety of concepts affecting several populations that may limit its usefulness to researchers. Future study is needed to either constrain the theory or explain the need for combining providers and patients in the same theory.

Research requires further theoretical development. Just as green theories prompted the development of new scientific professions and collaborative research models, healthcare theoretical development demands new technological and economic models to support global change. Improved patient care will involve improving research tools like search engines and larger databases and standardizing systematic search methodologies. Today's nurse researcher needs to experiment, not just observe. Educators can teach research methodologies as part of daily practice. Nurses willing to learn from other professions and to advocate for nurse methodologies will advance the state of the science. Rural evidence-based practice is built on the publication of rural experimental studies using midrange contextual theories as well as grand conceptual theories.

REFERENCES

Baernholdt, M., Jennings, B. M., & Lewis, E. J. (2013). A pilot study of staff nurses' perceptions of factors that influence quality of care in critical access hospitals. *Journal of Nursing Care Quality, 28*(4), 352–359. doi:10.1097/NCQ.0b013e31829fad73

Barrett, A., Terry, D. R., Quynh, L., & Ha, H. (2015). Rural community nurses: Insights into health workforce and health service needs. *International Journal of Health, Wellness & Society, 5*(3), 109–120.

Bennett, A. D. (2009). *Project genesis: Community assessment of a rural southeastern Arizona border community* (Doctoral dissertation). Retrieved from http://citeseerx.ist.psu.edu/viewdoc/download?doi=10.1.1.503.8367&rep=rep1&type=pdf

Bopp, M., & Fallon, E. A. (2013). Health and wellness programming in faith-based organizations: A description of a nationwide sample. *Health Promotion Practice, 14*(1), 122–131. doi:10.1177/1524839912446478

Bratt, M. M., Baernholdt, M., & Pruszynski, J. (2014). Are rural and urban newly licensed nurses different? A longitudinal study of a nurse residency programme. *Journal of Nursing Management, 22*(6), 779–791.

Bunce, M. (2003). Reproducing rural idylls. In P. J. Cloke (Ed.), *Country visions* (p. 14). Harlow, UK: Pearson.

Burdette, L. (2012). Relationship between self-care agency, self-care practices and obesity among rural midlife women. *Self-Care, Dependent-Care & Nursing, 19*(1), 5–14.

Bushy, A. (2000). *Orientation to nursing in the rural community.* Thousand Oaks, CA: Sage.

Bushy, A. (2004). Creating nursing research opportunities in rural healthcare facilities. *Journal of Nursing Care Quality, 19*(2), 162–168.

Bushy, A. (2013). Health disparities in rural populations across the life span. In C. A. Winters (Ed.), *Rural nursing: Concepts, theory, and practice* (4th ed., pp. 225–239). New York, NY: Springer Publishing.

Bushy, A., & Winters, C. A. (2013). Nursing workforce development, clinical practice, research and nursing theory: Connecting the dots. In C. A. Winters (Ed.), *Rural nursing: Concepts, theory, and practice* (4th ed., pp. 449–467). New York, NY: Springer Publishing.

Chinn, P. L., & Jacobs, M. K. (1978). A model for theory development in nursing. *Advances in Nursing Science, 1*(1), 1–11.

Cloke, P. (2003). Knowing ruralities. In Cloke, P. (Ed.), *Country visions* (pp. 1–13). Harlow, UK: Pearson.

Croyle, R. T. (2005). *Theory at a glance: A guide for health promotion practice* (2nd ed.). Washington, DC: U.S. Department of Health and Human Services, National Institutes of Health.

Hanan, K. (2013). Systematic reviews and beyond. *Online Journal of Rural Nursing and Health Care, 13*(2), 2–5. Retrieved from http://rnojournal.binghamton.edu/index.php/RNO/article/view/298

Hartley, D. (2005). Rural health research: Building capacity and influencing policy in the United States and Canada. *Canadian Journal of Nursing Research, 37*(1), 7–13.

Hurme, E. (2009). Competencies for nursing practice in a rural critical access hospital. *Online Journal of Rural Nursing & Health Care, 9*(2), 67–81. Retrieved from http://rnojournal.binghamton.edu/index.php/RNO/article/view/88

Jackman, D., Myrick, F., & Yonge, O. (2012). Putting the (R)ural in preceptorship. *Nursing Research & Practice, 2012*, 1–7. doi:10.1155/2012/528580

Jackman, D., Yonge, O., Myrick, F., Janke, F., & Konkin J. (2016). A rural interprofessional educational initiative: What success looks like. *Online Journal of Rural Nursing and Health Care, 16*(2). doi:10.14574/ojrnhc.v16/2.41

Kitchen, K. K., Andren, M. S., McKibbin, C. L., Wykes, T. L., Lee, A. A., Carrico, C. P., & Bourassa, K. A. (2013). Depression treatment among rural older adults: Preferences and factors influencing future service use. *Clinical Gerontologist, 36*(3), 241–259. doi:10.1080/07317115.2013.767872

Lee, H. J. (Ed.). (1998). *Conceptual basis for rural nursing.* New York, NY: Springer Publishing.

Lee, H. J., & Winters, C. A. (2004). Testing rural nursing theory: Perceptions and needs of service providers. *Online Journal of Rural Nursing & Health Care, 4*(1), 10. Retrieved from http://rnojournal.binghamton.edu/index.php/RNO/article/view/212

Lee, H. J., Winters, C. A., Boland, R. L., Raph, S. J., & Buehler, J. A. (2013). An analysis of key concepts for rural nursing. In C. A. Winters (Ed.), *Rural nursing: Concepts, theory, and practice* (4th ed., pp. 469–480). New York, NY: Springer Publishing.

Long, K. A. (1999). Reflections on "Rural nursing: Developing the theory base." *Scholarly Inquiry for Nursing Practice, 13*(3), 275–279.

Long, K. A., & Weinert, C. (1989). Rural nursing: Developing the theory base. *Scholarly Inquiry for Nursing Practice, 3*(2), 113–127.

Long, K. A., & Weinert, C. (1991). *Rural nursing: developing the theory base.* (NLN Publications 21-2408) (pp. 389–406). New York, NY: National League of Nursing.

Long K. A. & Weinert, C. (2013). Rural nursing: Developing the theory base. In C. Winters, (Ed.). *Rural nursing: Concepts, theory, and practice* (4th ed., pp. 1–14). New York, NY: Springer Publishing.

Mallow, J. A., Theeke, L. A., Barnes, E. R., Whetsel, T., & Mallow, B. K. (2014). Using mHealth tools to improve rural diabetes care guided by the chronic care model. *Online Journal of Rural Nursing & Health Care, 14*(1), 43–65. doi:10.14574/ojrnhc.v14i1.276

McNeely, A. G., & Shreffler, M. J. (1998). Familiarity. In. H. J. Lee (Ed.), *Conceptual basis for rural nursing* (pp. 89–109). New York, NY: Springer Publishing.

Molinari, D. L. (2011). Rural nurse transition-to-practice programs. In D. L. Molinari & A. Bushy (Eds.), *The rural nurse: Transition to practice* (pp. 23–34). New York, NY: Springer Publishing.

Molinari, D. L., & Bushy, A. (2012). *The rural nurse: Transition to practice.* New York, NY: Springer Publishing.

Molinari, D. L., Jaiswal, A., & Hollinger-Forrest, T. (2011). Rural nurses: Lifestyle preferences and education perceptions. *Online Journal of Rural Nursing & Health Care,*

11(2), 16–26. Retrieved from http://rnojournal.binghamton.edu/index.php/RNO/article/view/27

Molinari, D. L., Jaiswal, A. R., & Peterson, T. (2012). Rural nurse perceptions of organizational culture and the intent to move. In D. Molinari & A. Bushy (Eds.), *The rural nurse: Transition to practice* (pp. 61–70). New York, NY: Springer Publishing.

Molinari, D. L., Monserud, M., & Hudzinski, D. (2008). A new type of rural nurse residency. *Journal of Continuing Education in Nursing, 39*(1), 42–46. doi:10.3928/00220124-20080101-05

Nakamura, Y., Lipschitz, D. L., Donaldson, G. W., Kida, Y., Williams, S., Landward, R., . . . Tuteja, A. (2017). Investigating clinical benefits of a novel sleep-focused mind-body program on Gulf war illness symptoms: A randomized controlled trial. *Psychosomatic Medicine, 79*(6), 706–718. doi:10.1097/PSY.0000000000000469

Ortiz, J., Bushy, A., Zhou, Y., & Hong, Z. (2013). Accountable care organizations: Benefits and barriers as perceived by Rural Health Clinic management. *Rural and Remote Health, 13*(2), 2417. Retrieved from https://www.rrh.org.au/articles/showarticlenew.asp?ArticleID=2417

Parsons, T. (1961). *Theories of society: Foundations of modern sociological theory.* New York, NY: Free Press of Glencoe.

Pierce, L., Thompson, T., Govoni, A., & Steiner, V. (2012). Caregivers' incongruence; Emotional strain in caring for persons with stroke. *Rehabilitative Nursing, 37*(5), 258–266. doi:10.1002/rnj.35

Poland, B., Lehoux, P., Holmes, D., & Andrews, G. (2005). How place matters: Unpacking technology and power in health and social care. *Health & Social Care in the Community, 13*(2), 170–180.

Reblin, M., Clayton, M. F., Xu, J., Hulett, J. M., Latimer, S., Donaldson, G. W., & Ellington, L. (2017). Caregiver, patient, and nurse visit communication patterns in cancer home hospice. *Psycho-Oncology, 26*(12) 2285–2293. doi:10.1002/pon.4361

Rohatinsky, N., & Ferguson, L. (2013). Mentorship in rural healthcare organizations: Challenges and opportunities. *Online Journal of Rural Nursing & Health Care, 13*(2), 149–172. Retrieved from http://rnojournal.binghamton.edu/index.php/RNO/article/view/273

Ross, J. (2008). *Rural nursing: Aspects of practice.* Dunedin, New Zealand: Rural Health Opportunities.

Scharff, J. E. (2006). The distinctive nature and scope of rural nursing practice: Philosophical bases. In H. J. Lee & C. A. Winters (Eds.), *Rural nursing: Concepts, theory, and practice* (2nd ed., pp. 179–196). New York, NY: Springer Publishing.

Sellers, S. C., Poduska, M. D., Propp, L. H., & White, S. I. (1999). The health care meanings, values, and practices of Anglo-American males in the rural midwest. *Journal of Transcultural Nursing, 10*(4), 320–330.

Seright, T. J. (2011). Clinical decision-making of rural novice nurses. *Rural and Remote Health, 11*(3), 1726. Retrieved from https://www.rrh.org.au/journal/article/1726

Shookner, M., Scott, C. M., & Vollman, A. R. (2008). Creating supportive environments for health: Social network analysis. In A. R. Vollman, E. T. Anderson, & J. McFarlane (Eds.), *Canadian community as partner: Theory & multidisciplinary practice* (2nd ed.). Philadelphia, PA: Lippincott Williams & Wilkins.

Skillman, S. M., Palazzo, L., Hart, L. G., & Butterfield, P. (2007). Changes in the rural registered nurse workforce from 1980 to 2004. *Rural Health Research Center.* Retrieved from http://depts.washington.edu/uwrhrc/uploads/RHRC%20FR115%20Skillman.pdf

Swan, M. A., & Hobbs, B. B. (2017). Concept analysis: Lack of anonymity. *Journal of Advanced Nursing, 73*(5), 1075–1084. doi:10.1111/jan.13236

Williams, M. A. (2012). Rural professional isolation: An integrative review. *Online Journal of Rural Nursing & Health Care, 12*(2), 3–10. Retrieved from http://rnojournal .binghamton.edu/index.php/RNO/article/view/51

Winters, C. A., Lee, H. J., Besel, J., Strand, A., Echeverri, R., Jorgensen, K. P., & Dea, J. E. (2007). Access to and use of research by rural nurses. *Rural and Remote Health, 7*(3), 758. Retrieved from https://www.rrh.org.au/journal/article/758

Winters, C. A., Thomlinson, E. H., O'Lynn, C., Lee, H. J., McDonagh, M. K., Edge, D. S., & Reimer, M. A. (2006). Exploring rural nursing theory across borders. In H. J. Lee & C. A. Winters (Eds.), *Rural nursing: Concepts, theory, and practice* (2nd ed., pp. 27–39). New York, NY: Springer Publishing.

Yonge, O., Myrick, F., & Ferguson, L. (2011). The process of developing a framework to guide rural nurse preceptors in the evaluation of student performance. *Nurse Education in Practice, 11*(2), 76–80. doi:10.1016/j.nepr.2011.01.001

Yonge, O., Myrick, F., Ferguson, L., & Grundy, Q. (2013). Multiple lenses: Rural landscape through the eyes of nurse preceptors and students. *Journal of Rural and Community Development, 8*(1), 145–159.

Yonge, O., Myrick, F., Ferguson, L., & Grundy, Q. (2015). Lessons about boundaries and reciprocity in rural-based preceptorship. *Quality Advancement in Nursing Education, 1*(2). doi:10.17483/2368-6669.1002

CHAPTER 6

Lack of Anonymity: Changes for the 21st Century

Marilyn A. Swan and Barbara B. Hobbs

DISCUSSION QUESTIONS

- Lack of anonymity involves being known and connected to others. According to the text, lack of anonymity is greater in rural settings and can influence nurses' care. However, the Internet and use of social media are creating new relationships that can affect patients' healthcare knowledge and access. As a rural nurse, what factors might influence a patient to use the local healthcare services rather than distant providers (Internet or place-bound)?
- Lack of anonymity and privacy issues can arise with Internet use and social media. How has social media use affected your anonymity and privacy? How has your need for privacy and anonymity affected your social media use?
- Confidentiality is an ethical principle for nursing. Regardless of the setting, nurses are expected to maintain confidentiality; however, lack of anonymity found in the rural setting can add to the challenge. How would you, or have you, addressed a breach in confidentiality?
- In the rural setting, nurses may have a hard time setting work and family boundaries for their privacy. What strategies could be used to set boundaries?
- Understanding the challenges nurses encounter in rural settings, what factors, traits, behaviors, and beliefs do you think make a good rural nurse? What factors, traits, behaviors, and beliefs might limit your effectiveness?
- Have you ever been faced with caring for a patient you know on a personal basis? What was your experience and how has that experience informed your practice?
- If you were a rural nurse, what measures would you use to foster and support professional and personal privacy for yourself and others?

Strike up a conversation in any rural diner and it will not take long to learn from the locals how everybody knows everybody else. Being known and named is an ever-present reality of daily life in rural communities and commonly described in rural literature (Lee, 1998). Rural nursing investigators identify lack of anonymity as an aspect of rural life and experienced by rural nurses in their personal and professional lives (Hegney, 1996; Long & Weinert, 1989). As a concept, lack of anonymity is firmly established in rural life; however, lack of anonymity is often described in literature alongside privacy, confidentiality, and familiarity. Being closely related concepts, it makes sense that they are discussed together. However, these four concepts are not synonymous, and there is benefit in examining each concept to gain understanding about how the concepts differ from each other, and how they influence rural nursing practice.

Rural dwellers, people who live in rural and remote areas, are interconnected to each other and their community. Rural nurses, like rural dwellers, experience this interconnectedness in their personal and professional lives. Being known as a rural nurse has been described as "life in a fishbowl," where you are recognized and observed in and out of work (Rosenthal, 2010). Still, being known and connected within a rural community means the rural nurse has social capital (Lauder, Reel, Farmer, & Griggs, 2006). Social capital is described as social connection within a community that bridges people and builds trust (Whitley & McKenzie, 2005). Trust is necessary in relationships that involve privacy and confidentiality. In rural areas, trusting relationships develop and grow even in the presence of lack of anonymity. Through the experience of lack of anonymity, rural nurses are uniquely placed to impact health and well-being of rural dwellers and their communities.

The purpose of this chapter is to take a 21st-century view by beginning to reconsider our thinking on lack of anonymity. We begin by defining and describing the related concepts, and propose a model of how the concepts may be associated with lack of anonymity. Gaining an understanding of the concepts is necessary as we explore how the concepts affect rural nursing practice. We end with case studies and questions that highlight the different concepts in hypothetical situations experienced by a rural nurse.

LACK OF ANONYMITY AND RELATED CONCEPTS

The focus of this section is to provide a summative overview of four concepts that are foundational to the discussion on lack of anonymity. We begin with concepts, as the relationship between concepts and knowledge development helps us to better understand nursing practice (Rodgers, 2000). The more insight we have into a concept related to rural practice environments, the better prepared we can be for rural nursing practice.

Lack of Anonymity and Anonymity

It is beneficial to understand anonymity when discussing lack of anonymity; understanding what a concept is not can aid in understanding the concept. Lee defines lack of anonymity as "a condition in which one cannot remain nameless or unknown" (Lee, 1998, p. 77). In contrast, Marx (1999) defines anonymity as "a person cannot be identified" (p. 100) which is similar to Zimbardo's (1969) description of anonymity as the loss of individual uniqueness or characteristics. Essentially, anonymity means a person is not known. In rural health literature, discussion on anonymity is often limited. The ability to be anonymous, or unknown, is to be alone and without relationship with others. And here is where we need to begin our rethinking. Since anonymity means an individual is not known, and lack of anonymity is being known, this means there is a relational quality to lack of anonymity. In essence, we cannot be anonymous by ourselves; we need the presence of another person.

The relational quality of lack of anonymity is described in literature. Stewart Fahs (2017) described leaders in rural healthcare as embedded within a community. Rolland (2016) captured the lack of anonymity experienced by rural emergency department (ED) nurses as they provided care to people known to them. Kozica et al. (2015) identified lack of anonymity as a barrier rural woman face when considering whether to participate in a healthy lifestyle class. Swan and Hobbs (2017) maintain that individuals are identifiable and interconnected to communities. These examples support the contention that lack of anonymity, in its variation and contexts, is about being relational.

Anonymity has significant societal implications. Bodle (2013) suggested that anonymity is fundamental to freedom of expression and privacy rights. Anonymity can allow individuals to speak freely in opposition to an idea, policy, or government without retaliation, social exclusion, or loss of personal privacy (*McIntyre v. Ohio Elections Commission*, 1995). For example, the influential Federalist Papers were written anonymously to encourage support for the ratification of the U.S. Constitution by New York citizens (Congress.gov, n.d.). The U.S. Supreme Court has ruled on several cases that involve anonymity and afford protections under the U.S. Constitution for those who may take unpopular stances in society (*McIntyre v. Ohio Elections Commission*, 1995). Significant discussions are occurring regarding the practice and ethics of anonymity versus nonanonymity, particularly in online environments (Bodle, 2013). Being anonymous frees an individual of the accountability, reputation, and responsibility associated with lack of anonymity (Swan & Hobbs, 2017). This contributes to the positive side of anonymity, including free expression of ideas, truth-telling, and self-disclosure of private information not normally shared (Bodle, 2013; Novak, 2014). For example, an anonymous informant, or participant, may share information that might not otherwise be known, such as in a research study or journalistic inquiry. The benefits of anonymity, as previously described, are compelling and worth protecting; however, anonymity has drawbacks.

Contemporary discussions on anonymity center on digital technology and online environments. A debate persists between those seeking online anonymity, including the use of pseudonyms, versus a growing online culture that requires user identification, such as Facebook and Google+ (Bodle, 2013). There is ample documentation that anonymous online environments provide opportunity for criminals to conceal their identities from an unsuspecting public, and have depersonalization effects resulting in aggressive, hateful speech (Bodle, 2013; Novak, 2014). When someone believes that they are protected by anonymity, they may act in more aggressive ways, or in ways that they would not act if they were known. The relational quality of lack of anonymity implies some presence of trust; trust is common in rural communities. Insider status and trusting relationships found in many rural communities may insulate rural dwellers from the negatives of anonymity. Because rural dwellers have trusting relationships with people they know, they may be at greater risk for being preyed upon through the Internet. Taking time to consider the role of anonymity in society is an important exercise as we reflect on the lack of anonymity experienced in rural communities.

So, what does this have to do with rethinking lack of anonymity? Lack of anonymity is inherent in a rural environment, and occurs without an individual's consent. This means that the rural nurse and the rural dweller both experience lack of anonymity in healthcare encounters. The relational quality of lack of anonymity places rural nurses in practice environments where trusting relationships are commonplace. Anonymity is one way to protect privacy rights, but anonymity is not synonymous with privacy.

Privacy

Privacy issues are commonly reported with lack of anonymity (Novak, 2014). Although closely related, the concepts are distinctly different; by definition, privacy involves concealment, individuals attempting to keep something to themselves. Individuals manage privacy by not sharing personal information with another, or, by self-disclosing private information to another with the expectation that the information will not be shared. In the latter, a trusting relationship is an essential component of privacy (Townsend, 2009). Privacy is largely personal, with an acceptable level of disclosure varying from person to person.

Since privacy is personal, there is a misperception that privacy is fully under an individual's control. For example, a simple "like" in Facebook shares posted information with friends of a friend, and so forth. Once personal information is shared in a public forum, individual control may be lost. Complicating this further is that an individual may not know, or have control over, what is shared about him or herself on social media websites. Privacy issues are a reality in rural healthcare and research. Noone and Young (2009) identified breaks in privacy for adolescent females seeking contraceptives at a rural clinic by being seen and identified by people in the waiting room. Stein's (2010) ethnographic research into gay and lesbian civil rights in a rural community is upended when journalists reveal the name of the town used during the study. With the promised anonymity and confidentiality compromised, Stein was surprised to learn that the study participants were upset, not by being identified, but that their privacy was compromised (2010). These are examples of private information being disclosed without consent.

Like anonymity, privacy has societal implications. The U.S. Supreme Court established a *right to privacy* as implied in the Constitution in *Griswold v. Connecticut* in 1965 (Garrow, 2011). Following this decision, the right to privacy was further supported in *Katz v. U.S.* and *Roe v. Wade* (Fradella, Morrow, Fischer, & Ireland, 2011; Rausch, 2012). Privacy, particularly as it pertains to digital and online communication, remains in the public and political forum. As of this writing, the Email Privacy Act passed by the U. S. House of Representatives is awaiting action by the Senate (Congress.gov, 2017). The Trump administration recently reversed the Internet privacy protections implemented under the Obama administration; telecommunication companies can now track people's personal Internet information without consent (Lohr, 2017). Privacy and individual rights to privacy will continue to be topics of national conversation. The ongoing debate of what is private, or not, may lie in the variability between individuals on what is acceptable to disclose to others.

As we consider how to rethink lack of anonymity, we need to recognize that the concepts of lack of anonymity and privacy are not synonymous. Privacy issues can arise with or without the presence of lack of anonymity. Lack of anonymity may be experienced without loss of privacy. Privacy appears to be connected to how rural dwellers manage boundaries of the personal and public self (Long & Weinert, 1989; Swan & Hobbs, 2017).

Confidentiality

Confidentiality is often linked to privacy and anonymity. The linkage to anonymity is commonly related to journalistic protection of sources, or the use of anonymity in research to ensure confidentiality of study participants (Novak, 2014). In research, confidentiality is maintained by de-identifying, or making study participants, or situations, anonymous. In the strictest sense, study participants are never truly anonymous, as the researcher knows who participated (Novak, 2014). Confidentiality is relational and requires trust in, or with, another individual (Novak, 2014; Townsend, 2009). In healthcare, confidentiality is a central belief of ethical care; nurses have a duty to protect information known about or disclosed by a patient during the provision of care (American Nurses Association, 2015).

Townsend (2009) suggests that confidentiality works differently within the intimate nature of rural communities. The close relationships and contact at social and community events may place the rural nurse in situations where patients are encountered outside of the healthcare setting. Therefore, rural nurses must be hypervigilant in maintaining confidentiality. In contrast, nurses working in urban settings are less likely to meet patients in social settings; thus, confidentiality is maintained.

Familiarity

In their concept analysis on familiarity, McNeely and Shreffler (1998) defined familiarity as a "friendly relationship or close acquaintance, intimacy, informality, and the exhibited familiarity is welcome or unwelcome" (p. 98). The definition of familiarity is expansive, encompassing relationships that range from friendly to intimate and including relationships that include components of being welcome and unwelcome. Unlike privacy and confidentiality, trust is not necessarily an element of familiarity. It is possible to be familiar with someone and not trust them; the *unwelcome* element of familiarity may intersect with personal privacy and boundaries.

Support for the familiarity definition can be located in literature. Ryan and McKenna (2013) studied the factors that rural family caregivers considered before placing an older adult in a nursing home. The study identified that familiarity with the nursing home owners, staff, residents, and the rural community was a factor in making the decision about nursing home placement. The personal relationship with the nursing home owners and staff reveals a welcomed, friendly relationship containing easy, informal communication. Ryan and McKenna (2013) suggest that familiarity was a source of social support for the older adult placed in the nursing home, and the family. Further, they suggest that rural nurse's social capital plays a role in the social networks and relationships in rural communities. Social capital is known to be about trusting relationships and connectivity to others and the greater community. As suggested by Ryan and McKenna, the familiarity experienced by rural family caregivers, and the social capital identified, indicates that the relationship extends beyond simply being able to identify someone.

What does this have to do with rethinking lack of anonymity? Lack of anonymity and familiarity are often discussed together, and the difference between the two concepts is not always clear. Both concepts are relational and center on knowing about another person or entity. Swan and Hobbs's (2017) analysis identified familiarity as a consequence of lack of anonymity. Thus, experiencing lack of anonymity contributes to the development of familiarity.

PROPOSED MODEL OF LACK OF ANONYMINITY

The purpose of examining concepts is to gain insight into how the concepts affect nursing practice. The previous review defines, describes, and provides a high-level overview of each concept from current literature. To explain proposed linkages between lack of anonymity with the concepts of privacy, confidentiality, and familiarity, we propose a Model of Lack of Anonymity (see Figure 6.1).

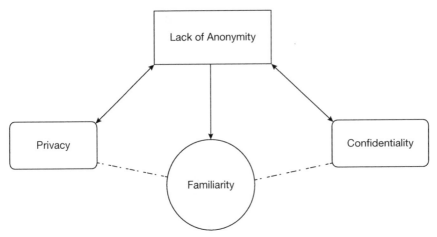

FIGURE 6.1. Proposed model of lack of anonymity.

The one-way arrow from Lack of Anonymity to Familiarity indicates that familiarity is a consequence of lack of anonymity (Swan & Hobbs, 2017). Lack of anonymity and familiarity are both relational and occur through individual interactions with others. Based on evidence in the literature, the bidirectional arrows from Lack of Anonymity to Privacy and Confidentiality suggest that there is a relationship and influence between the concepts. For example, a rural nurse who experiences high lack of anonymity may encounter more issues with privacy and confidentiality in his or her personal and professional life. A dash line from Familiarity to Privacy and Confidentiality indicates that the evidence is not clear on the relationship of the concepts to each other; however, since familiarity is a consequence of lack of anonymity, this suggests that there may be a relationship. The proposed model is not validated and requires further research be done to fully understand the relationship between the concepts; additionally, there may be other concepts not considered in this review that require inclusion.

IMPLICATIONS

Rural Nursing Practice

Lack of anonymity is a reality in rural environments, affecting the rural nurse and the rural dweller. Rural dwellers experience relationships with others in a community; familiarity provides opportunity to make friends, and have meaningful relationships. People can call others by name, and can identify each other's unique qualities and characteristics. Experiencing lack of anonymity by being identifiable and known can be challenging for rural nurses. Rural nurses report issues with personal privacy that may require navigating professional issues and relationships in a community setting. Establishing personal and professional boundaries will help rural nurses with maintaining personal privacy.

Accountability and responsibility are characteristics of rural dwellers; rural dwellers generally engage in honest communication that promotes trusting relationships. Rural nurses provide care to people whom they know and with whom they may have significant relationships. Thus, rural nurses may know medical and personal information about a patient that an urban nurse may not know. Similarly, this knowledge may afford rural nurses the opportunity to establish a trusting relationship prior to a health encounter. A preexisting trust relationship may prompt the sharing of confidential information with a rural nurse. Rural nurses have reported challenges in maintaining confidentiality while maintaining personal and professional boundaries (Swan & Hobbs, 2017). Establishing these boundaries may well be one of the most difficult challenges for rural nurses who experience lack of anonymity in their everyday lives. Future research into how rural nurses manage confidentiality in rural and remote communities may reveal strategies that could be taught or implemented across disciplines in rural healthcare facilities. Gaining knowledge on confidentiality supports ethical nursing practice for rural nurses.

Rural dwellers may also know their nurse, a situation that may or may not be comforting. Noone and Young (2009) describe the paradoxical nature of lack of anonymity; some rural dwellers find comfort in knowing their healthcare providers on a personal level, whereas others do not. There is ample evidence in the literature that rural dwellers find comfort in knowing their nurse, but rural nurses should not assume that all rural dwellers are comfortable *being known* by their nurse. Some rural dwellers may have concern that private health information may be made public. This paradoxical nature may explain some of the variation in privacy expectations among individuals. Rural nurses need to consider how being known to their patient may potentially affect the information disclosed by the patient. Extra care and attention to privacy and confidentiality may be warranted as reassurance to rural dwellers.

The Internet, communication technology, and telemedicine increase access to health information and healthcare providers outside of a rural community. Researchers at the Pew Research Center (2015) report that 87% of U.S. citizens are using the Internet. Greater connectivity and access to health information may act to bridge rural dwellers to outside healthcare resources and information, thus affecting the social capital of rural nurses. Additionally, recognizing that care may be obtained outside of the rural community, specific health history questions should be asked to verify patients' knowledge and ensure their understanding is consistent with the best evidence and current health information.

This review supports that familiarity has an important function in the life of rural dwellers, by providing social support, particularly during challenges and life transitions (Ryan & McKenna, 2013). The concept of social capital and how social capital functions in familiar relationships are not understood and require further exploration and research (Lee & McDonagh, 2013). The connectedness that rural nurses experience in practice positions them to positively impact health (Lauder et al., 2006). Lack of anonymity is often portrayed as a negative of rural communities; however, there is growing evidence that lack of anonymity plays a positive role in relationships and the development of familiarity. Understanding these positive aspects of lack of anonymity will provide greater insight into the role and function of social capital and support in rural communities.

Privacy is a personal issue that may be experienced in rural environments. Lack of anonymity, or being known, can limit privacy. For example, rural dwellers may opt out of mental health services to prevent being recognized by their car parked in the clinic lot (Graber, 2011; Kitchen Andren et al., 2013). In this case, the health and well-being of the patient is being affected out of concern for personal privacy. Rural nurses may need to ask specific questions regarding patients' concerns and seek to understand how privacy issues may affect healthcare choices.

Nursing Research

The concepts described are closely related, but are not synonymous or interchangeable. Clearly defining concepts is essential to ensure that the right concept is being studied and measured; without clear definitions, findings may be inconsistent, and conceptual clarity may be diminished. For example, a rural nurse may experience lack of anonymity but have issue with a lack of privacy. Since lack of anonymity, to some degree, is present in a rural environment, the central issue may be the rural nurse's expectation of personal privacy. Thus, privacy is the concept of interest, not necessarily lack of anonymity. Care must be taken to prevent lack of anonymity from being a catchall term; rethinking lack of anonymity and how it influences a rural environment may well reveal new concepts requiring exploration. The state of rural nursing science will advance with the use of common definitions of rural concepts.

In addition, further research on privacy and lack of anonymity is needed to help to identify and delineate the personal issues of privacy from the relational components of lack of anonymity. This delineation is critical to ensure that we are asking research questions appropriate to the concept. Future studies exploring the rural dwellers' expectations of personal privacy would add greater depth to our understanding. Further, it is unknown if the expectation of personal privacy in rural environments is different than the expectation of those living in urban environments.

CASE STUDIES

The following case studies have been developed to demonstrate how the concepts of lack of anonymity, privacy, confidentiality, and familiarity are encountered in the daily work of a rural nurse.

Karen is a registered nurse in a small rural community. She grew up on a farm outside of town and is related to or knows most of the people in the community. Karen, her husband, and their two school-aged children live in town. Karen and her family are active in youth sports and church activities.

Karen met Leah in the sixth grade, after Leah and her family moved to town. Karen and Leah were friends and used to hang out together. That changed in high school, when Leah began to "party" and experiment with alcohol, marijuana, and other drugs. Karen was not interested in partying with Leah, and the two drifted apart. Today, Leah is a part-time waitress at the local diner. Leah is divorced, mother to three school-aged children, and rents an apartment in town.

Case Study 1

Karen provided nursing care to Leah's child during a recent hospitalization that provided time for Leah and Karen to visit and catch up on their life activities. A couple of weeks after the child was discharged, Karen stopped at the grocery store after work to pick up a few groceries. The store was busy and Karen was pressed for time. While shopping, Karen ran into Leah, who stopped her and started to ask detailed questions related to her child's condition and medical care received during the hospital stay.

How should Karen respond?

What concept is best represented in the case study? How do you recognize the concept?

Case Study 2

Karen was walking down the hallway that connects the hospital and clinic and found Leah in the hallway holding one child and trying to entertain the other two. Karen greeted Leah and asked if she needed any help. Leah declined help and said that she did not want to sit in the waiting room and be seen by others. Leah expressed concern that people would determine that she was here to see a visiting specialist, who came to the clinic once a month, and guess at why she needed care. Leah stated, "I don't want people knowing anything about me."

(continued)

CASE STUDY 2 (*continued*)

How should Karen respond?

What concept is best represented in the case study? How do you recognize the concept?

CASE STUDY 3

Karen cared for Leah's child a third time in the ED. During the encounter, Karen learned that Leah's child had a serious, chronic health condition. Leah wept as she shared the diagnosis; she shared the challenges of being the sole parent responsible for the care needs of her family and the financial hardship of paying the medical bills along with living expenses. Karen felt compassion for Leah and connected Leah to the local social service and volunteer agencies for additional support. Leah was appreciative and gave Karen a hug and thanked her for providing great care. A few days later, Karen received a friend request from Leah on a social network. Karen thought this might be a good way to support Leah and accepted the friend request. In reviewing the social network postings, Karen learned that Leah's child was responding well to a medicine listed in the post that Karen knew had been prescribed on discharge from the ED. Karen was excited for Leah and posted a comment that she was glad that the medicine from the ED visit was helping. The next day, Karen was pulled into her manager's office and was told that she violated patient confidentiality.

How should Karen respond?

What concept is best represented in the case study? How do you recognize the concept?

CASE STUDY 4

Leah's child has had a series of recent hospitalizations and Karen has been involved in providing nursing care. Leah is always pleased to see Karen and initiates conversations about their children and mutual interests. During the most recent hospitalization, Leah was struggling with making a treatment decision for her child. Over several shifts, Karen was assigned to Leah's child and had many conversations with Leah about treatment options. Leah told Karen that she appreciated her thoughts and education on different treatment options, and shared how the information Karen provided helped her to decide on the best treatment option for her child.

How should Karen respond?

What concept is best represented in the case study? How do you recognize the concept?

CONCLUSION

Lack of anonymity is relational and a reality of rural life. Rural dwellers are identifiable and will become known to others in the community. Likewise, as a rural nurse, being known and recognizable is expected. As a result, rural nurses may need to manage aspects of their personal and professional lives to control their privacy. Trusting relationships exist in rural communities and extend into rural practice settings. As such, rural nurses need to recognize how breaking a trusting relationship will influence the ability to ensure patient privacy and confidentiality. Likewise, sharing confidential or private information about another can also affect the patient–nurse trusting relationship.

The analysis prompts us to rethink how we view lack of anonymity, and consider how lack of anonymity influences, both positively and negatively, rural nursing practice. The relational quality of lack of anonymity, confidentiality, and familiarity reflect the interconnectedness found in rural communities. These stand in contrast to the personal nature of privacy. These four concepts help us to understand rural nursing practice. A proposed model of lack of anonymity suggests that more research is needed to fully understand how the concepts, and possibly others, are related.

Rural nurses are uniquely positioned to influence health and well-being in rural communities. Rethinking lack of anonymity for the 21st century requires us to look deeply into rural concepts in order to open up new possibilities for research and to further our understanding and advance rural nursing science.

REFERENCES

American Nurses Association. (2015). *Code of ethics for nurses with interpretive statements.* Washington, DC: American Nurses Publishing.

Bodle, R. (2013). The ethics of online anonymity or Zuckerberg vs. "Moot." *Computers and Society, 43*(1), 22–35. doi:10.1145/2505414.2505417

Congress.gov. (n.d.). *About the federalist papers.* Retrieved from https://www.congress.gov/resources/display/content/About+the+Federalist+Papers

Congress.gov. (2017, February 7). *H. R. 387-Email Privacy Act.* Retrieved from https://www.congress.gov/bill/115th-congress/house-bill/387

Fradella, H. F., Morrow, W. J., Fischer, R. G., & Ireland, C. (2011). Quantifying Katz: Empirically measuring "reasonable expectations of privacy" in the fourth amendment context. *American Journal of Criminal Law, 38*(3), 289–373.

Garrow, D. J. (2011). The legal legacy of Griswold v. Connecticut. *Human Rights, 38*(2), 24–25.

Graber, M. A. (2011). Virtual mentor. *American Medical Association Journal of Ethics, 13*(5), 273–277.

Hegney, D. (1996). The status of rural nursing in Australia: A review. *Australian Journal of Rural Health, 4*, 1–10. doi:10.1111/j.1440-1584.1996.tb00180.x

Kitchen Andren, K. A., McKibbin, C. L., Wykes, T. L., Lee, A. A., Carrico, C. P., & Bourassa, K. A. (2013). Depression treatment among rural older adults: Preferences and factors influencing future service use. *Clinical Gerontologist, 36*(3), 241–259. doi:10.1080/07317115.2013.767872

Kozica, S. L., Harrison, C. L., Teede, H. J., Ng, S., Moran, L. J., & Lombard, C. B. (2015). Engaging rural women in healthy lifestyle programs: Insights from a randomized controlled trial. *Trials, 16*, 413. doi:10.1186/s13063-015-0860-5

Lauder, W., Reel, S., Farmer, J., & Griggs, H. (2006). Social capital, rural nursing and rural nursing theory. *Nursing Inquiry, 13*(1), 73–79. doi:10.1111/j.1440-1800.2006.00297.x

Lee, H. J. (1998). Lack of anonymity. In H. J. Lee (Ed.), *Conceptual basis for rural nursing* (1st ed., pp. 76–88). New York, NY: Springer Publishing.

Lee, H. J., & McDonagh, M. K. (2013). Updating the rural nursing theory base. In C. A. Winters (Ed.), *Rural nursing: Concepts, theory, and practice* (4th ed., pp. 15–33). New York, NY: Springer Publishing.

Lohr, S. (2017, April 3). *Trump completes repeal of online privacy protections from Obama era.* Retrieved from https://www.nytimes.com/2017/04/03/technology/trump-repeal-online-privacy-protections.html?_r=0

Long, K. A., & Weinert, S. C. (1989). Rural nursing: Developing the theory base. *Scholarly Inquiry for Nursing Practice: An International Journal, 3*(2), 113–127.

Marx, G. T. (1999). What's in a name? Some reflections on the sociology of anonymity. *The Information Society, 15*, 99–112.

McIntyre v. Ohio Elections Commission, 514 U.S. 334 U.S. (1995). Retrieved from https://www.law.cornell.edu/supct/html/93-986.ZO.html

McNeely, A. G., & Shreffler, M. J. (1998). Familiarity. In H. Lee (Ed.), *Conceptual basis for rural nursing* (1st ed., pp. 89–101). New York, NY: Springer Publishing.

Noone, J., & Young, H. M. (2009). Preparing daughters: The context of rurality on mothers' role in contraception. *The Journal of Rural Health, 25*(3), 282–288. doi:10.1111/j.1748-0361.2009.00231.x

Novak, A. (2014). Anonymity, confidentiality, privacy, and identity: The ties that bind and break in communication research. *Review of Communication, 14*(1), 36–48. doi:10.1080/15358593.2014.942351

Pew Research Center. (2015, October 8). Social media usage: 2005–2015. Retrieved from http://www.pewinternet.org/2015/10/08/social-networking-usage-2005-2015

Rausch, R. L. (2012). Reframing Roe: Property over privacy. *Berkley Journal of Gender, Law & Justice, 27*(1), 28–63.

Rodgers, B. L. (2000). Philosophical foundations of concept development. In B. L. Rodgers & K. A. Knafl (Eds.), *Concept development in nursing* (2nd ed., pp. 7–37). Philadelphia, PA: Saunders.

Rolland, R. A. (2016). Emergency room nurses transitioning from curative to end-of-life care: The rural influence. *Online Journal of Rural Nursing and Health Care, 16*(2), 58–85. doi:10.14574/ojrnhc.v16i2.396

Rosenthal, K. A. (2010). The rural nursing generalist in the acute care setting: Flowing like a river. In C. A. Winters & H. J. Lee (Eds.), *Rural nursing concepts: Theory and practice* (3rd ed., pp. 269–283). New York, NY: Springer Publishing.

Ryan, A., & McKenna, H. (2013). 'Familiarity' as a key factor influencing rural family carers' experience of the nursing home placement of an older relative: A qualitative study. *BMC Health Services Research, 13*, 252. doi:10.1186/1472-6963-13-252

Stein, A. (2010). Sex, truths, and audiotape: Anonymity and the ethics of exposure in public ethnography. *Journal of Contemporary Ethnography, 39*(5), 554–568. doi:10.1177/0891241610375955

Stewart Fahs, P. (2017). Leading-following in the context of rural nursing. *Nursing Science Quarterly, 30*(2), 176–178. doi:10.1177/0894318417693317

Swan, M. A., & Hobbs, B. B. (2017). Concept analysis: Lack of anonymity. *Journal of Advanced Nursing, 73*(5), 1075–1084. doi:10.1111/jan.13236

Townsend, T. (2009). Ethics conflicts in rural communities: Privacy and confidentiality. In W. A. Nelson (Ed.), *Handbook for rural health care ethics: A practical guide for professionals* (1st ed., pp. 128–141). Lebanon, NH: University Press of New England.

Whitley, R., & McKenzie, K. (2005). Social capital and psychiatry: Review of the literature. *Harvard Review of Psychiatry, 13*(2), 71–84. doi:10.1080/10673220590956474

Zimbardo, P. G. (1969). The human choice: Individuation, reason and order versus deindividuation, impulse and chaos. In W. Arnold & D. Levine (Eds.), *Nebraska Symposium on Motivation* (1st ed., Vol. XVII, pp. 237–307). Lincoln: University of Nebraska Press.

CHAPTER 7

A Program of Research in Rural Settings[*]

Clarann Weinert, Elizabeth Nichols, and Jean Shreffler-Grant

DISCUSSION TOPICS

- Identify several challenges experienced by the research team in the course of their "journey."
- How did the research team overcome some of the challenges identified in question #1?
- Discuss how the national focus on health literacy was utilized by the research team as an opportunity to advance their program of research.

Sustaining a program of nursing research in a rural setting is a journey with many opportunities and challenges. The purpose of recounting the story of our journey is to share how a program of nursing research can thrive despite being conducted in low nursing research resource environments, across geographic distances, and with a limited patchwork of funding. We attribute our success to an active and astute research team, a topic of interest to all team members, the ability to work across long distances, and a large dose of persistence. In telling this story, only the highlights of our studies are presented. The full descriptions of these studies have been published previously.

THE RESEARCH TEAM

The early phase of this journey was launched by a senior administrator at the University of North Dakota (UND) and a senior investigator from Montana State University (MSU), institutions separated by 800 miles. A master's student

*From Weinert, C., Nichols, E., & Shreffler-Grant, J. (2015). A program of nursing research in a rural setting. *Online Journal of Rural Nursing and Health Care, 15*(1), 100–116. doi:10.14574/ojrnhc.v15i1.343. Reprinted with permission.

and junior faculty member at UND rounded out the original team. Shortly into the research adventure, these two junior individuals moved on—the master's student into a doctoral program in another state, the faculty member to clinical practice. To replace the lost team members and enrich this two-institutional research team, the two senior investigators then sought additional members from each institution who were junior in their research roles but interested and competent. A junior investigator from MSU with an interest in complementary and alternative medicine (CAM) and previous rural research joined and was quickly mentored into the role of principal investigator. In addition, a senior faculty member from UND joined the team. These four researchers began a research collaboration that has continued for almost 20 years.

Depending on the needs of the research program, other investigators have joined the team for specific tasks. For example, two senior MSU investigators were hired: one to conduct interviews in an early study, and one to collect data in a more recent study. Graduate and undergraduate students enriched the research team and engaged in library searches, assisted with data collection and management, and helped with the preparation of manuscripts and presentations.

A significant challenge to the team was working over long distances—not only across states but also within the state of Montana. For example, the principal investigator's location is 200 miles from the main campus of MSU and the second MSU investigator. The key to successfully meeting this challenge has been ongoing and frequent communication among the members of the team, utilizing a variety of strategies. The increased ease of electronic and telephone communication facilitated productive meetings. Highly important were annual face-to-face meetings that promoted team cohesion, allowed for concentrated group work time, and resulted in the production of grant applications, publications, and presentations.

Over the course of the journey, the core research team has adapted to a variety of changes: new academic roles/status, the relocation of one of the North Dakota team members to Montana, and the death of the other North Dakota colleague. The remaining three core members continue to work successfully as an engaged research team.

IDENTIFYING THE FOCUS OF RESEARCH

Central to our program of research has been an emphasis on examining strategies for enhancing the health of older rural adults. Our early studies on the use of CAM by older rural dwellers were driven by the interests of the initial junior team members and that meshed well with the broader research endeavors of the senior investigators. Further, the cutting-edge studies by Eisenberg et al. (1993) and Eisenberg et al. (1998) on CAM use did not differentiate between urban and rural populations, our area of interest.

During the late 1990s and early 2000s, several well-known national studies were conducted that demonstrated the use of CAM among the general U.S. population was more common than previously thought. Further, researchers found that often there was limited communication between consumers and providers about treatment options and the consumers' use of CAM (Astin, 1998; Eisenberg et al., 1993). Researchers noted that CAM therapies were used more often for chronic than acute health problems. Use was more common among women, younger adults, those with higher incomes, more education, and those living in the western United States (Astin, Pelletier, Marie, & Haskell, 2000; Cherniack, Senzel, & Pan, 2001; Eisenberg et al., 1998). These investigators tended not to differentiate between rural and urban populations. However, when studies were designed to focus on the use of CAM among rural dwellers, the results were inconsistent. Vallerand, Fouladbakhsh, and Templin (2003) found that CAM use was less prevalent among rural dwellers than among urban. Yet, Harron and Glasser (2003) reported that the use of CAM was more common among rural residents. Conversely, other researchers found that the prevalence of use among rural and urban dwellers was similar (Arcury, Preisser, Gesler, & Sherman, 2004).

Initial Studies on the Research Journey

The initial research on our journey included a series of studies with older adults living in rural areas to further understand the role of CAM in health decisions. The primary purpose was to explore the use of, and satisfaction with, CAM from the perspectives of older rural people. The team also sought to gain a better understanding of why CAM was used and what sources were used to obtain information about CAM therapies. Throughout these early studies, participants were recruited from counties in Montana and North Dakota that met the federal definitions for "rural" and "frontier." All studies discussed in this journey were approved by the universities' institutional review boards for protection of human subjects.

In the first study, 325 randomly selected older adults in 19 rural communities were interviewed by telephone. Participants had a mean age of 72 years and most (67.7%) reported having one or more chronic illnesses. Only 17.5% reported using complementary providers, while 35.7% used self-prescribed CAM practices, such as home remedies, nutritional supplements, and herbal products. Participants most often learned about the therapies from relatives and friends or consumer marketing rather than from healthcare professionals. Those most likely to use CAM were women who were fairly well educated, not currently married, and in their early older years. They had one or more significant chronic illnesses and lower health-related quality of life (Shreffler-Grant, Hill, Weinert, Nichols, & Ide, 2007; Shreffler-Grant, Weinert, Nichols, & Ide, 2005). From this survey, the research team gained an overview of who used

CAM and what type they used, but it did not provide information about why they used CAM, or how much they knew about what they used.

To obtain more in-depth information, 10 older rural adults with a chronic illness who had reported using CAM in the initial interview were reinterviewed. Six of the 10 participants were women; eight were between the ages of 70 and 80; and two were between 60 and 70 years. Their mean education level was 12.5 years. They used self-prescribed CAM therapies primarily to compensate for perceived dietary deficiencies. For the most part, they were satisfied with the results they attributed to the CAM. It was clear, however, that some participants used the therapies in an inconsistent manner and did not understand the purpose of the products.

Participants attempted to use reputable sources for information; yet, few sought information from their allopathic providers due to a perception that the providers were too busy to answer their questions about CAM (Nichols, Sullivan, Ide, Shreffler-Grant, & Weinert, 2005).

It was of interest to the team that most of the respondents in the original study did not interact with CAM providers. The team questioned whether this phenomenon was related to the availability of providers in rural areas and concluded it merited further study. Internet and telephone directory searches were used to locate CAM resources in 20 small rural communities in Montana and North Dakota. Seventy-three providers, representing a wide variety of CAM therapies, were identified in these communities. The team also sought to ascertain the contribution of one type of CAM provider, naturopathic physicians to rural healthcare (Nichols, Weinert, Shreffler-Grant, & Ide, 2006), through an online survey. Most naturopaths were located in population centers, but some offered outreach clinics to rural communities.

In summary, participants in all of these early studies tended to use self-directed or self-prescribed CAM rather than therapies provided by practitioners. Local availability of practitioners did not appear to be a factor in the use of CAM by older rural residents. The residents gleaned information about the therapies primarily by word of mouth or from the media. Some respondents used CAM inconsistently; others did not seek information about the effects or risks, and when they did, the information sources used were those generally considered unreliable.

CAM Health Literacy—A Detour

As on any journey, it is wise to be aware of changing circumstances and respond appropriately. On a road trip, if there is construction indicated ahead, one needs to be prepared to slow, stop, or perhaps take a detour. On our research journey, we became astutely aware of the growing national focus on the role of health literacy, that is, "the degree to which individuals have the capacity to obtain, process, and understand basic health information and services needed to make appropriate health decisions" (U.S.

Department of Health and Human Services, 2000). Creating a health literate populace had become a major priority in the nation's public healthcare policy, research, practice, and education arenas. The Institute of Medicine (IOM) included health literacy as one of 20 priority areas and noted that it is fundamental to improving self-management of health conditions (IOM, 2004). The IOM cited a critical need for more rigorous work to develop appropriate, reliable, and valid measures of health literacy (IOM, 2004). More specific to the teams' program of research, the IOM also noted that there was very little research on how American consumers obtain, understand, and evaluate information about the various CAM therapies (IOM, 2005). With the advent of these critical documents, there was a clear need for research in the area of CAM health literacy. It was evident to our team that a detour from our focus on informed CAM use was needed. In order to develop and test an intervention to enhance health decision making related to CAM, a measure of CAM health literacy was essential. Prior to developing a measure, it was critical to have a definition and conceptual model of CAM health literacy.

CAM Health Literacy Model Development

The team's working definition of CAM health literacy was the information about CAM that individuals need to make informed health decisions. The MSU Conceptual Model of CAM Health Literacy was constructed from a comprehensive review of the literature, the team's prior research, the definition of CAM health literacy, and input from national experts (Shreffler-Grant, Nichols, Weinert, & Ide, 2013). There are three major components to the model: antecedents, structure, and outcome. The primary outcome of the model is informed self-management of health. Antecedents are factors that can affect the structural component. Four concepts, dose, effect, safety, and availability, compose the structural component and were the focus for the subsequent CAM health literacy instrument development. The MSU Conceptual Model of CAM Health Literacy is the first known attempt to conceptualize the essential elements of health literacy regarding CAM. Health literacy, in this model, is expanded in a context different from allopathic healthcare and goes beyond reading and computational skills (see Figure 7.1). The development and refinement of the model was thoroughly discussed in an earlier publication (Shreffler-Grant, Nichols, Weinert, & Ide, 2013).

Instrument Development

Following the articulation of the conceptual model, the next segment of our research journey was the development of a measure of CAM health literacy. DeVellis' well-established and tested eight-step process for scale development was used to guide our efforts (DeVellis, 2012; see Table 7.1.)

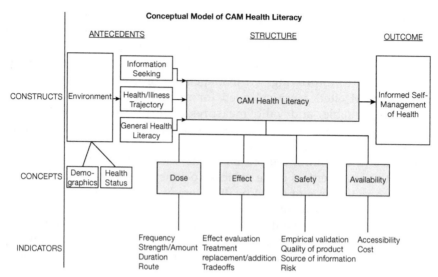

FIGURE 7.1. Montana State University (MSU) conceptual model of Complementary and Alternative Medicine (CAM) health literacy.
Source: Shreffler-Grant, J., Nichols, E., Weinert, C., & Ide, B. (2013). The Montana State University conceptual model of complementary and alternative medicine health literacy. *Journal of Health Communication, 18*(10), 1193–1200. doi:10.1080/10810730.2013.778365

TABLE 7.1 DeVellis's Guidelines for Scale Development

Step 1	Construct Determination
Step 2	Generate item pool
Step 3	Determine measurement format
Step 4	Review of item pool
Step 5	Consider validation items
Step 6	Administer to development sample
Step 7	Evaluate items
Step 8	Optimize scale length

The structural component of the newly developed model provided the constructs and concepts necessary to initiate the instrument development process. Empirical indicators were identified for each of the four majo concepts, and two to seven items for each indicator were generated. A six-point Likert scale response format with equally weighted items was selected to allow for a summed single scale score. To ensure that the items were clear and understandable, plain language principles (Plain Language, 2013) were used and medical jargon was avoided. Items were written at an eighth grade or less reading level based on the Flesch–Kincaid grade level (Readability Formulas, 2013).

To refine the item pool, a panel of experts in the areas of tool development and CAM therapy generously reviewed the items for consistency with the model and clarity of wording. They also suggested additional items. A revised item pool and response set was reviewed and critiqued by four focus groups. Two focus groups were composed of community dwelling senior citizens and two of allopathic and complementary healthcare providers. Recommendations from the experts and the focus groups resulted in the team's careful rereview of the item pool. At this point in the journey, the initial instrument consisted of 54 items with two versions of the measure. One version had a dichotomous response option of "agree/disagree"; the other version had a four-point response set with anchors of "agree strongly" to "disagree strongly."

Refining the Instrument

A professional research interview company was hired to administer the draft CAM health literacy instruments, obtain basic demographic data including CAM use, and a single item health literacy measure included for validity assessment: the participant's ease of completion of medical forms (Chew, Bradley, & Boyko, 2004). Interviews were conducted with a random sample of 1,200 adults over the age of 55 from households in nonmetropolitan areas of the northwestern quadrant of the United States. One half of the sample ($n = 600$) completed the version with the four-point response set, the other half with the dichotomous response option.

Decision Point

The availability of resources required a team decision as to how to proceed with the initial data analysis. We had the skill and statistical programs necessary to analyze the four-response data set. However, to appropriately analyze the two-response set required different statistical resources and personnel. In addition, DeVellis, a consultant on the project, recommended focusing on the four-point response set. Thus, the decision was made to initially analyze only the four-point response set version. The analysis procedures were conducted on one half of that sample ($n = 300$), and then were validated by comparing the results with results of duplicate analyses from the second half of that data set. The procedures were then run on the data from the entire sample ($n = 600$). Standard exploratory factor analysis procedures with the number of factors (three) based upon parallel analysis were used. Principal components extraction with oblimin rotation was used to determine factors and item loadings. Items with weak loadings or that loaded on more than one factor were deleted. The reliabilities of each factor as well as each item's contribution to that alpha were also examined to determine which items to retain. This process continued until a stable solution with an adequate alpha was obtained. The final 21-item four-response set instrument had a Cronbach's alpha of 0.75. The correlation between the CAM Health Literacy Scale and the medical forms completion item was 0.174 ($p = .003$) (Shreffler-Grant, Weinert, & Nichols, 2014).

Validation Study

The final leg of the instrument development detour was to conduct a study to further assess validity by comparing CAM Health Literacy Scale scores with those on a general health literacy measure. The validation procedures were implemented with a convenience sample of 110 community-dwelling older adults (average age 68). The data collection packet included the MSU CAM Health Literacy Scale and two health literacy measures: the Newest Vital Sign (Osborn et al., 2007) and one question about ease of completion of medical forms (Chew et al., 2004). Also included were basic demographics, CAM use information, and presence of chronic illness. Sixty-six percent of the sample were women, 75% had more than a high school education, and 51% were currently married. Eighty-two percent indicated that they used CAM, and 51% said that they had no significant health problems. The alpha on the CAM Health Literacy Scale in this sample was 0.73. The correlation with the Newest Vital Sign was 0.221 ($p = .002$) and with the single medical forms completion question was 0.277 ($p = .004$) (Shreffler-Grant et al., 2014). Now, with an instrument in hand, the team was ready to return to the main trail—how to improve the CAM health literacy of older rural dwellers and thus enhance the information they bring to bear on the management of their health.

FUNDING THE JOURNEY

Ideally, a program of research is continuously funded; however, life is not always ideal. Yet, there are times when the "financial planets" do align! The launching of our journey fortuitously coincided with the National Center for Complementary and Alternative Medicine becoming a funding agency. This center funded our first exploratory study and also our most recent work to develop the CAM Health Literacy Scale. Between the two grants, the research journey was sustained by small intramural grants, investigator dedication, the generosity of time and expertise donated by our nursing and nonnursing research colleagues, and the ongoing commitment of the team members. At times, we felt like "the little engine that could!"

LESSONS LEARNED ON THE JOURNEY

This research program has been a journey filled with twists and turns that are likely to continue as we travel down the CAM health literacy path. The success of this research team can be attributed to active, committed investigators, a topic of interest that has engaged all members, and, at least, occasional funding. Maintaining sufficient continuity in the research team while also being open to enlist help from additional investigators was critical to the development and sustainability of this program of research.

The importance of building from one study to the next was an ever-present precept. We invested significant time and energy reflecting, discussing, and "cogitating" about the results of each step of the research program in order to tease out the meaning from the data and identify remaining questions to be answered along with the most appropriate approaches to answer them.

Being alert to historical events that have relevance to the program of research is critical. The CAM health literacy "detour" was inspired by the IOM report that indicated a critical need for more rigorous work to develop appropriate, reliable, and valid measures of health literacy (IOM, 2004). In retrospect, what we thought was a detour may have been a main road on the map. From the outset of our research endeavors, the overall goal was the promotion of informed healthcare choices by older rural dwellers. Addressing the definition, model, and measurement of CAM health literacy has enlightened and enhanced our research program and is a genuine fit with our goal.

This research journey has not been without obstacles. The several definitions of health literacy complicated the task of developing the model of CAM health literacy. Further, it became clear that there were no markers on the trail, other than our own model, to guide the writing of items and the selection of the response option anchors. An additional challenge was the lack of an appropriate and mature measure of general health literacy against which to validate the MSU CAM Health Literacy Scale. Additional obstacles were the geographic distance between team members along with limited and inconsistent funding.

Reviewing the journey of a team of researchers over time, including the original intent, the challenges, and the detours, can be instructive to other teams as they travel on their own research journeys. The way is seldom straight nor paved with continuous funding, but persistence, a meaningful goal, and good working relationships have kept this team on task and energized.

ACKNOWLEDGMENTS

Research supported by: National Institutes of Health/National Center for Complementary and Alternative Medicine R15 AT095-01, R15 T006609-01; National Institutes of Health/National Institute of Nursing Research 1P20NR07790-01; Montana State University College of Nursing Block Grant; University of North Dakota College of Nursing Intramural Grant. Acknowledgment also to Bette Ide, PhD, RN, FAAN, Lompoc, CA, a former research team member (deceased).

REFERENCES

Arcury, T., Preisser, J., Gesler, W., & Sherman, J. (2004). Complementary and alternative medicine use among rural residents in western North Carolina. *Complementary Health Practice Review, 9*(2), 93–102. doi:10.1177/1076167503253433

Astin, J. (1998). Why patients use alternative medicine: Results of a national study. *Journal of the American Medical Association, 279*(19), 1548–1553. doi:10.1001/jama.279.19.1548

Astin, J., Pelletier, K., Marie, A., & Haskell, W. (2000). Complementary and alternative medicine use among elderly persons: One-year analysis of a Blue Shield Medicare supplement. *Journal of Gerontology Series A, Biological Sciences and Medical Sciences, 55*(1), M4–M9.

Cherniack, E., Senzel, R., & Pan, C. (2001). Correlates of use of alternative medicine by the elderly in an urban population. *Journal of Alternative and Complementary Medicine, 7,* 277–280. doi:10.1089/107555301300328160

Chew, L. D., Bradley, K. A., & Boyko, E. J. (2004). Brief questions to identify patients with inadequate health literacy. *Family Medicine, 36*(8), 588–594.

DeVellis, R. (2012). *Scale development: Theory and applications* (3rd ed.). Thousand Oaks, CA: Sage.

Eisenberg, D., Davis, R., Ettner, S., Appel, S., Wilkey, S., Van Rompay, M., & Kessler, R. (1998). Trends in alternative medicine use in the United States, 1990–1997; Results of a follow-up national survey. *Journal of the American Medical Association, 280*(18), 1569–1575. doi:10.1001/jama.280.18.1569

Eisenberg, D., Kessler, R., Foster, C., Norlock, F., Calkins, D., & Delbanco, T. (1993). Unconventional medicine in the United States. *New England Journal of Medicine, 328,* 246–252. doi:10.1056/NEJM199301283280406

Harron, M., & Glasser, M. (2003). Use of and attitudes toward complementary and alternative medicine among family practice patients in small rural Illinois communities. *Journal of Rural Health, 19*(3), 279–284. doi:10.1111/j.1748-0361.2003.tb00574.x

Institute of Medicine. (2004). *Health literacy: A prescription to end confusion.* Washington, DC: The National Academies Press.

Institute of Medicine. (2005). *Complementary and alternative medicine in the United States.* Washington, DC: The National Academies Press.

Nichols, E., Sullivan, T., Ide, B., Shreffler-Grant, J., & Weinert, C. (2005). Health care choices: Complementary therapy, chronic illness, and older rural dwellers. *Journal of Holistic Nursing, 23*(4), 381–394. doi:10.1177/0898010105281088

Nichols, E., Weinert, C., Shreffler-Grant, J., & Ide, B. (2006). Complementary and alternative providers in rural locations. *Online Journal of Rural Nursing and Health Care, 6*(2), 40–46. Retrieved from http://rnojournal.binghamton.edu/index.php/RNO/index

Osborn, C. Y., Weiss, B. D., Davis, T. C., Skripkauskas, S., Rodrigue, C., Bass, P. F., & Wolf, M. S. (2007). Measuring adult literacy in health care: Performance of the newest vital sign. *American Journal of Health Behavior, 31*(Suppl. 1), S36–S46. doi:10.5993/AJHB.31.s1.6

Plain Language. (2013). Plain Language and Information Network (PLAIN), U.S. General Services Administration. Retrieved from http://www.plainlanguage.gov

Readability Formulas (2013). *The Flesch Grade Readability Formula.* Retrieved from http://www.readabilityformulas.com/flesch-grade-level-readability-formula.php

Shreffler-Grant, J., Hill, W., Weinert, C., Nichols, E., & Ide, B. (2007). Complementary therapy and older rural women: Who uses and who does not? *Nursing Research, 56*(1), 28–33. doi:10.1097/00006199-200701000-00004

Shreffler-Grant, J., Nichols, E., Weinert, C., & Ide, B. (2013). The Montana State University conceptual model of complementary and alternative medicine health literacy. *Journal of Health Communication, 18*(10), 1193–1200. doi:10.1080/10810730.2013.778365

Shreffler-Grant, J., Weinert, C., & Nichols, E. (2014). Instrument to measure health literacy about complementary and alternative medicine. *Journal of Nursing Measurement, 22*(3), 489–499. doi:10.1891/1061-3749.22.3.489

Shreffler-Grant, J., Weinert, C., Nichols, E., & Ide, B. (2005). Complementary therapy use among older rural adults. *Public Health Nursing, 22*(4), 323–3311. doi:10.1111/j.0737-1209.2005.220407.x

U.S. Department of Health and Human Services (2000). *Healthy People 2010, Section 11-2: Health Communication Objective.* Retrieved from http://www.healthypeople.gov.

Vallerand, A., Fouladbakhsh, J., & Templin, T. (2003). The use of complementary/alternative medicine therapies for the self-treatment of pain among residents of urban, suburban, and rural communities. *American Journal of Public Health, 93,* 923–925. doi:10.2105/AJPH.93.6.923

Rural Nursing Practice

The section opens with the chapter by Jane Ellis Scharff, "The Nature and Scope of Rural Nursing Practice: Philosophical Basis," which has appeared in the previous editions of this book. This classic work is followed by a qualitative study using phenomenological methods of the lived experience of rural nurses working in critical access hospitals in Montana and Vermont.

Using nurse practitioners as healthcare providers is the premise of the chapter written by a director of a Family Nurse Practitioner program. The authors of Chapter 11 provide examples of the use of telehealth technology to overcome the problems encountered in access to care because of distance and weather, particularly in chronically ill patients living in rural and remote areas. Exploration of the experience of nurses living in rural and frontier areas who chose to commute to urban medical centers for practice is the subject of Chapter 12.

The melding of two middle-range theories, rural nursing theory and the Synergy Model for Patient Care, is proposed by the authors of the Chapter 13 . The latter, a nursing practice model developed by the American Association of Critical Care Nurses, describes the relationship between patient and nurse and is worthy of further exploration and research.

Assessment is the focus of Chapters 14, 15, and 16. Being able to assess resilience in older frontier women is the focus of Chapter 14 while recognizing cultural differences in management of bereavement in rural settings is highlighted in Chapter 15. Revision and expansion of the framework of the Symptom–Action–Timeline process (SATL; Buehler, Malone, & Majerus, 1998) to the Symptom–Action Process (SAP; O'Lynn, 2010), and then to the Health-Needs–Action Process (HNAP) through extensive literature review is the focus of Chapter 16.

REFERENCES

Buehler, J., Malone, M., & Majerus, J. (1998). Patterns of responses to symptoms in rural residents: The symptom-action-time-line process. In H. Lee (Ed.), *Conceptual basis for rural nursing* (pp. 153–162). New York, NY: Springer Publishing.

O'Lynn, C. (2006). Updating the symptom-action-time-line process. In H. Lee & C. A. Winters (Eds.), *Rural Nursing: Concepts, Theory, and Practice* (2nd ed., pp. 138–152). New York, NY: Springer Publishing.

CHAPTER 8

The Distinctive Nature and Scope of Rural Nursing Practice: Philosophical Bases

Jane Ellis Scharff

DISCUSSION QUESTIONS

- Describe from your perspective what it means to "be a rural nurse." Compare and contrast your meaning of being rural with your colleagues' meaning of being an urban nurse. How are they similar? How are they different?
- Design a project to explore rural nursing. How does rural nursing today compare with rural nursing described by Scharff?

Plenty and little have changed in 10 years. Rural nursing practice seemed a dichotomous set of the routine and the extraordinary to me back then, as it does now. I was an insider, if not an old-timer, and my findings, although remarkable to some, seemed simply confirmatory to me. Already a budding pragmatist and not yet fully a scientist, I thought, at the time, it was enough to have empiric validation for the practice that I had known and in which my former workplace colleagues continued. For that reason and so many others, I did not publish the findings of my master's thesis in 1987. Subsequently, I have been cited frequently, misrepresented occasionally, and poached a time or two when it comes to references about the world of rural nursing. It is time to uphold my responsibility to nursing science and to set the record straight. The nature and scope of rural nursing is distinctive. I am now willing to be quoted on that. Furthermore, rural nursing can now be given a definition based on that distinctiveness.

Rural nursing practice, be it hospital practice, private practice, or community health practice, is distinctive in its nature and scope from the practice of nursing in urban settings. It is distinctive in its boundaries, intersections, dimensions, and even in its core. Ten years ago, I was loath to claim distinctiveness within rural nursing's core. It seemed too bold to proclaim that at the very level of essence, and not attributable to setting alone, rural nursing could be so different. Today, I am determined to claim it: The core of all nursing is care, and care is the substance of the relationship between nurse and patient; consequently, what happens at the core of rural nursing is something apart from what happens at the core of nursing anywhere else.

I am still a pragmatist; my job is to get readers as close to the experience as I can. Thankfully, my growth as a scientist makes the job easier than it was some years back. Although no longer in the practice, I understand rural nursing better today than I did then. The importance of rural nursing has not decreased as my worldview has expanded. On the contrary, the more I dissect and reconstruct my thoughts about life and truth and nursing science, the more clearly I see the beauty emanating from the nature and scope of rural nursing, and the more clearly I appreciate its relevance to all of nursing science.

From an ontological viewpoint, I will share some information about what it means to "be" a rural nurse, and from an epistemological viewpoint, I will express a little of what it means to "know" rural nursing practice. What came as primary expression to me, because I lived it, breathed it, and studied it, is secondary expression as I write it; I will do my best to translate the experience through common language. However, the story I tell will require imagination to transcend time and space and to gain a sense of the reality of rural nursing practice. The information for this chapter comes from my ethnographic study of rural hospital nurses in the Inland Northwest, completed in 1987, from dialogue with key informants before then and up until today, and from my personal experiences within rural healthcare systems over the past 20 years.

In the past 10 or 15 years, I have made some presentations about portions of this work to nurse clinicians, nurse researchers, and nonnurse healthcare audiences. Inevitably, following such presentations, I was approached by one or two individuals who had been rural nurses who wanted to tell me that the presentation struck a chord. I understood their need, which stemmed from the human desire to be recognized and understood. It stems from the frequent, albeit unintended, distortion of truth about rural nursing communicated by those who do not fully understand what it means to walk a mile in a rural nurse's duty shoes. I may not be able to change that, but I offer my perspective nonetheless.

CONCEPTUALIZING RURAL NURSING PRACTICE

Being Rural

There was a wonderful line in the 1984 science fiction film *The Adventures of Buckaroo Banzai: Across the Eighth Dimension* (Rausch, 1984). The line was delivered by the main character, Buckaroo, a multiskilled neurosurgeon, particle physicist, rock musician, and Zen warrior who, in the midst of chaos matter-of-factly declared, "No matter where you go, there you are." If this sounds simple, I would caution that it is hardly simple. Buckaroo was talking about being in the moment, so imagine for a moment what it means to have "gone rural." What of rural nursing identity? While the imagery may seem silly or surreal, the truth is real, authentic, important, credible, respectable, and as serious as any nursing practice anywhere. However, as indicated earlier, rural nursing practice is also distinctive from nursing anywhere else. Although I use the analogy of Buckaroo Banzai, hoping it will bring a smile, rural nurses will recognize the script of playing a cool and noble professional, simultaneously enacting multiple roles, and managing the continual transition from one part to another with the frankness of Buckaroo.

Being rural means being a long way from anywhere and pretty close to nowhere. Being rural means being independent or perhaps just being alone. Being a rural nurse means that when a nurse saves a life, everyone in town recognizes that she or he was there; and when a nurse loses a life, everyone in town recognizes that she or he was there. Being rural means turning inward for answers, because there may be nobody to turn to outward. Being rural means that when a nurse walks into the emergency department (ED), it may be her or his spouse or child who needs a nurse, and at that moment, being a nurse takes priority over being anyone else. Being a rural nurse means being able to deal with what she or he has got, where she or he is, and being able to live with the consequences.

Knowing Rural

Certainly, every reader has heard that a little knowledge can be a dangerous thing. The adage was probably modified from what Alexander Pope (1711, as cited in Evans, 1978) said in the 17th century: "A little learning is a dangerous thing." I dispute it now and say that a little knowledge can be a lifesaving thing. The demarcation between danger and safety is the difference between having knowledge and *using* knowledge. From time to time, I have had conversations with academic colleagues about dangerous nurses. In these conversations, we have agreed that dangerous nurses are not those who know they do not know what they are doing—although there is certainly an element of danger in that scenario, which ultimately must be addressed. The greater danger, however, emerges with those nurses who think they do know, but actually do not know, what they are doing. Although I have no statistics on the prevalence of such nurses, it is my belief that they hide more easily in urban settings than they do in rural settings.

Knowing rural means knowing that what one knows may be all one has. Knowing rural means personally knowing everyone with whom one works and having knowledge about nearly everyone for whom one cares. As a rural nurse, knowing means sharing knowledge in an informal yet crucially important exchange with other professionals, where the addition of one mind can mean expanding the knowledge base by 100%. Although *whom* one knows can be important in any setting, the distinction between rural and urban dynamics of whom one knows is that in the urban setting whom one knows is more likely to be related to competitive advantage, whereas in the rural setting whom one knows is more likely to be related to cooperative advantage. Knowing rural means that knowledge can mean the difference between perishing, surviving, and thriving, and therefore knowing is inextricably connected to *being* when one is rural.

THE NATURE AND SCOPE OF NURSING

For practicality, a framework for the study of the nature and scope of rural nursing practice was sought to identify and describe the distinctive characteristics of practice in rural settings. The American Nurses Association (ANA) Social Policy Statement (1980) provided the framework for a logical sequence of investigation into details of rural nursing practice. The policy statement includes an organized and systematic approach to studying nursing nature and scope.

- *Nursing's Nature.* Within the policy statement, the nature of nursing is characterized as a relationship between the nursing profession and the society that is mutually beneficial, and nursing itself is deemed an essential outgrowth of the society that it serves. Nursing is described as existing in response to society's needs. From that standpoint, my study of rural nursing was based on assumptions that rural nursing emerges from and is essential to rural society, and distinctions of rural nursing are due, in part, to distinctive interests and needs of rural society.
- *Nursing's Scope.* The scope of nursing includes four definitive characteristics: intersections, dimensions, core, and boundary (ANA, 1980). These four characteristics became conceptual foundation blocks for my study of rural nursing.
  - *Intersections.* Nursing intersects with other professions involved in healthcare. These intersections are points at which nursing meets and interfaces with other professions and expands its practice into the domain of other professions as necessary.
  - *Dimensions.* Characteristics such as philosophy, ethics, roles, responsibilities, skills, and authority are examples of nursing dimensions. These are qualities that add depth to nursing practice. They are characteristics underscored and influenced by interpersonal relationships and intimacy as well as the intrapersonal quality of nursing.
  - *Core.* The concept of the core of nursing is complex and somewhat more difficult to discuss than are the other concepts. It is oversimplification to say that the needs of people are the core of nursing, although such is true. Nursing exists to deal with human response to health issues, and

human response can be equated to human need with respect to health. The patients' *needs* and their responses are outgrowths of who they are as human *beings*. The nursing care we provide is an outgrowth of who we are as human *beings*. The core of nursing is the dynamic of nursing care juxtaposed with human response.

- *Boundaries.* Nursing's boundaries change and expand in direct reflection of the intersections, dimensions, and core of practice. Boundaries are nebulous, unseen, intangible lines of demarcation between what is clearly within the nature and scope of nursing and what is questionably within nursing's scope. Unlike physical boundaries, nursing's boundaries are metaphysical, are relationally and contextually based, and sometimes have origins outside the control of nursing.

METHODS

In an effort to describe the nature and scope of rural nursing, it was determined that an ethnographic method, using participant observation and interviewing techniques, would yield the most pertinent data for analysis. Data were gathered throughout several stages of conceptualization concerning rural nursing phenomena. Field notations, printed news media, and taped interviews were employed. The study of rural hospital nurses included an exploratory phase in which eight rural nurses from northwest Montana were interviewed. These interviews were audiotaped, and from initial open-ended questions, a more refined interview guide was developed that contained both closed and open-ended questions. Twenty-six rural hospital nurses in one of four rural towns in eastern Washington, northern Idaho, or western Montana were interviewed. All interviews were audiotaped and then transcribed verbatim. The findings reported in this chapter are related to many aspects of rural nursing practice and are based on the responses of all 34 rural nurses, as well as several other key rural informants and my own observations. All samples were convenience, and all informants elected to be included in the studies.

FINDINGS

Informant Demographics

All of the informants were women ranging in age from 25 to 61 years with an average age of 40 years. The number of years actively employed as a RN was 3 to 35 years. The mean number of years spent working in rural hospitals was 8 years and, for most informants, was roughly half the total of their active nursing years. Most informants were originally diploma-prepared, seven were baccalaureate graduates, and four were associate graduates. Two inform-ants had achieved a master's degree in nursing. Although informants were not asked about marital or parental status, nearly all said during the interview that they were married and were parents.

Most of the informants worked full time, and those who worked part time averaged 23 hr/wk. In addition, many were placed "on call" if they were not working. On-call status could be attributed to low census, high census, operat-ing room call, cardiac care call, or emergency department call. Most informants reported 1 or 2 days of overtime per month. In almost every case, informants indicated a need to be flexible about their working schedules with regard to the events of the rural practice setting. Turnover rates were low at all facilities, and the most senior nurses had been on staff from 16 to 25 years.

Hospital Demographics

Information about the hospitals was obtained through interviews with nursing, fiscal, administrative, or other personnel, as well as from public records and the participant observation process. The hospital organizations were between 20 and 60 years in existence, the present structures were between 3 and 35 years old, and all had undergone some renovation over time. Ownership of the hos-pitals was stated as nonproprietary, public district, or community. Each hos-pital was governed by a board of directors of three to 10 individuals who held fiduciary and decision-making authorities and to whom the administration was accountable. Board membership was either self-perpetuating or community elected. One facility was accredited by what was then the Joint Commission on Accreditation of Healthcare Organizations (JCAHO). Administrative personnel said that there was little to be gained by small rural hospitals having JCAHO accreditation, especially in light of what the JCAHO charged for the process.

The hospitals had licensure ranging from 20 to 44 acute care beds, zero to three intensive or cardiac beds, five to seven newborn bassinets, and three to five swing beds for extended care. In every case, occupancy was at a fraction of licensure, and occupancy figures averaged to be about 20% to 40% for acute care beds. There was some variability in the use of the other services at each facility. Two had fairly active use of the cardiac or intensive care beds. Two had fairly active obstetrical departments. Three had active surgical departments. Emergency cases at these hospitals ranged from three to 13 per 24-hour day during the previous fiscal year. One relied on the constant occupancy of swing beds to maintain financial solvency. The number of physicians on medical staff ranged from three to 17. Typically, physicians who held admitting privilege at a given facility did not necessarily live within the community. Undoubtedly, the variety of medical practitioners on staff impacted the occupancy of each facility. Usually, nurses were expected to be able to float from medical–surgical areas to emergency, obstetrical, and intensive care areas, but not to the operating room, which seemed to be the one sacrosanct specialty area.

The Rural Communities

At the time of the study, I spent several weeks traveling to and about four separate communities in western Montana, northern Idaho, and eastern Washington to gather information regarding the nature and scope of rural nursing. Each of these towns fits the operational definition of being geographically isolated and of having less than 5,000 residents. Upon arrival in each community, time was taken to drive about, observe the local terrain, look for indicators of economy, walk around town to observe the pace and lifestyle, note the casual conversations taking place in public areas, and read each community's local weekly newspaper.

There were many similarities and few differences between the communities in terms of how they appeared to the outsider. Each town was located near railroad tracks, all of which were currently used. Three of the towns were on a river in forested mountain terrain and were logging or lumber mill towns. The fourth town was on an expansive plain and was an agricultural community. Each town was inhabited mostly by White residents, and each was laid out in typical western fashion with one main street and several auxiliary streets at which the center of the business district was found. Each town boasted the typical hardware stores, grocery stores, restaurants, farm or logging machinery shops, tool shops, post office, drug store, employment office, beauty shops, ice-cream stands, feed stores, junk shops, small motels, bars, and churches. Each town had a well-kept appearance, although each had a few empty buildings or storefronts in the business district.

Residents in these communities were friendly and helpful. They recognized me as an outsider, and, although willing to answer my questions, were curious and wanted to know the purpose of my presence in their town. When I explained myself, the residents registered sincere interest and pleasure that their community had been targeted for this study. They acted like they felt privileged and eagerly conveyed their high regard for nurses in general and *their* nurses specifically. Never did these residents express animosity toward the community of nurses. Most of them had a story to tell about how a friend or relative's life was saved at the local hospital.

Rural Hospital Nurses

The rural nurses I observed and interviewed were a dynamic group of women who could certainly be called "expert generalists." They moved quickly, and for the most part easily, from one role to another as circumstances required. They explained that most rural nurses have a great deal of knowledge regarding a variety of nursing practice areas. When beginning work in a rural hospital, many nurses suffer reality shock due to the variety of demands placed on them. One seasoned nurse told me, "Although you might start out and you don't have that wide knowledge, you better get it quickly." A relative newcomer nurse expressed admiration about the knowledge level of her rural colleagues, calling them "impressive." The nurses I interviewed routinely worked in three or four different specialty areas of nursing practice every week, and sometimes every day. When talking with one respondent about this phenomenon and how easy certain nurses made it look, she said, "The ones who are experienced in rural nursing seem to be very comfortable in switching back and forth between specialties."

Nursing Staff Tenure and Group Acceptance

At all facilities, nurses were heard to use the terms "new" or "newcomer" and "old" or "old-timer" in reference to a given nurse's tenure on the staff. There was no particular time limit identified when a nurse makes the transition from new to old, nor how one arrives at a level of acceptance. However, tenure of less than 2 years was apparently definitely considered "new," and tenure of 3 to 5 years in combination with competence generally constituted acceptance. Tenure beyond 10 years was considered "seasoned," and in special cases of achieving high proficiency or social acceptance, one of these nurses might be called an "old-timer," but usually this term was reserved for someone who had been around for 20 or more years. What I discerned was some gray area depending on a nurse's tenure, level of proficiency, and sociability related to group fit. It seemed that a nurse who was very skillful, flexible, and likeable might reach old-timer status sooner than a nurse who was lacking one of those characteristics.

Although I cannot pinpoint a "typical" rural nurse, certain characteristics were confirmed as traits of distinctive advantage for a rural nurse's success. For example, good common sense, good judgment ability, the ability to set priorities, good physical assessment skills, and physical and emotional strengths were considered of survival significance to these nurses, due, in part, to the aloneness of their practices. They made comments such as, "You have to make all your own decisions. There's no one to do that for you." "You have to be able to be autonomous." "You can't go to somebody for concurrence with decision making." "At any time during your shift, your assignment may change drastically." "You can make the difference between life or death—the judgment calls are yours." All informants were adamant that the prevalent feeling of aloneness and serious responsibility were distinctive to the rural setting. None would concede that the feeling was anything like that experienced in an urban setting. These nurses expressed a very real and pervasive sense of responsibility that rural nurses bear for their patients. The nurses who do not have the ability consistently to carry the burden of such decisional responsibility are the ones who do not survive as rural nurses. Old-timers claimed they could often tell right away, or within a few weeks, if a newcomer was going to catch on or not. Old-timers based such predictions on their assessments of a newcomer's characteristics as mentioned earlier, combined with evidence of adaptation to the new environment.

Education and Professional Development

The burden for self-responsibility of education is greater in the rural setting than in the urban setting, and most rural nurses accept this burden. There is a wide variety of sources from which rural nurses receive their continuing education, such as out-of-town workshops or conferences, in-service education, journals, textbooks, practice sessions, physicians, and other nurses. The greatest educational needs voiced were in cardiac, trauma, maternal/child, and complex medical nursing.

Informants indicated a thirst for knowledge in accredited professional continuing education. Several respondents reported attending more than 10 continuing education events in a year. Most attended between three and 10 events annually. These events were developed and held locally, developed elsewhere but held locally, or developed and held in urban settings. Although expenses were a factor, they were not the central factor in respondents' attending continuing education events.

Nearly all informants also relied on journals for new information, read journals regularly, and reported the most popular journals to be *Nursing, American Journal of Nursing, RN, Journal of Nursing Administration*, and *Nursing Management*, in that order. Current journals were visible in each facility, and notations were seen hanging on bulletin boards in nursing report rooms or locker rooms with a suggestion from one nurse to others that everyone review a given recent journal article germane to a given current case.

Rural nurses, in fact, identify one another as their most important single source of information and education. This was often explained as information being imparted from a peer when it was needed most, so that learning occurred while doing, which tended to heighten the memory. Comments that supported these phenomena included, "We try to share everything we can with each other." "New nurses sometimes come in with great new information or real current ideas. It helps a lot." "Sometimes the new girls expect you to know things, and I don't, and it can be embarrassing. So, we look it up together." "When you've been around for a while, you develop camaraderie. We know what we can expect from each other."

Out-of-town workshops were identified as the next most important source of continuing education to rural nurses. Informants qualified this by stressing that the topic or presentation needed to be relevant to the rural environment. One informant said, "It's got to be meaningful. You know, you go up to the city and they tell you how to do something, and they don't realize how different the setup is."

Interpersonal Relationships and Nursing Practice

Rural nurses know everyone who works at the hospital, all of the physicians, and most of their patients. Rural nurses say that the interpersonal closeness of knowing everyone with whom they work and for whom they care generally has a positive influence on their practice. The intensity of this interpersonal dynamic is unique to the rural setting. Although it is likely that nurses in any setting develop close relationships, rural nurses are in the distinctive situation of being personally acquainted with all of those around them, so that the depth of interaction is potentially greater, and the accountability for interpersonal exchange is a constant that is simply not present in other settings. An informant explained the bond she felt with coworkers by saying, "It's nice to know the people you're working with. You work more together, you try harder, and you work closer." Another nurse shared that among many rewarding qualities of rural nursing, "The cooperation of the other nurses and the cohesiveness of the group is probably the biggest."

An old-timer at one hospital said, "I don't have to explain when I say something. They believe me, and they do it without wasting time." It was easy to verify this through observation. Certain old-timers could communicate a virtual reassignment of responsibilities through the tone of their voices as they disappeared momentarily to deal with a risen crisis, such as the admission of trauma victims in the ED. On occasions, it was like watching a dance, the motions of which were so well understood, each dancer so valued and respected, that without missing a step, workers would change places based on available expertise and would back each other up without visible cues. Even physicians were seen deferring to old-timer nurses at such times. Yet, the choreography depended heavily on the direction of the one in charge; and on other occasions, with an inexperienced newcomer directing, the dance was frantic and the flow chaotic.

Practicing Medicine

Rural nurses are understandably reluctant to admit that they practice medicine, but they know their boundaries are sometimes stretched by circumstance. "You take it upon yourself and do what has to be done to make sure the patient's stable before you can call the doctor," said one nurse to me. When patient crises occur, calling the physician is considered important, but it simply does not rank at the top of the list. The nurses I interviewed and watched used a standard A-B-C (airway, breathing, circulation) order of setting priorities to respond to patient needs. Thus, they often began written or unwritten medical protocols while the aide would be sent to summon the physician. Physician response times varied from 5 to 30 minutes at the rural hospitals, resulting in nurses being responsible for considerable decision making during the time lapse. At each site, I heard or saw variations on the themes of nurses stabilizing cardiac or trauma victims and nurses managing precipitous births without the benefit of physicians present. In interviews, nurses were adamant that they had a responsibility to the patients to do whatever was required during an emergency, and although it sometimes felt uncomfortable, inaction would have constituted neglect.

The words of one nurse summarize the collective opinion, "We do it because we have to, because it would be wrong if we didn't."

There were also circumstances of newcomer physicians relying on seasoned nurses for insight into or even direction regarding a given patient case. Per physician request, the nurse would literally advise what medications and treatments to order in cases where the doctor did not have the familiarity with a patient's history that the nurse did. This was especially true in after-hours situations of physicians covering for another's patients. My assessment of these circumstances is that each party acted within unseen lines of mutual trust and understanding with the dynamic of trust specific to a given relationship.

Another observation I made at these facilities, which struck me then and which I have informally reconfirmed on multiple occasions since, is that rural physicians seem more likely to read and respond to nurses' notes about patients than do urban physicians. Doubtless there is great individual variability, yet it is tempting to hypothesize that rural professionals have a better grasp than do their urban counterparts of pertinent information that is necessary to communicate to the healthcare team. Certainly, further study would be required to confirm the probability.

Rural Expertise: Aces and Pinch Hitters

Rural nurses generally believe that no one can be an expert in every area of rural nursing practice. However, a few nurses are extremely proficient in all clinical areas, and these nurses become role models and mentors to the other nurses with whom they work. At two study sites, many informants identified a colleague or two who fit this category. Interestingly, those who were identified by others as "aces" did not identify themselves as such. Each nurse was very modest about her own capability, but the pride toward aces among the staff was obvious. I was aware that talking to or watching these aces in action was as much an honor for the locals as it was for me as an investigating outsider.

All rural nurses interviewed agreed that they must be competent in more than one clinical area to be considered an acceptable staff member. The top four clinical areas deemed to be most important for competency were emergency nursing, obstetrical nursing, intensive or coronary nursing, and medical–surgical nursing. A supervisory nurse told me, "There's a difference between competent and expert. I think everybody who works in this hospital should be able to walk into any specialty area and function." But there was an expectation held by all informants that they be clinically strong, if not expert, in at least two of the above-named areas and be able to float to any other department and still function well in a pinch.

With regard to functioning in a pinch, in the early 1980s two rural Montana nurse executives who are admitted baseball fans coined the Pinch Hitter Theory of Rural Nursing. One of those persons, Jean Shreffler, now an academic, is author of other chapters in this book. The second person, Maura Fields, was then and remains today the nurse executive at a rural hospital in Montana and is arguably one of the most innovative and masterful nurse leaders I have ever had the good fortune to know. Her rendition of the theory went like this:

> In rural nursing, you have to be like a pinch hitter. You may not perform a task or procedure or work on a very specialized case but once a year. But when you go to do it, you have to do it like you do it every day. In baseball, a batting average of 300 is good. But the pinch hitter, well, you want them to be better than that, really, you want them to bat a thousand. That's what it's like for a rural nurse, when they go to work, you want them to bat a thousand. (Maura Fields, 1983, personal conversation)

For those readers who are doubting that there can be that many instances in which the aforementioned theory becomes important, rest assured that it happens all the time. Industrial and recreational traumas are frequent in these communities. Rural citizens experience their share of severe burns, drug overdoses, cardiac arrests, head injuries, freak accidents, and critical illness. Although transfer to larger medical centers is sometimes preferred, stabilization is necessary first, and transfer is sometimes not possible. One hospital in this study is 90 road miles from the nearest medical center of any size and 150 road miles from a trauma center. Rotary blade or fixed wing aircraft are often used to transport cases that require more care than can be delivered locally, but northwest mountain weather conditions can be a significant factor in keeping aircraft grounded.

Although rural nurses do not expect an easy routine, frustration is common surrounding the conflict of trying to achieve expertise in such a complex practice. Boredom is rare as they face the constant variety of demands. One informant related the example of the prior day's evening shift. The informant was one of two RNs on duty at the time, assisted by one aide. The scenario she described began after change of shift report and went like this:

> Just yesterday evening there were seven patients in the house with nothing going on. Within an hour, there was one admitted with a depression state, an OB came in, and there were four or five cases in the ER, one being a child with rectal bleeding, which makes you wonder about child abuse.

Although two nurses and an aide would have no difficulty caring for seven stable medical–surgical patients, the admission of the depressed patient was a wrench in the works. Mental health diagnoses are among those for which rural nurses feel least appropriately prepared, and they lack confidence in rural physicians' ability to treat mental health patients appropriately, as well. The depressed patient required suicide precautions for a period of time, which meant that the aide was assigned to remain with the patient at all times. The pediatric patient in the ED required careful documentation, delicate interaction, and a social services consultation. The obstetrical patient admission required nurse assessment and individual care until it was determined that the patient was in early labor. One nurse moved back and forth between the ED and the general care unit; the other moved back and forth between the labor room, the depressed patient, and the general care unit.

Here is an account from another informant about another evening shift where three RNs were on duty but without assistance from an aide:

> Not long ago we had an OB with a bad baby, small for gestational age; and at the same time, we got two ambulances 5 minutes apart, and they were both cardiacs with chest pain. While that was happening, there was surgery going on, and there was somebody in the unit. I don't know if God is watching you or what, but, for the most part, things seem to come out okay in the end.

In this case, one nurse was already assigned to the intensive care unit, and one was required to remain with the obstetrical patient to do monitoring and other procedures. When the first ambulance arrived, the third nurse was dispatched to the ED. Fortunately, some ambulance crew members were emergency medical technicians and could help with continued patient monitoring and calling in the physician, laboratory, and respiratory personnel. Also, fortunately, the physician arrived within 10 minutes and was designated to care for both patients. The final good fortune is that nothing went wrong on the general care unit while hell was breaking loose elsewhere.

Knowing Patients Personally

Most rural nurses subscribe to the belief that when they know patients personally, they can give better care. The possibility of experiencing fear when caring for family members or best friends notwithstanding, the rewards are considered rich. A gradual loss of anonymity occurs to rural nurses as they become immersed in and assimilated into rural society, making anonymity nonexistent for old-timers. "I can be more supportive emotionally when I know them," one said, and another elaborated, "Let's say in the ER, with chronic lungers, you know them, and they feel secure because they know we remember them." I saw instances of rural nurses informally calling to check on patients after discharge. As far as I know, patients were always glad to have these calls. The loss of anonymity is generally considered reassuring for those professionals who are comfortable with rural life, but it can be constricting as well. It should not be assumed, however, that negative aspects of anonymity loss are necessarily related to poor patient outcomes. On the contrary, one informant told me,

> I know of several situations where knowing my OB patients who had poor outcomes made a difference to them, where I was really able to help them

get through the experience. It's a real emotional drain, but you're ahead of the game because the trust is there.

The argument could be made that patients perceive their care to be better based on the close personal contact that is often made in the rural setting. A nurse who believes that her relationship to a patient made a difference in the patient's outcome said,

> I recovered my little neighbor girl after her surgery. Most little kids are scared when they wake up, but when she woke up she knew me and wasn't afraid and recovered really fast. Because fear generates pain, but she wasn't afraid, she recovered faster than usual.

It is a cultural expectation of many rural people to be taken care of by someone they know. This differs from the expectation in urban settings. For the most part, informants agreed that rural people do expect to have their medical needs met, even though they live far from a major medical center. However, one informant said that rural patients often wait until they are "half dead" before they seek intervention and are "grateful for what they get." Another nurse said, "People have told me they were glad I was on when they were here, that if I said it was going to be okay, then it was going to be okay."

Nearly all rural nurses could confirm that sometimes they had patients from out of town who had previously experienced urban hospital admissions. These patients, whether vacationing in the rural setting or passing through the rural area, ended up in rural hospitals for reasons not important to this story. Their comments about the care they received in rural hospitals are important. The nurses were told by these patients that the care was of better quality, that they felt more cared for, that the rural nurses took more time to listen, that care was accomplished more quickly and smoothly, and that they felt more like people and less like numbers in the rural hospital than they did in any urban hospital. The outsider patients often expressed surprise at the high level of competence they encountered in the rural setting.

DISCUSSION

Rural Nursing's Distinctive Nature and Scope

Analyses of the reports of rural nurses show that the nature and scope of rural nursing are clearly distinctive. Using a framework to focus the discussion, the distinctions can apparently be categorized as those pertaining to rural nursing's nature, as well as the four components of rural nursing's scope, those being intersections, dimensions, core, and boundary.

THE NATURE OF RURAL NURSING

Most rural nurses have difficulty in defining their practice, although they can describe it. Their descriptions are a variety of rich, thoughtful, colorful, and articulate responses. Rural nursing is generalist nursing, not to be mistaken for mundane, and includes an intensity of purpose that makes it distinctive. Rural nurses may feel misunderstood and poorly recognized by the larger nursing community, but they are nonetheless a proud lot.

THE SCOPE OF RURAL NURSING

The intersections of rural nursing are distinctively marked and fluid. Rural nurses consistently and necessarily practice well within the realm of other healthcare disciplines, the most notable being respiratory therapy, pharmacy, and medicine. The intersection between nursing and medicine has the most extensive implications. It is a gray area that hinges on circumstances and relationships, and the most complex intersections occur during emergent situations, "until the doctor gets there." Some rural nurses embrace this intersection more willingly than others, but none do it casually. Reflective concern is apparent in comments related to this intersection. One informant said, "It means putting your neck out there on the line, but you have to make the judgment and go on." Another told me, "It sometimes feels uncomfortable, but it's part of my responsibility to the patient."

It is evident that the practice of rural nursing is dimensionally distinctive. Rural nurses embrace an ethic of openness and honesty that is pervasive. The dimension of interpersonal knowing is viewed as a positive feature of rural practice, and it exists between nurses and patients as well as among coworkers. A nurse administrator shared with me that, "in terms of practice outcomes, your accountability is right in front of your face." Rural nurses talked about being able to accomplish goals more quickly with their patients and said that guidance, teaching, and counseling behaviors are automatic to their practice in the rural environment. Communication patterns in the rural setting are more direct and suffer less obfuscation than do those in urban settings. There are fewer barriers to go through when imparting messages from one to another. As a result, there are probably fewer errors of omission and commission related to practice in the rural setting than there are in the urban setting. Confronting and managing conflict is more common in the rural setting, avoidance being an unacceptable dynamic for group cohesiveness that stems from mutual concern and regard for one another. Independent decision making is given in rural practice, but rural nurses are aware of their limitations. One said, "You have to know when you don't know, and you have to know where to go to find out." Rural nurses are mindful, if not fully informed, about the legal dimensions of their practice. However, with respect to questions of patient safety and survival, rural nurses sometimes decide that their ethical obligation to do what is right for their patients carries more weight than their legal responsibility to uphold the law. These cases generally become lessons of learning, are scrutinized and discussed by the group, and are entered into memory for future reference.

Human responses, which nurses diagnose and treat, are the core of nursing. Some sources have suggested, and informants in this study agreed, that rural dwellers are known to delay health seeking and tend to define health as the ability to get out of bed and go to work. Thinking in terms of nursing diagnosis, one might call this behavior "dysfunctional perceptual orientation to health," which requires distinctive intervention at nursing's core. Rural nurses are faced with determining an appropriate line of demarcation between a rural dweller's rugged individualism and stubborn disregard for health. Inextricable from rural nursing's core are the relational issues of what it means to be rural. As noted earlier in this chapter, from an ontological standpoint, rural nursing is distinctive at its very core.

Boundary being dependent on the intersections, dimensions, and core of nursing, there can be no question as to rural nursing's distinctive boundary. Rural nursing is constantly changing in response to complex intersections and dimensional intricacies distinctive to rural society. The boundary is therefore neither smooth nor even static. When nurses come to a rural setting from an urban setting, they are very aware that the boundary of their practice changes. The transitional period for these nurses is not always easy, and boundary expansion can be accompanied by ambivalence, anxiety, and frustration. Newcomers must become adjusted to the rural culture to function effectively, and not all survive. Rural experts can play a key role in the success of newcomer transition, and those aces who invest themselves in the orientation and mentoring of newcomers know the importance of the payoff.

DEFINING RURAL NURSING

Rural nursing is a special variety of nursing in which the nurse must have a wide range of advanced knowledge and ability, in combination with commitment, to practice proficiently in multiple clinical areas simultaneously along the career trajectory. The practice requires constant and continual personal and professional adaptation in developing identity. A rural nurse has both an ontological sense of being and an epistemological sense of knowing that connect the nurse with the surrounding community, and through which the rural nurse creates a reality of rural professional nursing practice. In no other setting is a nurse's practice so thoroughly and integrally a constant factor in a nurse's life. In a society where separating one's private life from one's professional life is considered obligatory, rural nurses are singularly challenged, stripped of their own anonymity while simultaneously charged with protecting their patients' privacy.

CLOSING THOUGHT

The newcomer practices nursing in a *rural setting*, unlike the old-timer who practices *rural nursing*. Somewhere between these spectral extremes lies the transitional period of events and conditions through which each nurse passes at her or his own pace. It is within this temporal zone that nurses experience rural reality and move toward becoming professionals who understand that having gone rural they are not less than they were, but rather they are more than they expected to be. Some may be conscious of the transition and others may not, but in the end, a few will say, "I am a rural nurse."

REFERENCES

American Nurses Association. (1980). *Nursing: A social policy statement.* Publication No. NP-63 20M 9/82R. Kansas City, MO: Author.

Evans, B. (Ed.). (1978). *Dictionary of quotations.* New York, NY: Avenel Books, Delecorte Press.

Rausch, E. M. (Screenplay Author). (1984). *The adventures of Buckaroo Banzai: Across the eighth dimension* [Film]. Stamford, CT: Vestron Video.

CHAPTER 9

Understanding the Lived Experiences of the Rural Bedside Nurse

Judith M. Paré, Polly Petersen,
and Dayle Boynton Sharp

DISCUSSION QUESTIONS

- The findings from these two qualitative studies have implications for nursing practice in rural areas. Analyzing the themes that emerged from each of the studies, propose strategies that will support a foundation of emergent leadership among rural nurses. What strategies should healthcare administrators implement to support the recruitment and retention of rural nurses?
- How can mobile technology be better utilized in rural settings to enhance options for continuing and advanced education of rural nurses? What are the three potential funding sources that would support the costs of these technologies?
- The concept of a situation or locale specific theory and its relationship to the larger body of nursing knowledge must be seriously considered (Winters, 2013). Reflect on the geographical locality of each of these studies. How did or did not these locations influence the emergent themes?

In 1997, federal legislation was enacted as part of the Balanced Budget Act that authorized states to create a State Flex Program. The State Flex Program allowed certain hospitals located in rural areas to become designated as critical access hospitals (CAHs) to receive cost-based reimbursement from Medicare. CAHs are usually farther than 35 miles from another CAH or larger tertiary care center and have an average daily census of less than 25 patients. Nurses who provide care in these settings are often required to take workload responsibilities with minimal staffing and technology supports. Nurses who work in CAHs are faced with the daily challenges of delivering care to a patient population that ranges in ages encompassing the life span and possess a plethora of acute and chronic healthcare needs.

There are gaps in the literature related to the lived experiences of nurses working in CAHs. Although we know that rural RNs are expected to care for a variety of patients who are also their family and friends in many different special circumstances, it is important to acknowledge the phenomenon of rural nursing practice. This chapter explains the use of a phenomenological approach to examine the lived experience of nurses working in critical access/rural settings.

GAINING INSIGHT THROUGH THE LENS OF PHENONMENOLOGY

Quantitative researchers seek answers to questions through calculable means. Qualitative researchers seek answers to phenomena that often require a deeper understanding of that phenomena. Phenomenology is both a philosophy and a scientific research methodology (Grove, Burns, & Gray, 2013). Phenomenologists embrace that challenge to achieve congruence between empirical facts and principles. To achieve the balance between the scientific process and an understanding of essences, psychologists agree that knowledge acquisition is the ultimate goal.

Phenomenology is an existential philosophy that is grounded in the belief that decision making is not based on knowledge; rather knowledge is an output of decision making (Butts & Rich, 2018). Researchers who seek to understand the meaning of lived experiences often select phenomenology as a theoretical foundation for research that examines the meaning of human experiences. For instance, a psychologist asks why a patient with third-degree burns who rates the pain as a number 8 on a scale of 1 to 10 should be treated differently than another patient with third-degree burns who rates the pain a 4 on the same scale. He or she asks why the constant of pain is viewed as an isolated event. In effect, the psychologist is asking why a qualitative difference exists when the "actual" difference is merely quantitative. This lived experience is ideally understood through the lens of phenomenology.

Paul Colaizzi was an existential phenomenologist who believed that to understand a human experience, researchers must view that experience simultaneous to the individuals who are living that experience (1973). He believed that the initial step in the research process involved the researcher's own examination of preconceived notions and biases related to the human phenomenon that was the focus of the research. The process of questioning these biases about a phenomenon can illuminate new insights, hypotheses, values, and attitudes that provide a foundation for the formulation of research questions and greater support for the human condition (Paré, 2015).

Acquiring this knowledge may be achieved through processes such as observation, imagination, critical reasoning, or problem solving. However, confirming the validity of that knowledge must at some point involve the art and science of experimentation. The validity of the findings, which are summarized in this chapter, was confirmed by the nurses who were participants in the research study.

Phenomenology provides an ideal foundation for nursing research because of its close alignment with nursing and health science theories, which value creativity and the uniqueness of the human condition as well as knowledge of personal meaning articulated through verbal communication (Kim & Kollack, 2005). Phenomenologists support the belief that the essence of a phenomenon resides in the daily experiences of individuals. The events that individuals share are, in fact, the essence of truth. Phenomenology explores the truths of life experiences through a detailed process of reflection and self-discovery (Sokolowski, 2000).

Colaizzi's Seven Procedural Steps

After interviews have been completed, Colaizzi recommends seven standardized steps to complete the analysis of the data. Step I involves reviewing subjects' responses; each response is identified as a "protocol." The review process affords the researcher an opportunity to gain a depth of understanding of the meaning behind the words used by the participants. On completion of the initial review of each subject's protocol, the next step requires a second perusal of the information to begin the process of extracting the impact of the data.

Step II requires a laborious review of each protocol. The goal of this second review is for the researcher to extrapolate significant statements made by participants during the interview process. The significant statements are defined as those statements having influence on the phenomenon being investigated (Paré, 2015). A possible outcome of this process may be the discovery of a replication or recurrence of comments made by participants and, if that occurs, those duplicate statements can be eliminated. During this step in the analysis process, the researcher can analyze quotations that may refer to specific circumstances or emotions and adapt them to a more global interpretation.

Step III requires the researcher to assign a meaning for every substantive statement identified in each protocol. This is a very innovative process that requires a thorough analysis of the data. The outcome of this process is the identification of the true essence and intent of statements made by the participants to questions asked during the initial interview with the researcher.

Step IV includes a process of clustering all the established meanings from those statements that the researcher identified as significant into categories that reflect a trend or theme. Each theme must then be labeled or coded to capture all possible meanings related to that theme. Once that process is finalized, groups of themes must be assimilated to create a new construct of those themes. This step requires that all themes possess internal commonalities and external variances.

Step V requires the identification of all emerging themes into a comprehensive depiction of the phenomenon that is the focus of the study. Once the complete depiction has emerged, the global configuration of the phenomenon becomes evident. At this point in the process, Colaizzi (1973) recommends the researcher collaborate with another phenomenological researcher to review the identified themes and confirm the depth and comprehensiveness of the process.

Step VI involves the analysis and synthesis of a holistic description of the phenomenon of study in a clear and detailed statement of understanding as much as possible. Part of this stage may also involve making edits to clarify clear linkages between groups of themes and their reasoned meanings. An outcome of this process may be the elimination of some elusive constructions that do not add to the foundation of the entire description.

Step VII is the final step in the process. The goal is affirmation of the study findings. This process mandates the researcher to contact the study participants and request a review of their transcript and validation of the thoroughness and accurateness of the responses and information. During this process, the participants can provide additional information or negate any potential errors in the transcription of the data (Paré, 2015).

REVIEW OF THE LITERATURE

The U.S. Census Bureau (Ratcliffe, Burd, Holder, & Fields, 2017) defines "rural" as those areas that encompass all population, housing, and territory not included within an urban area. Urban areas include geographical areas that are highly developed and populated with residential, commercial, and other nonresidential land uses. Nursing in a rural setting poses unique challenges that an urban nurse may not encounter or even be able to imagine. Nurses practice and reside in the same neighborhoods as the patients and yet it may take a nurse 2 to 4 hours to get to work due to precarious road or weather conditions (Bushy, 2003). A typical shift for a rural nurse working in an acute hospital setting may be 8 to 16 hours in length, depending on staffing patterns or emergent patient needs. Rural nurses report knowing how a patient will handle a hospital admission and the type of support he or she will have, if any, posthospitalization. If the patient is lacking a support network, a rural nurse will know what community resources can be alerted to provide essential care. This requires that rural nurses possess a broad knowledge base and a sense of resiliency regardless of the circumstances.

Rural nurses commonly express strong job satisfaction, stressing the realities of professional autonomy, the ability to serve a variety of patients with acute and chronic needs, and the ability to preserve close community ties (Bigbee, Gehrke, & Otterness, 2009). The lack of social boundaries and the related concepts of outsider/insider are valued by rural nurses who preserve their personal roots as rural residents (Long & Weinert, 2013).

Rural nurses must be skilled and ready to manage the care of any patient situation that presents in their practice setting (Paré, Peterson, & Sharp, 2017). They approach their professional responsibility with a general knowledge based primarily in an associate degree education (Newhouse, Morlock, Pronovost, & Breckenridge Sproat, 2011). Rural nurses are motivated by an unwavering desire to make contributions to a patient population that they often know as family, neighbors, and friends. However, lack of daily access to primary and secondary healthcare services such as mental health supports and disease prevention screenings can result in the rural nurse assuming multiple responsibilities they may not be trained or equipped to manage (Bushy, 2014).

Nurses practicing in CAH settings must be able to refocus and redirect their care priorities and skills to adapt to the dynamic nature of a rapidly changing patient population, culture, and acuity (Cramer, Jones, & Hertzog, 2011). Additionally, they may be working with minimal support from other members of the healthcare team who may be meeting the emergent needs of other patients simultaneously. Rural nurses are frequently required to cover various units and patient care departments based on census and acuity. This situation highlights the need for ongoing education and support for nurses supporting an increasingly fragile and robust patient population. Fiscal constraints often influence clinical practice, leading to obstacles for nurses and healthcare providers being able to participate in or sustain mentoring relationships because they simply are not sustainable outside of urban settings; thus there is no one to answer questions or provide clarification. These daily challenges may lead to increased issues of attrition as these nurses relocate to urban settings where they often experience salary increases and enhanced professional supports.

Rural nurses are also confronted with inconsistent physical and technological resources to manage and support positive patient outcomes (Hunsberger, Bauman, Blythe, & Crea, 2009). Expanding numbers of research studies (Estabrooks, Midozi, Cummings, & Wallin, 2007) have identified that lack of access to technology is one of the barriers rural nurses must cope with in order to provide current, evidence-based nursing care. Additionally, budgetary restrictions for advanced and continuing education for nurses and lack of medical libraries or access to improvements in patient care technologies present additional frustrations for rural nurses who struggle to maintain currency in their nursing practice (Koessl, Winters, Lee, & Hendrickx, 2013).

To address the gaps in the literature related to the lived experiences of rural nurses, understanding these phenomena is essential to determine strategies that will support nursing practice and address issues of recruitment and retention in rural and remote healthcare settings. The knowledge, attributes, and skills of rural and critical access nurses must be directed at making remote and rural healthcare a place where nurses not only desire employment but also chose to continue to work (Hegney, 2002).

THE LIVED EXPERIENCES OF RURAL NURSES

A New England View

The New England region has 40 acute care facilities that hold designations as CAHs. The requirements include the provision for 24-hour care, 7-day-a-week emergency care services for individuals across the life span who are experiencing varying types of physical and mental healthcare needs (Paré, 2015). Although most patients who seek care in these facilities are local residents, many of these facilities also serve a large percentage of travelers and vacationing tourists who experience injuries and traumas. The variety of patients and their acute and chronic care needs require that nurses possess a mastery of skills that can be as varied as the weather in New England.

SAMPLING METHOD

The sampling method that was chosen for the New England study was a convenience sample. The sample methodology allowed the researcher the ability to travel to the site for two initial recruitment meetings, data collection, and verification of participants' protocols. The RNs employed at the hospital were informed via a written flyer of the days and times for the information sessions. Information sessions were purposefully scheduled so that both weekday and weekend staff would have the same opportunity to attend and participate in the study. Copies of the Informed Consent document were distributed during the recruitment sessions and a portion of the presentation was dedicated as an open forum that allowed the participants opportunities to ask questions regarding the purpose, time commitment, and other study-related concerns. Four full-time RNs (Figure 9.1) agreed to participate in the study and each participant self-selected the day and time for his or her initial 20- to 30-minute interview.

DATA COLLECTION AND SURVEY QUESTIONS

The interview sessions and data collection were completed away from the clinical units in a private conference room. The nurses who agreed to participate in the study were apprised that the interviews would be audiotape recorded and then transcribed using Dragon NaturallySpeaking 13. During these initial interviews, the participants were asked to respond to the questions that appear in Box 9.1.

The second interviews were scheduled within 2 to 4 weeks of the initial interviews. During this time, the participants were provided with written copies of transcripts from their initial interviews and asked to validate the text and meaning of their responses. Two of the respondents asked to elaborate on the statements they had previously made and the other two participants confirmed the accuracy of the information.

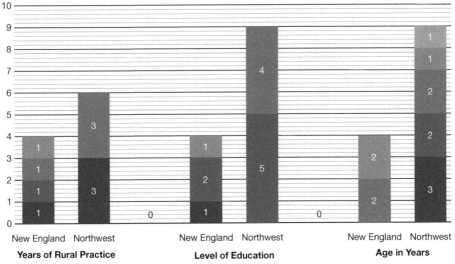

FIGURE 9.1. Demographics of participants.

BOX 9.1 Participant Questionnaire

- How many years of nursing experience do you have as a registered nurse?
- Can you describe the various settings in which you have worked other than your current position?
- What is your current position?
- How many hours per week do you work?
- What is it like to work in a critical access hospital?
- Tell me about your nursing practice. Using Benner's (1984) model of novice to expert, how often do you feel good about your experiences at work? Please explain.

FINDINGS

Themes were extrapolated using bracketing analysis. The process involved listing patterns of experiences from the transcribed protocols on index cards, identifying information that related to classified patterns, and tagging these patterns into trends (Paré, 2015). Coding and bracket analysis illuminated four essential themes:

- Responsibility
- Mentorship
- Isolation
- Spirituality

RESPONSIBILITY

Nurses related their thoughts of extreme responsibility for patients, family members, and colleagues while providing acute and chronic care to persons recovering from trauma, systemic disease, pregnancy, and end-of-life or palliative care. Nurses' protocols included:

> The persons who seek care in our hospital are friends, neighbors, colleagues, and sometimes, even our relatives. They are vital members of our town. It really takes a village to provide the best nursing care, and that is who we are. (Paré, 2015, p. 4)

MENTORSHIP

Nurses stressed the value of mentoring, despite the absence of an approved mentoring/preceptor program. Two nurses recalled events where they benefited by the mentoring of experienced nurses. Another nurse reported her satisfaction at being a mentor to a newly graduated nurse.

> I am one of the more senior members of the nursing staff and I consider myself an expert in several patient care specialties. I feel it is my responsibility to share what I have learned with younger nurses. I benefit as much as a novice nurse does when I can share my experiences. (Paré, 2015, p. 4)

ISOLATION

Nurses expressed feelings of isolation from both local and distant colleagues in the nursing community.

> I am very happy with my professional peer group, but there are times that I struggle to connect with them, especially in the bad weather. It simply isn't possible to attend a seminar or meeting of a professional organization if the roads are closed or if the hospital isn't adequately staffed. These are realities we deal with often but our peers who work in larger medical settings never experience.

SPIRITUALITY

Although the concept of spirituality was uniquely defined by each nurse participant, all nurses emphasized the importance of spirituality in their personal and professional lives. The nurses described how they draw on their own spiritual strength even during the most traumatic clinical situation. "At the end of each shift, I meditate on the care that I have provided to each patient and reflect upon how I can improve my practice." (Paré, 2015, p. 5)

Rural Nurses in the Northwest

In order to gain a deeper understanding of the lived experiences of rural nurses and the universality of that experience, a follow-up research study was conducted by the same researcher in the northwestern region of the United States. Recruitment efforts were conducted by posting flyers that highlighted the dates and times that researcher would be available to conduct interviews.

Nine full-time RNs (Figure 9.1) participated in the follow-up study. Interviews were conducted in person and audiotaped (Box 9.1). The transcribed protocols from these interviews were returned to the participants via an encrypted email server within 1 week. Participants were given the option to confirm the accuracy of their protocol via email, telephone, or Skype technology. These options were necessary due to the geographic distance between the researcher and the participants. Following the confirmation of the protocols, coding and clustering of information was completed and five central themes emerged. The only theme that emerged consistently in both studies was isolation. All other themes were distinctly different:

- Isolation
- Emergent leadership
- Self-reliance
- Social responsibility
- Empathy

ISOLATION

Rural nurses can experience isolation in a variety of ways. Isolation can be geographical, such as living in an area that is a great distance from family, friends, and services. Isolation can be professional, where the nurse is unable to contact other members of the healthcare community for consultation or support. Isolation can affect professional growth; nurses can experience limited access to continuing education opportunities.

> There are some, not a lot of opportunities to go to conferences. I want to get my CEN [emergency nursing certification] but [this year] there are no certification classes in Montana . . . to do that. Last year we had two and I scheduled myself to attend and we got snowed in and they shut the freeway down so I never made it. (Paré, 2015, p. 114)

Another form of isolation mentioned was the staffing levels that do not allow a nurse to actually leave the unit to participate in educational offerings at the CAH. They did not have the opportunity to view this offering within the unit or perhaps even access it at a convenient time.

It would be nice for the hospital, for example, to bring in a group of nurses to cover a floor so that a group of nurses could attend a conference and know that the floor and patient care needs were covered.

When the number of nurses is limited, the idea of exclusion from social and professional development situations only further contributes to a sense of isolation. One nurse mentioned that many times, if the Internet was compromised, there was no one to contact in the middle of the night; there was no IT support.

EMERGENT LEADERSHIP

The setting for this study had recently employed a new chief nursing officer (CNO). Although the nurses were accepting of changes that affected the quality of patient care, changes in leadership may have influenced the emergence of these themes. The staff educator spoke about the nurses trusting their new nursing administrator. She discussed nursing morale. She stated morale is better than it was since the change in nursing leadership and that there had been morale improvement throughout the facility since that leadership change.

SELF-RELIANCE

"Self-reliance" is defined as having the capacity to provide for one's own needs (Agich, 1993). It includes self-confidence and allows for a certain degree of freedom, providing the opportunity to make one's own decisions. Self-confidence allows an individual to make decisions necessary to complete daily tasks that are affected by changing circumstances (Chafey, Sullivan, & Shannon, 1998). Changing circumstances might include a change in job requirements, including floating to a different unit or a change in patient status. This is essential for the RN moving from novice to expert (Benner, 2001). As the nurse grows professionally and moves toward expert level, he or she will demonstrate autonomy in his or herr practice stimulating personal and professional growth (Hanson, Jenkins, & Ryan, 1990).

The study participants experienced barriers to their professional development that included a lack of a career ladder, promotion opportunities not correlated to advanced levels of education, and a lack of tuition reimbursement. One participant cited the issue of an equal pay scale for nurses with associate degrees and bachelor degrees as limiting motivation for advanced education: "There is no motivation to pursue an advanced degree at this facility. Your pay doesn't go up with additional degrees and they don't offer any educational assistance."

Despite limited funding and career advancement, they continued to feel an obligation to remain current in yearly competencies. They felt they were accountable for their own learning. As one study participant stated, "Each nurse must have self-motivation to want to stay current, improve, and learn. Each nurse should believe that they need to better herself in order to better serve her patients."

Nurses employed various techniques to continue their learning and to remain current in their skills.

> Everything that I learn . . . I write down in two little books. Because we are a small facility and I don't see everything, every day I write down everything . . . If you don't do these things every day it is easy for them to slip out of your mind.

Social Responsibility

Social responsibility is demonstrated by meeting the social and health needs of the community (International Council of Nurses, 2012) and having a sense of duty to help others. All nurses have a sense of this responsibility due to the association between social responsibility and professional values. Because of the close ties in rural communities, lack of extended services, and social injustice, it can be assumed rural nurses engage more with their patients and community than their urban counterparts. "Socially responsible nurses should have professional self-confidence" (Faseleh-Jahromi, Moattari, & Peyrovi, 2014, p. 292). Social responsibility contributes to the deep connectedness that rural nurses feel towards the patients they encounter. Often these individuals are friends, relatives, or others whom the nurse has known for many years.

One participant stated:

> We need to let our patients know that we want to know about them, what they do for a living, tell us what is bothering them; we need to show patients that we care enough to communicate and that their lives and health are important to us. Caring for the community expands to offering shelter to community members in need.

Empathy

Dinkins (2011) defines empathy "as understanding another's feelings, instincts, worries, or desires." Empathy was apparent in three areas: nurses' empathy for the community, their patients, and among the nurses. Nurses discussed that that they lived in "a small, intimate community" where "you . . . get to know the people and you have to be caring." Unfortunately, the caring continues when the patient is transferred to another hospital. One nurse demonstrated empathy for the families of patients who had been transferred to a hospital that was located 150 miles away. Because of the distance family members were not able to be with their loved ones during their illness or transition to death.

Nurses offered empathy to each other by supporting each other when necessary. When an emergency occurs or a unit is short staffed "we go and offer consult, support, and whatever we can to help. We are always a resource for the other departments especially if they have questions or if they need some extra help or some extra expertise."

CONCLUSION

Rural nursing is defined as "the provision of healthcare by professional nurses to persons living in sparsely populated areas" (Long & Weinert, 2013). Rural nursing theory supports the process of understanding commonalities and differences in rural care in order to support the delivery of evidence-based care to rural residents. The goal of this research was to understand the lived experiences of rural nurses who provide care to this increasingly fragile population of residents by understanding the phenomenon of the lived experience of the RN practicing in a rural healthcare setting. The findings from this research serves as a contribution to building a foundation that will support rural nurses to continue to excel in their practice and emerge as leaders in rural healthcare.

REFERENCES

Agich, G. J. (1993). *Autonomy of long-term care*. New York, NY: Oxford University Press.

Benner, P. (1984). *From novice to expert: Excellence to power in clinical nursing practice.* Menlo Park, CA: Addison-Wesley.

Benner, P. (2001). Creating a culture of safety and improvement: A key to reducing medical error. *American Journal of Critical Care, 10*(4), 281–284.

Bigbee, J. L., Gehrke, P., & Otterness, N. (2009). Public health nurses in rural/frontier one-nurse offices. *Rural Remote Health, 9*(4), 1282. Retrieved from https://www.rrh.org.au/journal/article/1282

Bushy, A. (2003). Considerations for working with diverse rural client systems. *Lippincott's Case Management, 8*(5), 214–223.

Bushy, A. (2014). Rural health care ethics. In J. Warren & K. Smalley (Eds.), *Rural public health* (pp. 41–53). New York, NY: Springer Publishing.

Butts, J. B., & Rich, K. L. (2018). *Philosophies and theories for advanced nursing practice* (3rd ed.). Burlington, MA: Jones & Bartlett.

Chafey, K., Sullivan, T., & Shannon, A. (1998). Self-reliance: Characterization of their own autonomy by elderly women. In H. L. Lee (Ed.), *Conceptual basis for nursing* (pp. 153–177). New York, NY: Springer Publishing.

Colaizzi, P. F. (1973). *Reflection and research in psychology: A phenomenological study of learning*. Dubuque, IA: Kendall Hunt.

Cramer, M. E., Jones, K. J., & Hertzog, M. (2011). Nursing staffing in critical access hospitals: Structural factors linked to quality care. *Journal of Nursing Care Quality, 26*(4), 335–343. doi:10.1097/NCQ.0B013e318210d30a

Dinkins, C. (2011, May 10). Ethics: Beyond patient care: Practicing empathy in the workplace. *OJIN: The Online Journal of Issues in Nursing, 16*(2), 11. doi:10.3912/OJIN.Vol16No02EthCol01

Estabrooks, C. A., Midozi, W. K., Cummings, G. G., & Wallin, L. (2007). Predicting research use in nursing organizations: A multilevel analysis. *Nursing Research, 56*(4, Suppl. 1), S7–S23. doi:10.1097/01.NNR.0000280647.18806.98

Faseleh-Jahromi, M., Moattari, M., & Peyrovi, H. (2014). Iranian nurses' perceptions of social responsibility: A qualitative study. *Nursing Ethics, 21*(3), 289–298. doi:10.1177/0969733013495223

Grove, S. K., Burns, N., & Gray, J. R. (2013). *The practice of nursing research: Appraisal, synthesis, and generation of evidence* (7th ed.). St. Louis, MO: Elsevier.

Hanson, C. M., Jenkins, S., & Ryan, R. (1990). Factors related to job satisfaction and autonomy as correlates of potential job retention for rural nurses. *Journal of Rural Health, 6*(3), 302–316. doi:10.1111/j.1748-0361.1990.tb00669.x

Hegney, D. (2002). Rural and remote area nursing: An Australian perspective. *Online Journal of Rural Nursing & Health Care, 3*(1), 24–38. Retrieved from http://rnojournal.binghamton.edu/index.php/RNO/article/view/240

Hunsberger, M., Bauman, A., Blythe, J., & Crea, M. (2009). Sustaining the rural workforce: Nursing perspectives on work life challenges. *Journal of Rural Health, 25*(1), 17–25. doi:10.1111/j.1748-0361.2009.00194.x

International Council of Nurses. (2012). *The ICN code of ethics for nurses*. Retrieved from http://www.icn.ch/images/stories/documents/about/icncode_english.pdf

Kim, H. S., & Kollack, I. (2005). *Nursing theories: Conceptual and philosophical foundations* (2nd ed.). New York, NY: Springer Publishing.

Koessl, B. D., Winters, C. A., Lee, H. J., & Hendrickx, L. (2013). Rural nurses' attitudes and beliefs toward evidence-based practice. In C. A. Winters (Ed.), *Rural nursing: Concepts, theory, and practice* (4th ed., pp. 275–291). New York, NY: Springer Publishing.

Long, K. A., & Weinert, C. (2013). Rural nursing: Developing the theory base. In C. A. Winters (Ed.), *Rural nursing: Concepts, theory, and practice* (4th ed., pp. 1–4). New York, NY: Springer Publishing.

Newhouse, R. P., Morlock, L., Pronovost, P., & Breckenridge Sproat, S. (2011). Rural hospital nursing: Results of a national survey of nurse executives. *Journal of Nursing Administration, 41*(3), 129–137. doi:10.1097/NNA.0b013e31820c7212

Paré, J. (2015). Understanding the lived experiences of nurses working in critical access hospitals. *American Research Journal of Nursing, 1*(5), 1–6. Retrieved from https://www.arjonline.org/papers/arjn/v1-i5/1.pdf

Paré J. M., Petersen, P., & Sharp, D. P. (2017). A story of emergent leadership: Understanding the lived experiences of nurses working in a rural hospital setting. *Online Journal of Rural Nursing and Health Care, 17*(2). doi:10.14574/ojrnhc.v1712.454

Ratcliffe, M., Burd, C., Holder, K., & Fields, A. (2017). Defining rural at the U.S. census bureau. Published December 8, 2016. Retrieved from https://www.census.gov/library/publications/2016/acs/acsgeo-1.html

Sokolowski, R. (2000). *Introduction to phenomenology*. New York, NY: Cambridge University Press.

Winters, C. A. (Ed.). (2013). *Rural nursing: Concepts, theory, and practice* (4th ed.). New York, NY: Springer Publishing.

CHAPTER 10

The Nurse Practitioner as Rural Healthcare Provider

Jana G. Zwilling

DISCUSSION QUESTIONS

- What are some barriers to full scope-of-practice for nurse practitioners (NPs) in rural areas? How might these differ by state? By healthcare system?
- Discuss the benefits and detriments to being an NP practicing in the rural area where you grew up.
- What economic benefits might be provided to rural areas with an NP-led primary care model? How might this benefit the patient? Community?
- Self-reliance and independence are a hallmark of the rural patient populations. Discuss benefits and detriments of this trait when attempting to provide chronic disease management. How might these differ with the provision of health promotion or prevention components?

In a keynote address to the National Organization of Nurse Practitioner Faculties (NONPFs), Dr. Loretta Ford stated, "Patients will be in control, as they always have been. This is something nurses have always understood" (Ford & Gardenier, 2015, p. 577). The rural patient population especially sees itself as self-reliant and independent. No one knows this better than an NP in a rural clinic. In these days of relative value units (RVUs) and quality measures (QMs) for healthcare reimbursement, there is something lacking: the patient. Yes, QMs attempt to put the patient's voice into some measurements, but health indicators measured by prescribed standards do not always demonstrate the high quality of care in a collaborative patient–provider relationship. For example, the American Diabetes Association (ADA) might recommend that a patient's A1C needs to be less than or equal to 6.5% (ADA, 2017). The NP in a rural setting might see a farmer present for a large wound obtained during harvest. The farmer needs to "get sewn up quick" so he can get back out in the fields. This farmer also happens to have type 2 diabetes and has not had an A1C checked for 2 years, his last one being 7.5%. The NP engages in a conversation and education regarding the patient's diabetes, while suturing the patient's wound. The patient agrees to have labs drawn prior to leaving the clinic and schedules an appointment for "after harvest." The fact that this farmer even had his labs drawn should be marked as a high QM. The give and take between the patient and the NP can make small, incremental improvements and greatly benefit the patient; however, these are not captured with the current QM model.

NPs have been steadily increasing in number and breaking down barriers to a full scope-of-practice. Evidence supports NPs in this role and looks for these advanced practice nurses to lead the way in formulating new and better primary care models. There have been many innovations over the past 50-plus years in the healthcare arena, none as disruptive as that of the NP. "If the natural process of disruption is allowed to proceed, we'll be able to build a new system that's characterized by lower costs, higher quality, and greater convenience than could ever be achieved under the old system" (Christensen, Bohmer, & Kenagy, 2000, p. 2).

Since Dr. Ford and Dr. Silver initiated this new role, NPs have been chipping away at barriers to the provision of affordable, accessible, quality care for the needs of the general healthcare consumer, especially those in rural and underserved populations. This chapter provides insight into the contributions of NPs as healthcare providers in the rural setting. This is accomplished through a brief background on NPs, a discussion on access to healthcare, and a look at the unique patient-centered care provided by NPs.

BACKGROUND

NPs have been recognized healthcare providers in the United States since 1965. The idea began with rural pediatric public health nurses in Colorado. These nurses were advocating for their patients and wanted to provide more services while out in the rural areas performing home visits. Often the only healthcare provider in the county, these nurses felt their patients should not have to wait on assessments or orders from a physician to obtain needed care. Thus, the first NP training program was born out of necessity to provide more and better services for the rural and underserved populations (American Association of Nurse Practitioners [AANP], n.d-b).

The NP role has continued to evolve since 1965, in both educational preparation and practice. Currently, NPs must have either a master's or doctor of nursing practice degree. Most NP programs require applicants to practice as an RN for a minimum of 1 year prior to applying for graduate school. Each NP must pass a state RN-licensing exam, and then pass a national certification exam to practice. There are also requirements for continuing education that differ based on the state and national certification organization. According to the AANP (n.d-a), "NPs assess patients, order and interpret diagnostic tests, make diagnoses, and initiate and manage treatment plans, including prescribing medications." Many NPs perform their roles as independent practitioners, without physician supervision or collaboration. NPs have fully independent practice in 22 states and the District of Columbia, with legislative efforts active in many other states (AANP, n.d-a).

There are presently 205,000 licensed NPs in the United States. Approximately 90% of these NPs are certified in a primary care area such as family or adult care. Approximately 66% of NPs work in communities with populations of less than 250,000, with 35% practicing in communities of less than 50,000 (Chattopadhyay, Zangaro, & White, 2015). NPs tend to care for rural and underserved populations. A study of the geographic distribution of primary care clinicians demonstrated an average of 5.8 more NPs per 100,000 patient population in rural areas versus urban while there were 24 less physicians per 100,000 patient population in rural versus urban areas (Graves et al., 2016).

RURAL HEALTHCARE ACCESS

Access to healthcare is defined as "the timely use of personal health services to achieve the best health outcomes" (Millman, 1993, p. 4). Getting "good access" to healthcare requires entrance into the healthcare system, access to facilities with necessary services, and providers who meet the individual needs of the patient. Access is measured by the presence of health insurance, physical healthcare facility, healthcare utilization measures, and patients' own assessment of how readily they can access care (Agency for Healthcare Research and Quality [AHRQ], 2011). Isolation and distance from other towns, neighbors, or healthcare tends to have a different definition when viewed from the inside as opposed to the outside of the rural population. Living in an urban area where all necessities and more are located within a few city blocks, one might view having to drive 100 miles for a healthcare appointment ludicrous. However, having grown up with your nearest neighbor 2 miles away, your mom driving an hour and a half to work 3 days per week, and your school bus ride taking 2 hours, 100 miles does not phase most rural persons. The view of healthcare accessibility, therefore, differs greatly by population. This subjectivity can be viewed in the measurement of access. A rural patient may construe very easy access and the effective receipt of "needed" services as one acute appointment during the year for which they drove 50 miles.

Rural Healthcare Providers

The United States has long attempted to attract healthcare providers, especially primary care physicians, to rural areas. Medicare provides a large sum of money for graduate medical education (GME). The Medicare Prescription Drug, Improvement, and Modernization Act of 2003, Pub. L. No. 108-173, 117 STAT. 2066 (2003), shuffled GME residency positions to attempt better distribution in rural areas and primary care specialties. A study conducted in 2013 showed that, of 3,000 residencies participating in this redistribution, only 12 were located in rural areas. The growth of primary care residencies did improve; however, specialty care residencies grew larger by twice the number of primary care (Chen, Xierali, Piwnica-Worms, & Phillips, 2013).

Less than 33% of physicians work in a primary care area defined as family medicine, general practice, internal medicine, pediatrics, and geriatrics (AHRQ, 2012). Only 11% of the physician population is located in rural areas (Rosenblatt, Chen, Lishner, & Doescher, 2010). Conversely, examinations into the NP workforce have illustrated a strong commitment to rural healthcare. Over 60% of NPs work in a primary care area defined as family medicine, pediatrics, or internal medicine (Chattopadhyay et al., 2015). Nationwide, approximately 15% of NPs practice in rural areas with a per-capita ratio of rural NPs at 2.8 per 10,000 population in those areas.

Rural locales demand an experienced clinician with a broad array of skills. Typically, the NP in rural areas is a family NP. Training as a family NP provides the broadest scope-of-practice, highly desired by rural healthcare systems to eliminate the necessity of multiple provider types. Rural NPs usually work more and longer hours, see more patients on an average day, perform more procedures, and refer significantly less than their urban counterparts (Brown, Hart, & Burman, 2009). Many NPs working in rural areas of the United States have additional privileges either not available or not necessary for their urban colleagues. In critical access hospital (CAH) or other small rural hospital settings, NPs likely have hospital admitting privileges as well as long-term care–admitting privileges and all the responsibilities associated with caring for those patients within those facility types.

Health Professions Shortage Areas, CAHs, and NPs

A CAH is a facility that has applied for and met specific criteria to gain CAH designation. Some requirements of this designation are having no more than 25 inpatient beds, maintaining an annual average length of stay no more than 96 hours for acute inpatient care, offering 24-hour, 7-day per week emergency care, and being located in a rural area at least 35 miles away from any other hospital or CAH (Social Security Administration, 2006). These requirements support a focus on common outpatient conditions and immediate needs of the patient, while referring other conditions to larger facilities with more resources. It is of utmost importance for CAHs to keep costs low. This focus on high quality care at a low cost is ideally met within the scope-of-practice of an NP. One particular case study identified significant cost savings, as much as 28% for a CAH, by employing salaried and benefitted NPs in their emergency department (ED) as opposed to contracting with either local or locum physicians (Henderson, 2006).

Health professional shortage areas (HPSAs) are roughly defined as a physician to patient ratio of 3,000:1 (or greater), and primary care providers are limited to physicians in general or family practice, general internal medicine, OB/GYN, or pediatrics (Salinsky, 2010). The HPSA numbers do not take any advanced practice registered nurse (APRN) roles, including NPs into consideration. Medicare and Medicaid, while beneficial for some populations, can even be detrimental to rural areas. Although the patient may be covered for health services, to some extent, reimbursement rates to rural healthcare facilities can be lacking. For example, NPs are reimbursed at 85% of the rate of physicians, even when providing the same service (Medicare Learning Network, Center for Medicare & Medicaid Services, and Department of Health and Human Services, 2016). With many rural healthcare facilities employing primarily, or only, NPs, this lower reimbursement rate can be crippling. Furthermore, primary care practices bill largely for outpatient office visits or consultations versus for numerous procedures such as those billed by specialists. Reimbursement rates for office visits are significantly lower than procedural costs, hence another barrier to income production for rural facilities (Zismer, Christianson, Marr, & Cummings, 2015). The 2017 Medicare Payment Advisory Commission (MedPAC) report cited negative average Medicare margins for rural healthcare facilities, with declines expected to continue (MedPAC, 2017).

For CAH status, a physician must be associated with the facility; however, there is no requirement for that provider to be on-site. In many cases, one physician is associated with multiple CAHs while NPs independently provide the ongoing care. As an exemplar, North Dakota has 36 CAHs spread across 69,000 square miles and a population distribution of 9.7 persons per square mile (U.S. Census Bureau, 2010). Based on a review of North Dakota CAH websites, NPs outnumber physicians approximately 2:1 and physician assistants 5:1 as permanent employees of these facilities. With full scope-of-practice, NPs would be poised to be the optimum primary care providers for rural communities across the nation.

Rural Patient-Centered Care

The rural patient population can be challenging to care for due to a multitude of reasons. This population tends to have older, lower income persons who are more dependent on Medicare or Medicaid, and are more likely to live in an HPSA (Rosenblatt et al., 2010). The rates of suicide and accidental death are also higher in the rural populations (Defriese & Ricketts, 1989). Farming and ranching are two major industries in rural locations of the United States. These industries have the fourth highest occupational fatality rate at 38.5 per 100,000 full-time equivalent (FTE; Bureau of Labor Statistics, U.S. Department of Labor, 2016). These industries also tend to have a large number of family-owned or private farms and ranches not always able to supply employer-paid health insurance. Geographic access or distances can also be a challenge for patients and providers alike. One study cited that rural patients, on average, travel 113 miles for a primary care visit with an NP (Brown et al., 2009).

The rural nursing theory outlines four primary concepts of rural populations that can affect healthcare (Long & Weinert, 1989). Rural persons tend to assess their own health based on their ability to perform their jobs or daily work activities. If they can work there should be no healthcare intervention necessary. The isolation and distance of rural populations could be construed as a barrier to healthcare access, but it has been found that rural inhabitants do not view themselves as isolated, nor do they see health services as inaccessible. The rural population is also construed as self-reliant and independent. Geographically, self-reliance can be a necessity in rural areas, but can be a challenge with health promotion and disease management. Finally, the lack of anonymity and outsider/insider concepts can affect the provision and acceptance of rural healthcare (Long & Weinert, 1989).

According to the AHRQ, "good access" includes "providers ... with whom patients can develop a relationship based on mutual communication and trust" (Bierman, Magari, Jette, Splaine, & Wasson, 1998, p. 17). With the cultural differences outlined in the rural nursing theory (Long & Weinert, 1989), provision of care with a trusting relationship where communication is paramount can be difficult. Nurses have ranked first in the Gallup Poll for honesty and ethics for the past 15 years (Norman, 2016). There has also been abundant evidence over the past several years demonstrating that NPs have superior interpersonal skills and can produce excellent patient outcomes (Caldwell, 2007; Horrocks, Anderson, & Salisbury, 2002; Leipert, Wagner, Forbes, & Forchuk, 2011).

"Culturally beneficial nursing care can only occur when cultural care values, expressions, or patterns are known and used appropriately and knowingly by the nurse providing care ... beneficial, healthy, satisfying, culturally based nursing care enhances the well-being of clients" (Leininger, 1991, pp. 44–45). Rural communities are often essentially a large family where everyone is involved in each other's lives. Healthcare providers entering the community for a short period of time, often demonstrated with HPSA or National Health Service Corps (NHSC) loan repayment participants, are frequently met with skepticism and mistrust as these providers traditionally enter and leave the communities quite frequently (Pathman, Konrad, Dann, & Koch, 2004). Much time is needed to integrate a new "family member." NPs commonly "grow where they are planted," meaning they are members of the community and work as RNs in the local healthcare facility. After obtaining their advanced degree, NPs stay in their home areas to care for their friends, neighbors, and family. Although it is not always the case that NPs have resided in the area in which they currently practice, the nursing model provides the NP a distinct advantage with the patient-centered care structure.

The insider–outsider conundrum of rural culture can be a difficult barrier to overcome, especially when attempting to gain trust and establish a productive provider–patient relationship. NPs were "brought up" viewing the whole person versus merely the disease process. This thought process is so ingrained that NPs are typically found to quickly establish a nurturing rapport. Horrocks et al. (2002) found NPs, overall, spent more time with their patients, provided more guidance on self-care and management, and provided better communication. Ultimately, patients were more satisfied with the NP encounter as compared to physician encounters (Horrocks et al., 2002). NPs can easily overcome the insider/outsider barrier typical of rural communities. Rural healthcare facilities could benefit from training their own RNs as NPs in order to provide culturally competent care to their local residents.

Madeleine Leininger (1991, p. 48) also proposed that health is defined as "a state of wellbeing that is culturally defined, valued, and practiced, and which reflects the ability of the individuals or groups to perform their daily role activities in culturally expressed, beneficial, and patterned lifeways." Dr. Leininger's definition provides the underpinnings in describing the phenomenon of health in rural populations. Culturally speaking, rural persons tend to view their own health in terms of their individual work ability. Essentially, if they can perform their regular daily duties, they do not need any healthcare intercession. However, if an illness or injury decreases or prohibits their ability to work, they will be first in line at the clinic. Numerous examples of this can be seen in a rural NP practice. A rural farmer whose wife is trying to get him to have his cholesterol checked, says it will have to wait until after planting is done. However, when the farmer's prize bull steps on his foot and thus cannot push the pedals in the tractor, that farmer wants a quick fix so he can get back into the fields. The NP, knowing the futility of discussing preventive care and health promotion with the farmer, treats the fractured foot and provides direction for self-care, including written instructions for care and follow-up the farmer can take to his wife. This is just one example when knowing the cultural background of a patient, as well as his or her personal concept of health, can befit proper treatment and lead to a continued beneficial relationship.

Encounters with rural patients are not always that simple. Often the NP will need to strike a bargain or make some sort of compromise with the patient. This, fortunately, can be advantageous for both parties. Working with the patient in a team-based approach versus a dictatorial relationship can be very encouraging to that patient. When patients are emboldened to participate in their own healthcare, often they feel more in control and may be more apt to adhere more closely to provider guidance, especially with rural populations where self-reliance and independence are a common theme. "Promoting involvement in self-care, for example, often depends on the nurse's ability to use communication to create an identity for the client as someone who is capable of active participation in healthcare" (Kasch, Kasch, & Lisnek, 1998, p. 276). As an example, a rural mail carrier who has had type 2 diabetes for over 5 years attends annual physical exams with his primary provider but his A1C has been steadily increasing. Originally, the NP had recommended he check his blood sugar twice each day. The patient admits to checking it "rarely" or "maybe once a week." The NP asks the mail-carrier about the schedule that would work best for him. The patient is rather taken aback by this as he is used to being reprimanded by healthcare providers and family members for not taking better care of himself. He decides he can easily check his sugars first thing in the morning, but "the rest of my day is usually up in the air." The pair compromises on daily fasting sugars and checking postprandial sugars twice each week. The NP is satisfied as the patient will be checking his blood sugar and the patient is satisfied because he was the one to set the schedule, making him feel more in control.

The best healthcare providers will recognize that "patients will always be in control" (Ford & Gardenier, 2015, p. 577). Certainly, patients need evidence-based guidance and best practices to assist their decision making, but ultimately, the decision is their own.

CONCLUSION

Guiding and supporting, as well as advocating for patients, have always been a hallmark of nursing. NPs advance this care to the next level. In this time of exploding healthcare expenditures, provider shortages, geographical distribution issues, and significant numbers of underserved populations, our system of healthcare is ripe for an upheaval. Christensen et al. (2000) apparently had a crystal ball to be so accurate about future "disruptive innovations" in healthcare. NPs are a definite innovation who can not only cut healthcare costs but also provide superior, patient-centered care while circumventing primary care provider shortages in rural America.

REFERENCES

Agency for Healthcare Research and Quality. (2011). *National healthcare quality report* (pp. 211–221). Rockville, MD: U.S. Department of Health & Human Services. Retrieved from https://archive.ahrq.gov/research/findings/nhqrdr/nhqr11/chap9.html

Agency for Healthcare Research and Quality. (2012). *The number of practicing primary care physicians in the United States*. Rockville, MD: U.S. Department of Health & Human Services. Retrieved from http://www.ahrq.gov/research/findings/factsheets/primary/pcwork1/index.html

American Association of Nurse Practitioners. (n.d.-a). All about NPs. Retrieved from https://www.aanp.org/all-about-nps

American Association of Nurse Practitioners. (n.d.-b). *Historical timeline*. Retrieved from https://www.aanp.org/about-aanp/historical-timeline

American Diabetes Association. (2017). Glycemic targets. *Diabetes Care, 40*(Suppl. 1), S48–S56. doi:10.2337/dc17-S009

Bierman, A. S., Magari, E. S., Jette, A. M., Splaine, M., & Wasson, J. H. (1998). Assessing access as a first step toward improving the quality of care for very old adults. *Journal of Ambulatory Care Management, 21*(3), 17–26.

Brown, J., Hart, A. M., & Burman, M. E. (2009). A day in the life of rural advanced practice nurses. *Journal for Nurse Practitioners, 5*(2), 108–114.

Bureau of Labor Statistics, U.S. Department of Labor. (2016). Farmers, ranchers, and other agricultural managers. *Occupational Outlook Handbook, 2016-17 Edition*. Retrieved from https://www.bls.gov/ooh/management/farmers-ranchers-and-other-agricultural-managers.htm

Caldwell, D. (2007). Bloodroot: Life stories of nurse practitioners in rural Appalachia. *Journal of Holistic Nursing: Official Journal of the American Holistic Nurses' Association, 25*(2), 73–80.

Chattopadhyay, A., Zangaro, G. A., & White, K. (2015). Practice patterns and characteristics of nurse practitioners in the United States: Results from the 2012 national sample survey of nurse practitioners. *Journal for Nurse Practitioners, 11*(2), 170–177.

Chen, C., Xierali, I., Piwnica-Worms, K., & Phillips, R. (2013). The redistribution of graduate medical education positions in 2005 failed to boost primary care or rural training. *Health Affairs, 32*(1), 102–110.

Christensen, C. M., Bohmer, R. M. J., & Kenagy, J. (2000). Will disruptive innovations cure health care? *Harvard Business Review, 78*(5), 102–112, 199. Retrieved from https://hbr.org/2000/09/will-disruptive-innovations-cure-health-care

Defriese, G. H., & Ricketts, T. C. (1989). Primary health care in rural areas: An agenda for research. *Health Services Research, 23*, 931–974.

Ford, L. C., & Gardenier, D. (2015). Fasten your seat belts—It's going to be a bumpy ride. *Journal for Nurse Practitioners, 11*(6), 575–577.

Graves, J., Mishra, P., Dittus, R., Parikh, R., Perloff, J., & Buerhaus, P. (2016). Role of geography and nurse practitioner scope-of-practice in efforts to expand primary care. *Medical Care, 54*(1), 81–89.

Henderson, K. (2006). TelEmergency: Distance emergency care in rural emergency departments using nurse practitioners. *Journal of Emergency Nursing, 32*(5), 388–393.

Horrocks, S., Anderson, E., & Salisbury, C. (2002). Systematic review of whether nurse practitioners working in primary care can provide equivalent care to doctors. *British Medical Journal, 324*(7341), 819–823.

Kasch, C. R., Kasch, J. B., & Lisnek, P. (1998). Women's talk and nurse-client encounters: Developing criteria for assessing interpersonal skill, including commentary by Moccia, P. *Scholarly Inquiry for Nursing Practice, 12*(3), 269–287.

Leininger, M. M. (1991). The theory of culture care diversity and universality. In M. M. Leininger (Ed.), *Culture care diversity and universality: Theory of nursing* (pp. 5–68). New York, NY: National League for Nursing.

Leipert, B., Wagner, J., Forbes, D., & Forchuk, C. (2011). Canadian rural women's experiences with rural primary health care nurse practitioners. *Online Journal of Rural Nursing & Health Care, 11*(1), 37–53. Retrieved from http://rnojournal.binghamton.edu/index.php/RNO/article/view/8

Long, K. A., & Weinert, C. (1989). Rural nursing: Developing a theory base. *Scholarly Inquiry for Nursing Practice: An International Journal, 3*, 113–127.

Medicare Learning Network, Center for Medicare & Medicaid Services, and Department of Health and Human Services. (2016). *Advanced practice registered nurses, anesthesiologist assistants, and physician assistants.* Retrieved from https://www.cms.gov/Outreach-and-Education/Medicare-Learning-Network-MLN/MLNProducts/Downloads/Medicare-Information-for-APRNs-AAs-PAs-Booklet-ICN-901623.pdf

Medicare Payment Advisory Commission. (2017). *Report to the Congress: Medicare payment policy* (pp. xi–xxiv). Retrieved from http://medpac.gov/docs/default-source/reports/mar17_entirereport224610adfa9c665e80adff00009edf9c.pdf?sfvrsn=0

The Medicare Prescription Drug, Improvement, and Modernization Act of 2003, 42 U.S.C. 1301 *et seq.* (2003). Retrieved from http://catalog.gpo.gov/fdlpdir/locate.jsp?ItemNumber=0575&sys=000560043

Millman, M. (Ed.). (1993). *Access to health care in America.* Washington, DC: National Academies Press.

Norman, J. (2016, December). Americans rate healthcare providers high on honesty, ethics. *Gallup.* Retrieved from http://news.gallop.com/poll/200057/americans-rate-healthcare-providers-high-honesty-ethics.aspx

Pathman, D. E., Konrad, T. R., Dann, R., & Koch, G. (2004). Retention of primary care physicians in rural health professional shortage areas. *American Journal of Public Health, 94*, 1723–1729.

Rosenblatt, R. A., Chen, F. M., Lishner, D. M., & Doescher, M. P. (2010). *The future of family medicine and implications for rural primary care physician supply.* Seattle, WA: WWAMI Rural Health Center. Retrieved from https://depts.washington.edu/uwrhrc/uploads/RHRC_FR125_Rosenblatt.pdf

Salinsky, E. (2010). Health care shortage designations: HPSA, MUA, and TBD [Background paper no. 75. *National Health Policy Forum.* Retrieved from http://www.nhpf.org/library/background-papers/BP75_HPSA-MUA_06-04-2010.pdf

Social Security Administration. (2006). *Compilation of the Social Security Laws, Medicare Rural Hospital Flexibility Program.* (Sec. 1820. [42 U.S.C. 1395i–4]). Retrieved from https://www.ssa.gov/OP_Home/ssact/title18/1820.htm

U.S. Census Bureau. (2010). Quick facts: North Dakota. Retrieved from https://www.census.gov/quickfacts/table/PST045215/38

Zismer, D. K., Christianson, J., Marr, T., & Cummings, D. (2015). An examination of the professional services productivity for physicians and licensed, advance practice professionals across six specialties in independent and integrated clinical practice: A report by the School of Public Health, University of Minnesota, for the Medicare Payment Advisory Commission. Retrieved from http://www.medpac.gov/docs/default-source/contractor-reports/an-examination-of-the-professional-services-productivity-for-physicians-and-licensed-advance-practic.pdf?sfvrsn=0

CHAPTER 11

Telehealth in Rural Nursing Practice

K. M. Reeder, Victoria Britson, and Mary Kay Nissen

DISCUSSION QUESTIONS

- What are the major influences of telehealth on rural and frontier nursing practice and healthcare?
- What are the advantages of using telehealth in rural and frontier environments?
- What is the role of the nurse in providing rural/frontier primary, urgent, and specialty care using telehealth modalities?
- How can nurses using telehealth help patients and families achieve desirable healthcare outcomes and enhance quality of life?

Telehealth nursing or telenursing involves the use of telecommunications and other technologies such as video conferencing for sharing information and providing patient care, education, public health, and administrative services over distances (Jones, 2012). Telehealth conceptually offers an approach to redesign and enhance nursing care outside of traditional healthcare settings, namely, hospitals and clinics (Fraiche, Eapen, & McClellan, 2017; HealthIT. gov, 2017; Health Resources & Services Administration [HRSA], 2016; Totten et al., 2016). Changes in healthcare policy, including reimbursement structures, can create uncertainty and increase risk for widening gaps in health among rural and frontier populations (Kusmin, 2016). Telehealth programs have been designed to address these and other rural health disparities by increasing access and improving safety and quality of care, as well as reducing healthcare costs.

Extant literature on telehealth is vast and varied. Interchangeable terms, including eHealth (electronic health), mHealth (mobile health), and telemedicine (medical care at a distance via various telecommunication technologies) were variably used to operationalize telehealth, making comparisons between studies difficult. In addition, evidence on cost and healthcare services use is sparse (HRSA, 2016). Thus, research is needed that examines patient outcomes and healthcare costs in rural and frontier populations with a variety of conditions and in a variety of contexts of care. Specifically, research is needed that examines patient and health services outcomes amenable to telehealth nursing interventions that will inform payers and policy-makers on digital healthcare delivery and value-based models that accommodate continued technology innovation and expanded roles, while supporting current practices and translation of new evidence (Graves, Ford, & Mooney, 2013; Knapp, 2016; Smith et al., 2015).

Historically, the uses of telehealth technologies by nurses were learned on the job, without formal training. Telehealth is increasingly being integrated into academic nursing curricula, signifying the importance of telehealth in nursing practice. In the current healthcare milieu, training and experience in telehealth by RNs and advanced practice registered nurses (APRNs) in rural and frontier environments is critical to providing effective nursing care. Despite widespread efforts by the American Academy of Ambulatory Care Nursing (AAACN; 2011) and American Telehealth Telemedicine Association (Gough et al., 2015) to provide evidence for telehealth use of standards of practice, there has been limited success in systematically implementing guideline-based telehealth care in clinical practice.

Providing healthcare using telehealth modalities differs from traditional nursing and advanced practice. Telehealth nursing requires collaboration and resourcefulness between on-site and distance-site colleagues, as well as patients and families receiving telehealth care to achieve positive outcomes. In addition to traditional skills that underpin the nursing process and advanced practice, telehealth nurses must be skilled in the use of telehealth technologies, including the use of peripheral equipment and troubleshooting interruptions in telehealth interactions and assessments due to a variety of potential equipment and technology issues. Examples of technological equipment nurses use in conducting telehealth encounters include the electronic stethoscope for auscultation, otoscope, and ophthalmoscope for ear and eye examinations, respectively, and a handheld camera to visualize and assess wounds and other visible alterations.

During telehealth encounters, healthcare providers must be mindful of camera presence, extraneous noise, body language, and backgrounds visualized on the video screen by patients, families, and other members of the healthcare team. Like face-to-face encounters, telehealth patient encounters require adherence to professional and legal standards of confidentiality, ethics, communication, and cultural considerations. Communication during telehealth encounters often present additional challenges in that there is frequently a slight delay in audio-visual transmission, resulting in an inadvertent talk-over audio effect during interactions, or pixelated or distorted visual effects. Thus, it is important to identify the need for repeated, or confirmatory collection of history and physical assessment information to account for potential disruptions in telehealth technologies and asymmetries in interactions that might otherwise result in inaccuracies.

In a Delphi study, van Houwelingen, Moerman, Ettema, Kort, and ten Cate (2016) identified essential telehealth activities used by nurses who provide remote healthcare to Dutch community-dwelling patients. Consensus on 14 nursing telehealth entrustable professional activities (NT-EPAs) was formed for telehealth nursing practice. Specific competencies were then selected for each NT-EPA that would be needed to carry out each activity. For example, the activity pertaining to coordination of care with the use of telehealth technology (NT-EPA #12) involves 14 competencies that address knowledge, communication, and clinical skills. Additional research is needed to validate the major nursing activities and their associated competencies in a variety of rural settings.

NEED FOR TELEHEALTH NURSING CARE IN RURAL POPULATIONS

Several factors specific to needs of rural and frontier populations have contributed to the growth and expansion of telehealth in rural nursing practice. Rural residents are more likely to report poor access to care and low perceived quality of care (Agency for Healthcare Research and Quality [AHRQ], 2015). In 2014, an estimated 46 million (15%) Americans lived in rural counties (Garcia et al., 2017; Kusmin, 2016; Moy et al., 2017). However, recruiting and retaining primary healthcare providers, specialists, and nurses in rural- and frontier-designated areas has been especially challenging.

The HRSA identified states and counties with medically underserved areas/populations (MUA/Ps). As illustrated in Figure 11.1, MUA/Ps are those areas identified as having (a) insufficient primary healthcare, dental, and mental health providers, (b) high infant mortality, extreme poverty levels, or (c) many elderly persons (HRSA, 2016).

Higher rates of cigarette smoking, hypertension, obesity, and leisure time physical inactivity were found in rural populations compared to those in urban populations (Garcia et al., 2017). In addition, social determinants of health such as education, income and poverty, and unemployment had a major influence on widening rural population health disparities (U.S. Department of Agriculture [USDA], 2016). Investigators recently illustrated that rural dwellers are more likely to have poorer health and live with more health risk factors and chronic conditions than their urban counterparts (Bolin, Bellamy, Ferdinand, Kash, & Helduser, 2015; Moy et al., 2017). In addition, persons who live in nonmetropolitan areas were at higher risk for death from the top five leading causes of death in the United States (Garcia et al., 2017; Moy et al., 2017).

Lack of health insurance and healthcare provider shortages for routine comprehensive care have contributed to widening gaps in primary care among

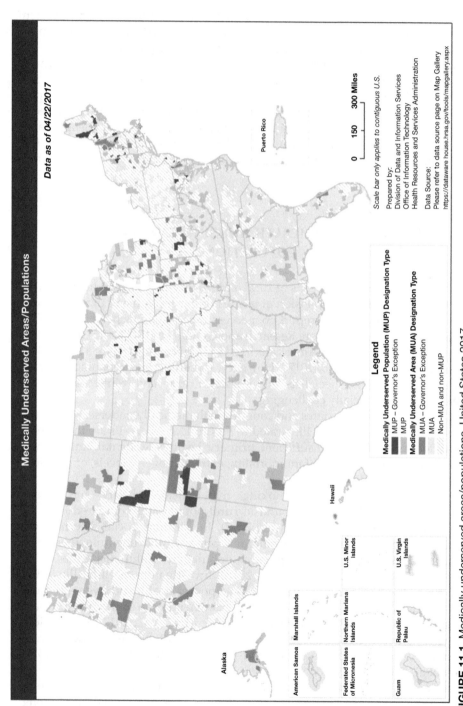

FIGURE 11.1. Medically underserved areas/populations, United States 2017.
Source: Health Resources & Services Administration—HRSA Data Warehouse (2017). Retrieved from https://datawarehouse.hrsa.gov/topics/shortageAreas.aspx.

rural populations. By 2015, there was an emerging trend, whereby rural states had slightly lower uninsured rates than the general U.S. population, and had similar primary care provider-to-patient ratios as the general population (Lee & Kaiser, 2016). These findings, however, must be interpreted with caution, as improvements in insured rates and patient-to-provider ratios might be related to increases in health insurance realized with promulgation of the Affordable Care Act in 2010, and warrant further examination on the potential impact and sustainability of subsequent policy changes.

Telehealth nursing care can help to bridge gaps in healthcare for persons in rural and frontier regions, and help patients gain local access to the necessary types and levels of healthcare providers distant sites to effectively address health concerns and optimize outcomes, including reducing mortality. When locally unavailable care or specialty consultations are needed, extensive travel to obtain these services may be required by patients and families. Transportation expense and time, delays in care and specialized treatments, and road conditions, especially during inclement weather, can be significant barriers to accessing care. In these and other similar situations, audio-visual telehealth technologies can be used to connect rural populations with needed healthcare services, thus providing continuity of care for patients in their local communities and improving patient outcomes. In an earlier study, patients who experienced a telehealth encounter reported increased satisfaction with telehealth visits due to decreased travel time for specialty care, improved communication and continuity of care with primary care providers, increased access to specialty providers, and prevention of unnecessary transfers to an emergency department or higher acuity level of care (Hofmeyer et al., 2016; Sabesan, Simcox, & Marr, 2012).

To illustrate the potential impact of telehealth on rural health outcomes, two telehealth nursing care approaches are described in hypothetical patient care scenarios using a commonly used method and a novel approach to telehealth care delivery as follows: institution-to-institution and direct-to-consumer approaches for a long-term care (LTC) facility resident and a rural community-dwelling resident.

Institution-to-Institution Telehealth Scenario

Mrs. Smith, an 82-year-old widow with a history of diabetes, heart failure, and depression was assessed by her LTC nurse, and was noted to be disoriented, pale, coughing, and slightly short of breath. Vital signs were as follows: body temperature = 100.4°, heart rate = 98/minute, respiration rate = 22/minute, and blood pressure = 114/78. Oxygen saturation via pulse oximetry was 91%. The LTC nurse contacted the telehealth provider at the remote hospital approximately 300 miles from the LTC facility for a consultation. After establishing a secure Internet connection with the remote site, a telehealth consultation encounter was initiated by the remote-site nurse practitioner who assessed Mrs. Smith with the on-site, in-person assistance of the LTC nurse.

After assessing Mrs. Smith, the APRN ordered lab work consisting of a complete blood count (CBC) with a differential and basic metabolic panel (BMP), and a chest x-ray, which were performed at the LTC facility. Oxygen by nasal cannula was administered at 2 L/minute, and albuterol nebulizer treatments were prescribed. After diagnostic test results were obtained, Mrs. Smith was diagnosed with a left lower lobe pneumonia and antibiotic therapy was initiated, followed by an echocardiogram and close monitoring of Mrs. Smith for signs and symptoms of worsening heart failure, which can be exacerbated by other conditions, such as pneumonia. With the appropriate and timely nursing interventions provided, Mrs. Smith's condition improved and hospitalization was avoided.

Direct-to-Consumer Primary Care Clinic Visit Telehealth Scenario

Tomar Lake is a small rural town on the border of two northern plains states, with 63 residents, and the seat for Fox County, a depressed region with less than 400 people. The township is known for harsh winter climate conditions, few community resources, and there is no available healthcare. The only public school and grocery store recently closed, leaving the town with only local gas station convenience store food items. With no viable jobs in town, most young people and families migrated to the nearest city, Coyote City (pop. 20,000), 90 miles west of town.

Mrs. Hutch is a 72-year-old widow, living alone on a fixed income in her small house in Tomar Lake. Most of her extended family migrated to Coyote City, where they have jobs. Mrs. Hutch's 23-year-old grandson, Ben, travels to Tomar Lake weekly to check on her and bring groceries to her from Coyote City. Mrs. Hutch does not drive, and depends on Ben to take her to physician appointments in Coyote City. Feeling that she is a burden on her grandson and other family members, Mrs. Hutch often delays, and even avoids altogether making and keeping needed follow-up blood pressure and diabetes care appointments at the clinic in Coyote City.

Mrs. Hutch's family recently voiced concerns about getting her to clinic visits, which have increasingly become more frequent due to her increased healthcare needs. Mrs. Hutch's family wants her to sell her house in Tomar Lake and move into an assisted living facility in Coyote City. Mrs. Hutch does not want to leave her home of over 50 years, her church, and her friends in Tomar Lake. Mrs. Hutch is active in community and church activities, and knows no one in the assisted living facility in Coyote City. She has become increasingly stressed over the pressure by family to relocate to Coyote City.

In their search for alternative options, Mrs. Hutch's family learned that the clinic in Coyote City recently integrated telehealth to its primary care service line aimed at providing local care to patients located in rural townships served by the clinic. While Mrs. Hutch possessed basic computer skills that she used to interact with her family and friends using email and an audio-visual communication program, her family replaced her computer with a newer, state-of-the-art computer, and her grandson, Ben, assisted her in setting up the computer and establishing her portal access system to the clinic. Ben provided step-by-step instruction for his grandmother on how to (a) operate her new computer, (b) access the Coyote City clinic using her secure patient portal, (c) how to enter requests to specific providers (i.e., nurse, pharmacist, physical therapist), and (d) how to troubleshoot common computer, Internet, and patient portal technology problems. Along with a technician from the clinic, Mrs. Hutch was also provided instruction on using the portal to access her healthcare provider and on use of computer attachments, or peripheral equipment and devices, such as a stethoscope for remote electronic auscultations, blood pressure cuff and measurement, and pulse oximeter, all of which can wirelessly transmit vital information to her healthcare provider and be entered in her eHealth record, instantly.

The addition of telehealth services for primary care allowed Mrs. Hutch to access her healthcare provider, clinic nurses, and pharmacist to discuss changes in health status and self-managed healthcare needs. With that, the direct-to-consumer telehealth services have given Mrs. Hutch the necessary human interaction with her nurse and other healthcare providers via the clinic's patient portal. While the learning curve for using the direct-to-consumer telehealth computer systems was steep, with the in-person support of Mrs. Hutch's grandson, Ben, she became comfortable in using the computer system and basic troubleshooting of connectivity issues. Mrs. Hutch's family is confident that she will receive safe and effective care in her home until she is unable to live independently, using telehealth care.

IMPLICATIONS OF TELEHEALTH FOR RURAL NURSING PRACTICE

Telehealth Program Implementation Considerations

Since promulgation of the Affordable Healthcare Act in 2010, proprietary and academic nurse-led clinics have increased in numbers due, in part, to increases in healthcare services demands. Telehealth services provided by nurse-led clinics are a novel method of healthcare delivery, but one that is growing and providing opportunities for nurses and other healthcare providers in multidisciplinary teams to render value-based care at a reasonable cost (National University, 2016). While the long-term impact of telehealth on healthcare costs and quality of care outcomes have yet to be realized, nurses are in a unique position to explore a variety of opportunities for delivering effective care in ways that acknowledge the changing consumer landscape (Lee & Kaiser, 2016). With the development and expansion of sustainable technologies that support the delivery of telehealth primary care services, nursing practice can further expand nursing care services to rural dwellers and underserved populations.

Prior to purchasing equipment, training providers, and going live in program implementation, a precise vision for achieving strategic healthcare goals for specific rural populations must be articulated. A need analysis can provide planners with a clear understanding of the nature and scope of unmet healthcare needs, provide a foundation for implementation, clarify objectives and shared expectations, improve coordination of services and resources, and provide support structures for program evaluation (Gough et al., 2015). Thus, the key to implementing a viable and sustainable telehealth care delivery program is thorough planning.

To deliver healthcare services using telehealth modalities, patient disclosures must be made and mechanisms must be in place to assure adherence to regulatory and accreditation requirements, regardless of type of provider (e.g., nurse, physician). At a minimum, healthcare providers must disclose or provide (a) specific services provided; (b) provider contact information; (c) licensure and qualifications of providers and associates; (d) fees for services and how payment will be made; (e) financial interests, other than fees charged; (f) appropriate uses and limitations of the site, including emergency health situations; (g) uses and response times for emails, electronic messages, and other communications transmitted via telehealth technologies; (h) to whom patient health information may be disclosed and for what purpose; (i) rights of patients with respect to protected patient health information; and (j) information collected and any passive tracking mechanisms used (Federation of State Medical Boards, 2014).

Scope of Practice

In primary care practice settings, many conditions are amenable to telehealth interventions. Conditions most sensitive to telehealth interventions are those with a reasonable level of certainty for establishing a diagnosis and generating a treatment plan, especially when visual information coupled with access to a medical record containing diagnostic studies and imaging results is available (American Telemedicine Association [ATA], 2014). Thus, chronic disease management is commonly an integral aspect of telehealth care.

Practice protocols and licensing requirements vary from state to state. In general, telehealth practice requires that nurse providers are licensed, or under the jurisdiction of the state board of nursing of the state in which the patients receiving telehealth care are located. Thus, the practice of nursing occurs at the location of the patient at the time telehealth technologies are used in the delivery of healthcare services.

Reimbursement for telehealth services is becoming standard in many states. Increasingly, states are implementing parity laws that require some payers to reimburse telehealth services to the same extent as in-person services. As of early 2017, 31 states and Washington, DC have private payer parity laws, and 20 states and Washington, DC have Medicaid parity laws (Gough et al., 2015). Rules for patients' locations (i.e., the originating site) during telehealth encounters are increasingly becoming more flexible to allow for patients' homes and schools to be authorized originating sites for reimbursable telehealth encounters. In 2016, Hawaii, Minnesota, and Washington state expanded reimbursement for real-time, audio-visual virtual telehealth visits with patients in their homes, and Hawaii and Missouri expanded reimbursement for virtual telehealth visits with patients at their schools (Gough et al., 2015). Thus, regardless of the type of nursing practice (e.g., clinic nurse, advanced practice nurse, nurse leader), understanding and adhering to scope of practice and other state regulations is critical to the success of implementing and sustaining telehealth nursing practice, and documenting outcomes.

CONCLUSION

Telehealth nursing is one of the fastest growing areas of healthcare, and has the potential to transform healthcare access, safety, and quality of healthcare for persons living in rural and frontier areas. Telehealth care trends currently shaping nursing practice include (a) transformation of the application of telehealth from increasing access to care to providing convenient sources of care and reducing healthcare costs; (b) expansion of telehealth from addressing urgent care episodes and chronic conditions; and (c) migration of telehealth from hospitals to satellite clinics to homes with mobile devices (Dorsey & Topol, 2016).

Future telehealth applications are boundless; from remote primary care visits to precise monitoring and treatment of patients, nursing care via telehealth is key to serving people where they live. Chronic care management of diabetes and precise monitoring, with adjustments in administration of insulin, for example, via electronic and virtual connections to patients' insulin pumps are possible. Telehealth technologies, including peripheral add-ons can be used to accurately and safely administer medications and to monitor untoward effects, reactions, therapeutic responses, toxicity, and incompatibilities (National Council of State Boards of Nursing [NCSBN], 2014). With vast and rapid changes in healthcare and healthcare technologies such as telehealth, it is imperative that nurses remain engaged and at the forefront of telehealth, as an ever-expanding care delivery system.

REFERENCES

Agency for Healthcare Research and Quality. (2015). *2014 national healthcare quality and disparities report: Chartbook on rural health care.* AHRQ Pub. No. 15-0007-9-EF. Rockville, MD: Author. Retrieved from https://www.ahrq.gov/sites/default/

files/wysiwyg/research/findings/nhqrdr/2014chartbooks/ruralhealth/
2014nhqdr-ruralhealth.pdf

American Academy of Ambulatory Care Nursing. (2011). *Scope & standards of practice for professional telehealth nursing* (5th ed.). Pitman, NJ: Author. Retrieved from https://www.aaacn.org/practice-resources/publications

American Telemedicine Association. (2014). *Practice guidelines & resources.* Retrieved from http://hub.americantelemed.org/resources/telemedicine-practice-guidelines

Bolin, J., Bellamy, G., Ferdinand, A., Kash, B., & Helduser, J. (2015). *Rural healthy people 2020* (Vol. 2). College Station: Texas A&M Health Science Center School of Public Health, Southwest Rural Health Research Center. Retrieved from http://sph.tamhsc.edu/srhrc/docs/rhp2020-volume-2.pdf

Dorsey, E. R., & Topol, E. J. (2016). State of telehealth. *New England Journal of Medicine, 375*, 154–161. doi:10.1056/NEJMra1601705

Fraiche, A. M., Eapen, Z. J., & McClellan, M. B. (2017). Moving beyond the walls of the clinic. *Journal of the American College of Cardiology: Heart Failure, 5*(4), 297–304.

Federation of State Medical Boards (2014). *Model policy for the appropriate use of telemedicine in the practice of medicine.* Retrieved from https://www.fsmb.org/Media/Default/PDF/FSMB/Advocacy/FSMB_Telemedicine_Policy.pdf

Garcia, M. C., Faul, M., Massetti, G., Thomas, C. C., Hong, Y., Bauer, U. E., & Iademarco, M. F. (2017). Reducing potentially excess deaths from the five leading causes of death in the rural United States, *Morbidity and Mortality Weekly Report Surveillance Summaries 2017, 66*(2), 1–7. Retrieved from https://www.cdc.gov/mmwr/volumes/66/ss/pdfs/ss6602.pdf

Gough, F., Budhrani, S., Cohn, E., Dappen, A., Leenknecht, C., Lewis, B., … Bernard, J. (2015). ATA practice guidelines for live, on-demand primary and urgent care. *Telehealth and e-Health, 21*(3), 233–241. doi:10.1089/tmj.2015.0008

Graves, B. A., Ford, C. D., & Mooney, K. D. (2013). Telehealth technologies for heart failure disease management in rural areas: An integrative research review. *Online Journal of Rural Nursing and Health Care, 13*(2), 56–83. Retrieved from http://rnojournal.binghamton.edu/index.php/RNO/article/view/282

Health Resources & Services Administration. (2016). Medically underserved areas and populations (MUA/Ps). Retrieved from https://bhw.hrsa.gov/shortage-designation/muap

Health Resources & Services Administration—HRSA Data Warehouse (2017). Shortage areas. Retrieved from https://datawarehouse.hrsa.gov/topics/shortageAreas.aspx

HealthIT.gov. (2017). What is telehealth? Retrieved from http://www.healthit.gov/providers-professionals/faqs/what-telehealth-how-telehealth-different-telemedicine

Hofmeyer, J., Leider, J., Satorius, J., Tanenbaum, E., Basel, D., & Knudson, A. (2016). Implementation of telemedicine consultation to assess unplanned transfers in rural long-term care facilities, 2012-2015: A pilot study. *Journal of Post-Acute and Long-Term Care Medicine, 17*(11), 1006–1010. doi:10.1016/j.jamda.2016.06.014

Jones, J. (2012). Telehealth. In J. J. Fitzpatrick & M. W. Kazer (Eds.), *Encyclopedia of nursing research* (3rd ed.). New York, NY: Springer Publishing.

Kaiser, L. S. & Lee, T. H. (2015). Turning value-based health care into a real business model. *Harvard Business Review.* Retrieved from http://www.medtronic.com/us-en/transforming-healthcare/aligning-value/turning-value-based-health-care-into-a-real-business-model-hbr.html

Knapp, T. R. (2016). *Legislative and policy recommendations for telehealth, telemedicine and digital healthcare delivery in the United States.* Unpublished paper, 1–6.

Kusmin, L. D. (2016). Rural America at a glance. *Economic Information Bulletin No. 162.* Washington, DC: U.S. Department of Agriculture. Retrieved from https://www.ers.usda.gov/webdocs/publications/80894/eib-162.pdf?v=42684

Moy, E., Garcia, M. C., Bastian, B., Rossen, L. M., Ingram, D. D., Faul, M., ... Iademarco, M. F. (2017). Leading causes of death in nonmetropolitan and metropolitan areas—United States, 1999–2014. *Morbidity and Mortality Weekly Report Surveillance Summaries 2017, 66*(1), 1–8. doi:10.15585/mmwr.ss6601a1

National Council of State Boards of Nursing. (2014). *The National Council of State Boards of Nursing (NCSBN®) position paper on telehealth nursing practice.* Retrieved from https://www.ncsbn.org/14_Telehealth.pdf

National University. (2016). National University nurse-managed clinic in Watts, Los Angeles collaborates with telehealth companies to expand access to virtual health care services. Retrieved from https://www.nu.edu/News/Expand-Access-to-Virtual-Health-Care-Services.html

Sabesan, S., Simcox, K., & Marr, I. (2012). Medical oncology clinics through videoconferencing: An acceptable telehealth model for rural health patients and health workers. *Internal Medicine Journal, 42*(7), 780–785. doi:10.1111/j.1445-5994.2011.02537.x

Smith, C. E., Spaulding, R., Piamjariyakul, U., Werkowitch, M., Yadrich, D. M., Hooper, D., ... Gilroy, R. (2015). mHealth clinic appointment PC tablet: Implementation, challenges and solutions. *Journal of Mobile Technology in Medicine, 4*(2), 21–32. doi:10.7309/jmtm.4.2.4

Totten, A. M., Womack, D. M., Eden, K. B., McDonagh, M. S., Griffin, J. C., Grusing, S., & Hersh, W. R. (2016). *Telehealth: Mapping the evidence for patient outcomes from systematic reviews* (Technical Brief No. 26, AHRQ Publication No.16-EHC034-EF). Rockville, MD: Agency for Healthcare Rsearch and Quality. Retrieved from https://www.ncbi.nlm.nih.gov/books/NBK379320/pdf/Bookshelf_NBK379320.pdf

U.S. Department of Agriculture. (2016). State fact sheets: South Dakota. Retrieved from https://data.ers.usda.gov/reports.aspx?State-FIPS=46&StateName=South%20Dakota&ID=17854#.VMk83GjF83l

van Houwelingen, C., Moerman, A., Ettema, R., Kort, H., & ten Cate, O. (2016). Competencies required for nursing telehealth activities: A Delphi study. *Nurse Education Today, 39*, 50–62. doi:10.1016/j.nedt.2015.12.025

CHAPTER 12

Experiences of Nurses Living in Rural Communities Who Commute for Employment

Laurie J. Johansen

DISCUSSION QUESTIONS

- List several circumstances that give rise to nurses experiencing a blurring of personal and professional boundaries as they live in a rural community.
- What are some challenges nurses face, related to their visibility and lack of anonymity, as they live and practice nursing in rural communities?
- How do the connections nurses make with their coworkers differ when working in a rural, healthcare facility, compared to working in a non-rural healthcare setting?
- Describe how RNs experience feeling valued as professional nurses in their rural, home communities.

In the United States, the rural population accounts for approximately 14% of the population residing on 72% of the landmass (U.S. Department of Agriculture [USDA], Economic Research Service, 2016). Benefits and challenges emerge with such demographically distinct features. One challenge faced by the rural population is a reduced ability to access healthcare due to various healthcare disparities. Factors affecting access to healthcare for the rural population are complex. However, one distinct factor affecting access to healthcare is a decreased availability of healthcare professionals, with a shortage of healthcare professionals creating barriers for rural dwellers to access healthcare services (National Rural Health Association [NRHA], 2016).

BACKGROUND

One factor that contributes to the lack of availability of healthcare professionals for the rural population is the increasing number of RNs driving away, or commuting away, from their rural, home communities for employment (Skillman, Palazzo, Keepnews, & Hart, 2006). Using 2004 data from the National Sample Survey of Registered Nurses (NSSRN), Skillman, Palazzo, Doescher, and Butterfield (2012) reported approximately 37% of RNs living in rural communities commuted for employment. In fact, the percentage of RNs commuting from rural, home communities for employment increased from 14% in 1980 to 37% in 2004. Further commuter trend data have not been published due to discontinuation of the NSSRN survey data collection. However, there is no evidence the commuter trend of RNs has stabilized or diminished. Additionally, in the literature, there is no focus on the impact of commuter trends of RNs on the availability of nurses working in rural healthcare settings.

Little is known about the experiences of RNs commuting for employment and the impact of those decisions. However, there are assumptions that higher wages in larger healthcare settings are a driving force of RNs' employment decisions (Skillman et al., 2012). It is known that the per capita rate of RNs residing in rural areas is lower than urban areas in the United States, with rural areas having 852.7 RNs per 100,000 people, compared to 934.8 RNs per 100,000 people in urban areas (Health Resources and Services Administration [HRSA], 2013). This per capita rate of RNs takes into account only the residences of RNs, not the per capita rate of RNs working in rural areas. When considering the rural population's access to healthcare, it is important to consider the impact of a continued trend of RNs commuting away from rural communities, adding to the potential for inadequate numbers of RNs practicing in rural healthcare settings. The looming nursing shortage (Snavely, 2016), coupled with decisions of RNs to commute for employment, potentially decreases access to quality healthcare in rural communities.

A qualitative study completed in 2017 explored the experiences of RNs living in rural communities who commuted to nonrural healthcare settings for employment. This chapter provides information about a portion of the findings from that study, which leads to greater understanding of RNs experiences and the potential implications for rural populations.

METHOD

A descriptive phenomenological study approach (Dahlberg, Nyström, & Dahlberg, 2008) was used to describe RNs' experiences living in rural communities while commuting to nonrural healthcare settings for employment. The sample selection process sought to recruit currently licensed RNs with varied experiences surrounding the phenomenon of commuting away. Specifically, RNs, living in rural communities with critical access hospitals located within those rural communities ("rural" defined as less than 2,500 residents), were sought, with those RNs commuting to nonrural healthcare settings for employment. Purposeful sampling with snowballing was used to seek variations in the RNs' experiences, including experiences practicing as a nurse, number of years practicing nursing, levels of education, types of worksites, length of residence in a rural community, and experiences with commuting for employment. In the end, 16 nurses participated in this study.

FINDINGS

The core meaning, or essence, of the phenomenon of commuting away for RNs who live in rural communities, and commute away to nonrural healthcare settings, was found to be *commuting to achieve personal and professional goals while being a nurse in a rural community*. One major component of the essence was identified as *being a nurse in a rural community*, which is the focus of this chapter.

Being a Nurse in a Rural Community

Nurses shared a wide array of experiences living in rural communities, some unique to each nurse and others similar to other nurses. However, whether the nurses had lived in their home communities their entirelives, or had recently moved to the rural community, all the nurses experienced *being a nurse in a rural community*. Discussion of these findings follows, weaving connections in the literature to the understanding of *being a nurse in a rural community*.

PRACTICING NURSING IN THE RURAL COMMUNITY

While *being a nurse in a rural community*, nurses had varying experiences working as healthcare professionals in rural, healthcare settings. Some had practiced in rural healthcare settings as a nurse, an emergency medical technician, or perhaps a nursing assistant, while others had never practiced as a healthcare professional in any rural healthcare setting. Irrespective of their previous experiences, they all had perceptions about what it would be like to be a rural nurse. Rural nurses were described as being "jacks of all trades" with diverse roles that required vast knowledge bases. Such role diffusion was supported within the rural nursing theory (Long & Weinert, 1989).

Nurses in this study had differing perceptions about the skills used by rural nurses, with some believing rural nurses used their professional skills more fully in rural healthcare settings, compared to skills used in nonrural healthcare settings. Other nurses had opposing perspectives, believing nurses would lose nursing skills if they practiced in rural healthcare settings because certain skills would not be used often enough. It is valuable to understand all perspectives about what it would be like to be a rural nurse. Differing perceptions surrounding the value of the roles of all nurses, including the rural nurse, have been found in the literature. Jackman, Myrick, and Yonge (2010) found the need for all roles of the nurse to be perceived, and represented, as important without diminishing the role of the rural nurse, in order to prevent negative influences on rural healthcare. Medves, Edge, Bisonette, and Stansfield (2015) went on to report the need to illuminate the opportunities for rural nurses to use all their nursing skills, as nurse specialists in rural nursing, in an effort to retain nurses in rural healthcare settings. In the end, differing perceptions were found, surrounding the perceived skills needed to practice rural nursing, and the subsequent impact on employment decisions.

As nurses shared their varying perspectives of skills needed to practice as rural nurses, it became evident that not all nurses felt comfortable with the role diffusion required to practice successfully as a rural nurse. Nurses shared their sense of discomfort and anxiety related to feeling unsure of their own ability to function as a rural nurse. The idea of leaving their practice in a nonrural healthcare setting to return to rural practice was daunting for some. Nurses in this study are not alone with such feelings. In 2009, Hunsberger, Baumann, Blythe, and Crea found similar findings, with nurses being uncomfortable and stressed practicing rural nursing with skills that they did not use on a routine basis. In the end, in this study, a wide range of experiences, perceptions, and feelings surrounding rural nursing came to be understood.

The type of care given to the people served in a rural healthcare settings was perceived to be different than care provided in nonrural healthcare settings. The rural environment was experienced as being more intimate, with nursing practice being more hands on in a caring and personal setting. One nurse said, "I just feel that it's not just numbers in and out . . . I love the more caring atmosphere that I think rural nursing brings to the table." Similar descriptions of care provided in rural healthcare settings were reported by Baernholdt, Jennings, Merwin, and Thornlow (2010) with rural nurses creating settings that made patients "feel at home" (p. 1350) where "nurses cared about me" (p. 1349). Individualized, hands-on patient care was found to be a hallmark of rural nursing for Baernholdt et al., as well as this study.

Caring for People You Knew and/or People Who Knew You in Rural Communities

As nurses practiced in rural healthcare settings, they experienced providing care for people they knew and people who knew them, with patients including community members, neighbors, friends, or family. Similar to the study by Scharff (2013), nurses working in rural healthcare settings within their home communities regarded themselves to be more connected to their home communities and the people served within those communities. Nurses got to know their patients better, noticing that patients were more receptive to them, finding, "Families could talk to me easier . . . They respond to you better." However, a lack of separation existed between the personal and professional lives of these nurses. Patients would ask about the personal life of the nurse, including information about who their family members were and details about their family as found in the rural nursing theory (Long & Weinert, 1989). The acceptance of the nurse was, at times, dependent on the concept of outsider/insider, with the familiarity between patients and their healthcare providers being a key component in the patient's acceptance of help from the medical professional.

One particular concern that surfaced about practicing rural nursing was the fear of caring for family and friends who were in need of urgent treatment. Being the primary person responsible for assisting a neighbor or family member in an emergency situation was daunting. Similar to the findings by Scharff (2013), fear also arose as the nurses contemplated future interactions that would occur in the community as the nurse communicated with family and community members. One nurse in this study shared:

> I don't want my neighbor and my family coming into the emergency room and I have to work on them [in rural, home community]. That scared me terribly. It still does. I don't want to be that first person that sees them and has to do that . . . And then you're seeing those people, whether it turns out good or bad, all the time, and it's hard . . . You're with those people all the time and so what if things don't go right? Then you have that where people hold you accountable for that whether you could have done something different or not, and I just think its way, way, way more personal and hard.

By the same token, findings revealed that not all nurses were comfortable knowing about patient outcomes in these situations, such as the death of a patient, before the family knew.

> Ninety-five percent of the patients you run into you know, both personally, community, you know them. That's very hard . . . always knowing the patients and you see them at vulnerable times . . . There is a death . . . You know before their family even knows.

Along with the connections experienced between nurses and patients came nurses' concerns surrounding the maintenance of patient confidentiality, due to a lack of separation between the personal and professional lives of rural nurses. Caring for someone with whom the nurse socially interacted in the community brought challenges maintaining privacy for patients. The feelings nurses experienced regarding the blurring of personal and professional lives in these situations ranged from contented or neutral feelings, to feelings of being uncomfortable.

Finally, due to the distinctive nature of the blurring of personal and professional lives between nurses and their patients in rural communities, nurses living in rural communities felt uncomfortable dealing with situations that involved legal aspects of the lives of their patients. One nurse shared:

> I had a situation where it was a neighbor . . . and there was alcohol involved. By law, I have to report it, and I knew that if I did, [the neighbor] would be in a lot of trouble again, and it was really hard . . . It was really hard . . . I was like, "I have no choice. I have to notify the police." I remember hugging [the neighbor's spouse], and I started crying . . . Sometimes the community would say, "How could you do that?" I'm like, "Oh, you just don't understand."

The providing of care to patients in rural healthcare settings is distinctive, as healthcare professionals care for people they know and people who know them. The beauty of this context parallels the challenges faced by nurses as they live *being a nurse in a rural community*.

CONNECTION TO COWORKERS

The blurring of the lines between nurses' personal and professional lives extended beyond patient care to include the connections nurses made with their coworkers, while working in a rural healthcare setting. Nurses knew everyone with whom they worked on a personal and professional level, creating a feeling of being a part of a family with these people, including medical providers and ancillary staff. Scharff (2013) summarized the connections between coworkers in rural settings, stating:

> Although it is likely that nurses in any setting develop close relationships, rural nurses are in the distinctive situation of being personally acquainted with all of those around them, so that the depth of interaction is potentially greater and the accountability for interpersonal exchange is a constant that is simply not present in other settings. (p. 250)

In this study, the resulting connections between coworkers in rural healthcare settings led to feelings of obligation to each other. One nurse in this study stated, "The relationship that you had with the rest of your staff, it was a tighter bond, because there were a smaller number of you, and you knew that you needed to be there for each other." Feelings of concern for their coworkers and patients followed the nurses into their personal lives and their time away from work. Also, with the nurses' residences being relatively close to the healthcare facility, it was convenient for nurses to get called back in to work when needed. It was not unusual for the nurses to feel obligated to go back in to work when needed during their time off because there were so few nurses working at the facility. MacKusick and Minick (2010) found that feelings of obligation were correlated with nurses leaving clinical practice due to nurses being called in to work on their time off and nurses feeling as though they never recover from the strain of working as a nurse. Similar feelings appeared in this study:

> When I worked in . . . [rural home community], it was almost too easy for me to pick up [hours] because I was too convenient, and that's where I burned myself out . . . because I was five blocks away. I was way too accessible . . . It was too easy for me to say yes, and I got too involved.

Thus, the experiences brought about by the connections to coworkers in rural healthcare settings had the potential to bring about feelings of obligation for the rural nurse. Just as the nurses' experiences working in rural healthcare facilities varied, nurses' feelings about connections to coworkers varied. Some nurses appreciated feeling like part of a family working in a rural healthcare facility, and missed those connections as they commuted to nonrural healthcare settings for employment. Other nurses appreciated feeling more disconnected from their coworkers as they commuted for employment, valuing a more distinct boundary between personal and professional lives and fewer feelings of obligation.

One last consideration found in this study regarding coworker connections in rural healthcare settings was the impact that currently employed people in a rural healthcare setting had on prospective employees. As nurses thought about seeking employment in a rural healthcare facility, they knew that they would be working with every professional in that healthcare facility. Thus, if there was an individual in that rural healthcare facility with whom the nurse would prefer not to work, their employment decision may have been swayed. One nurse discussed this, stating:

> There is also the fact that you know who works there [in rural facility], and you maybe don't want to necessarily work with them and you know you're going to work with them all the time . . . You don't want to go to work every day and just cringe to go to work . . . because there are only a few people that work there.

Nurses shared many experiences *Being a Nurse in a Rural Community*, including the blurring of the lines between their personal and professional lives. While working in rural healthcare settings, connections nurses made with their coworkers created varying feelings about the subsequent benefits, as well as challenges, in their personal and professional lives.

CONNECTIONS TO RURAL COMMUNITY

As nurses shared their experiences *Being a Nurse in a Rural Community*, they not only had a variety of experiences, or perceptions, of practicing nursing in a rural community, they also had a variety of connections to their rural communities.

All of the nurses in this study lived in a rural community. The nurses' social connections to their rural community were a key part of their lives, which is not exclusive to this sample of nurses. Historically, social networks in rural communities have been found to enrich the social well-being of nurses, as well as their job satisfaction in the rural community (Kulig et al., 2009). Richards, Farmer, and Selvaraj (2005) found that healthcare providers, which included nurses, who lived and practiced in a rural community felt like they were more a part of that community. However, as they commuted for employment to nonrural communities, they felt less connected to their home communities. Similar findings came from this study. As nurses in this study sample commuted for employment, they too experienced changes in their connections to their rural communities, feeling less tied to the community. Some nurses were saddened by this disconnect; others appreciated this experience. Understanding the nurse's experiences with connections to their rural communities led to the following themes.

Everybody Knows Everybody

A common statement made by many nurses was that, in a rural community, everybody knows everybody. People living in rural communities had a high level of information about their neighbors and community members. One nurse commented, "People knew everybody's business. They knew who came in [to the hospital] before you even did." Rural community members were also familiar with who the nurses were in their communities, as well as the nurses' families.

Rural community members knew how important the role of the nurse was to their community. Thus, due to the community members being familiar with the nurses and their families, they were willing to help care for the nurses' families. One nurse spoke about feelings of appreciation for such help, sharing the following experience:

> One time, there was an emergency, and I had to go in, and I didn't have anybody for my youngest, and he was three. So I just brought him with me, and the kitchen staff took him so I could help with the emergency . . . They just fed him brownies and juice for three hours. But that wouldn't happen in a different place.

Several nurses believed that the expectations of their community members required their professional roles as a nurse to extend into personal events, such as attending church or going to a ballgame. As one nurse said, "I'm a nurse in this community. So, at church when somebody faints, you know, everybody runs to me." Community members also came to the nurses' homes requesting assistance with their medical needs, such as assistance with a blood sugar check. Some nurses appreciated these interactions with community members, whereas others voiced discomfort. Community members did not always consider the areas of expertise that a nurse may, or may not have, when asking for assistance, and some nurses felt unprepared to offer assistance when it was out of their area of expertise. Then again, even if the community members were requesting assistance within an area of expertise for the nurse, the situation could be unnerving for the nurse, as one nurse shared:

> [In] rural communities . . . everybody knows what everybody does. So, your phone might ring. When I was getting my hair cut, she's like, "I told the . . . [medical provider] that if I go into labor, because I have quick labors, I was going to pick her up," and she said, "Oh no, you're not. You're going to pick up [nurse participant in this study] on the way because she's the one that does that." So you're like, "Are you really going to call me?" Just different things like that.

Even though the familiarity of community members with the nurse in the rural community was appreciated at times, for many nurses, this familiarity also created difficult situations. Nurses sensed judgments as well as social and professional expectations from community members, because of their role as a nurse in the community. Some social expectations interfered in the personal lives of the nurses and their families.

> When you work in the area you grew up in, you know almost all the people and their families, and certain situations are uncomfortable. And seeing them out—like, the older nurses never went to a bar. They never went to the VFW in town, because they worked at the hospital, and they wanted people to respect them. And I kind of felt the same way, so we just didn't go out.

Professional expectations from the rural community also surfaced about the nurses' employment decisions, with nurses feeling judged about their decisions to commute for employment elsewhere.

> The hospital needs help, why aren't you helping? Why are you going someplace else? You should be here. Quit your job and come here now, because that would be the thing that you should do. You get that strong opinion from the people that say that to you, "Why are you not here?"

The rural community members' familiarity with everybody not only exposed the nurse to judgments, but judgment fell on the nurse's family members as well, which leaked into the rural workplace. One nurse passed on the following experience:

> People know you, and they know who you are, and they know what kind of person you are . . . In a small town, people judge your kids based on your actions. If they like you, they like your kids. If they don't like you

or something that you did, they don't like your kids. Or if your kids did something that was way out in left field, you're going to hear about it first . . . I would hear things at work before I ever heard it from my kids or from anybody else.

In the end, within a rural community, the familiarity of everybody knowing everybody can create a kinship between community members, including nurses within those communities. However, concerns can arise regarding the role of nurses within the community, interfering in the nurses' personal lives.

FAMILY CONNECTIONS

Family connections to the rural community impacted the decision for many of the nurses to live in their rural community. Having family members in the community, some of the nurses had spent their entire lives in their rural community, while others nurses' residential histories ranged from having recently moved to the rural community, having lived in the rural community for several years, or having moved back after being gone for many years.

It was more of a personal, private, family decision that we wanted to have our kids raised in a smaller, safer town. We both are from . . . small towns . . . We definitely have always had that in the back of our minds that we want to be in a smaller town, not in a larger city . . . We wanted to get back closer to family.

The impact of family on the nurse living in a rural community is not new to the nurses in this study. Previous literature has supported the influence of family connections to nurses. Molanari, Jaiswal, and Hollinger-Forrest (2011) studied rural nurses' employment choices and lifestyle preferences, finding that ways of living found in rural communities impacted decisions to seek employment in rural communities. Being close to family was one lifestyle preference sought living in a rural community. Similarly, being close to family was a lifestyle consideration for many of the nurses in this study.

VISIBILITY IN THE RURAL COMMUNITY

With the familiarity of everybody knowing everybody in the rural community, nurses faced a lack of anonymity while living in a rural community. The inevitable blurring of boundaries between the nurses' personal and professional lives resulted in nurses facing challenges preserving anonymity and privacy, not only for themselves and their families but also their patients as well. Social interactions were common between nurses and community members. Community members frequently made contact with the nurses, asking for advice, opinions on health-related problems, or assistance with their medical needs. Such contacts may have been by phone, by community members stopping by a nurse's home, or while a nurse was out and about in the community.

> They can ask you a lot. "What do you think of this?" or "What should I do about that?" . . . "I was told this. What do you think?" or "This is what's happening," and they want you to say . . . They know you're a nurse . . . they expect you to know everything.

Frequently, confidentiality concerns arose when community members asked the nurses about patients in the rural communities. The nurses desired to maintain patient confidentiality for their patients, but found, "It's hard even when somebody says, 'How is so-and-so doing?' You can't say anything . . . They'll still ask, knowing that we can't say anything, but they'll still ask anyway, and it just makes it very difficult." Encounters with community members asking about patient information, or personal advice, occurred regularly at common locations within the community, such as the grocery store, church, or school activities. "You couldn't go to the grocery store without, 'Oh, did you work today? I saw you . . . [at work].' It was definitely a challenge."

Nurses also encountered their patients in their rural communities. At times, patients would disclose their own personal, medical information to the nurse and the group of people surrounding the nurse. In these circumstances, the nurses may have felt pleasure in the acknowledgement of the care they had provided. However, they were also put in a precarious position, as they continued to try to maintain their responsibility to assure patient confidentiality. One nurse explained:

> That's up to them if they want to come up to you in public and acknowledge that you were their nurse . . . It's that "thank you so much for your help" or "for helping my parents." There is that, too, which is kind of nice in a way because you know them and you've got that connection then.

Nurses faced an additional challenge of maintaining patient confidentiality. As nurses lived and worked in their rural, home community, they found it impossible to be able to come home and talk to family and friends about what had been taking place at work. The nurses knew that if they talked about work, even if they did not use specific names of people, the familiarity of everybody knowing everybody in the rural community could lead to family members or friends identifying who was being talked about. In the end, the nurses were unable to get the support they desired from those nearest and dearest to them, experiencing an inability to talk about the joys and burdens of their work. These nurses were not alone with these feelings, with Evanson (2006) finding similar experiences with public health nurses working in rural settings.

Lack of anonymity is a specific concept within the rural nursing theory (Long & Weinert, 1989) and has been commonly reported among other studies including rural nurses. In this study, nurses' feelings about their visibility in their communities ranged from neutral feelings, with a lack of anonymity just being part of a rural life, to this visibility being inconvenient and undesirable. For some nurses in this study, the discomfort with this visibility contributed to their decision to commute for employment outside of their rural, home communities. One nurse shared feelings of relief while commuting:

> I go home and nobody [patients] knows what I do at night after [I go home] . . . I like that people don't know what time I go home at night, and where I live, or what my home phone number is, or anything like that.

The blurring of the personal and professional lives of nurses in rural communities is commonplace. It is important to consider the implications of the visibility of nurses in rural communities and the impact a lack of anonymity may play in nurses' decisions to commute for employment.

RESPECT, TRUST, AND CONFIDENCE IN COMPETENCE

As stated earlier, all the nurses had different experiences living and practicing nursing in the rural community. One noteworthy finding from this study was that, whether the nurses had lived in the rural community their entire lives or had recently moved to the rural community, whether the nurses had worked in the rural community in the past or had never worked in the rural community, all the nurses in this study felt valued by their rural community members. The feeling of being valued came to be through the nurses' perceptions of being respected, trusted, and/or competent as nurses. By virtue of their roles as nurses and being members of the nursing profession, the connections to the close-knit rural community created a context where trust and respect developed.

> I feel like I'm respected, that's for sure. They trust you. Everybody's very trusting in a small town. When you make little connections and things like that in a small town, they remember you. Just the trust and the confidence that they have in you. Even though I was a new nurse at the nursing home, and I had like no experience whatsoever, they just trusted me. If something was wrong, they felt confident that they could tell me, and they felt confident that I would pass things on to the doctor or whoever to get resolved. Even the aides, I think they could sense that too. Families could talk to me a lot easier than some of the pool nurses that were coming in . . . They just trust you a lot more, and they know that you know what they're talking about, and you know kind of their background better . . .

Definitely I feel that people trust me being a nurse, and the confidence they put in me is really nice, too.

Nurses appreciated this sense of feeling valued. For some nurses, this sense of value continued within their rural, home communities even as they commuted for employment. However, this was something that was not experienced within the communities to which the nurses commuted for employment.

Beyond Being a Nurse in a Rural Community

The findings from this study revealed *being a nurse in a rural community* to be one key component of the essence of *commuting to achieve personal and professional goals while being a nurse in a rural community*. The remainder of the study results are not described in detail in this chapter. However, to summarize, although nurses experienced *being a nurse in a rural community*, there was an inability to get all of their personal and professional goals met in their rural, home communities. This, along with some of the experiences nurses faced by *being a nurse in a rural community*, led to nurses commuting to nonrural communities for employment, allowing them to experience different professional connections.

CONCLUSION

Nurses living in rural communities have rich personal and professional experiences. Understanding the complex layers of living as a nurse in a rural community adds depth to the understanding of nurses' decisions to commute away from their rural home communities for employment. This new knowledge can be used to create future recruitment and retention strategies for nurses practicing in rural settings. Successful interventions can alleviate the potential for a scarcity of RNs in the rural United States, diminishing barriers the rural population face accessing healthcare.

REFERENCES

Baernholdt, M., Jennings, B. M., Merwin, E., & Thornlow, D. (2010). What does quality care mean to nurses in rural hospitals? *Journal of Advanced Nursing, 66*(6), 1346–1355. doi:10.1111/j.1365-2648.2010.05290.x

Dahlberg, K., Nyström, M., & Dahlberg, H. (2008). *Reflective lifeworld research.* Lund, Sweden: Studentlitteratur.

Evanson, T. A. (2006). Intimate partner violence and rural public health nursing practice: Challenges and opportunities. *Online Journal of Rural Nursing and Health Care*, 6(1), 7–20. Retrieved from http://rnojournal.binghamton.edu/index.php/RNO/article/view/162

Health Resources and Services Administration, Bureau of Health Professions, National Center for Health Workforce Analysis. (2013). *The U.S. nursing workforce: Trends in supply and education.* Retrieved from https://bhw.hrsa.gov/sites/default/files/bhw/nchwa/projections/nursingworkforcetrendsoct2013.pdf

Hunsberger, M., Baumann, A., Blythe, J., & Crea, M. (2009). Sustaining the rural workforce: Nursing perspectives on worklife challenges. *The Journal of Rural Health*, 25(1), 17. doi:10.1111/j.1748-0361.2009.00194.x

Jackman, D., Myrick, F., & Yonge, O. (2010). Rural nursing in Canada: A voice unheard. *Online Journal of Rural Nursing and Health Care*, 10(1), 60–69. Retrieved from http://rnojournal.binghamton.edu/index.php/RNO/article/view/74

Kulig, J. C., Stewart, N., Penz, K., Forbes, D., Morgan, D., & Emerson, P. (2009). Work setting, community attachment, and satisfaction among rural and remote nurses. *Public Health Nursing*, 26(5), 430–439. doi:10.1111/j.1525-1446.2009.00801.x

Long, K. A., & Weinert, C. (1989). Rural nursing: Developing the theory base. *Research and Theory for Nursing Practice*, 3(2), 113–127.

MacKusick, C. I., & Minick, P. (2010). Why are nurses leaving? Findings from an initial qualitative study on nursing attrition. *MEDSURG Nursing*, 19(6), 335–340. Retrieved from http://amsn.inurse.com/sites/default/files/documents/practice-resources/healthy-work-environment/resources/MSNJ_MacKusick_19_06.pdf

Medves, J., Edge, D., Bisonette, L., & Stansfield, K. (2015). Supporting rural nurses: Skills and knowledge to practice in Ontario, Canada. *Online Journal of Rural Nursing and Health Care*, 15(1), 7–41. Retrieved from http://rnojournal.binghamton.edu/index.php/RNO/article/view/337

Molanari, D. L., Jaiswal, A., & Hollinger-Forrest, T. (2011). Rural nurses: Lifestyle preferences and education perceptions. *Online Journal of Rural Nursing and Health Care*, 11(2), 16–26. Retrieved from http://rnojournal.binghamton.edu/index.php/RNO/article/view/27

National Rural Health Association. (2016). About rural health care. Retrieved from http://www.ruralhealthweb.org/go/left/about-rural-health

Richards, H., Farmer, J., & Selvaraj, S. (2005). Sustaining the rural primary healthcare workforce: Survey of healthcare professionals in the Scottish Highlands. *Rural and Remote Health*, 5(1), 1–14. Retrieved from http://www.rrh.org.au/publishedarticles/article_print_365.pdf

Scharff, J. E. (2013). The distinctive nature and scope of rural nursing practice: Philosophical bases. In C. A. Winters (Ed), *Rural nursing: Concepts, theory, and practice* (4th ed., pp. 243). New York, NY: Springer Publishing.

Skillman, S. M., Palazzo, L., Doescher, M. P., & Butterfield, P. (2012). *Characteristics of rural RNs who live and work in different communities.* Retrieved from http://depts.washington.edu/uwrhrc/uploads/RHRC_FR133_Skillman.pdf

Skillman, S. M., Palazzo, L., Keepnews, D., & Hart, L. G. (2006). Characteristics of registered nurses in rural versus urban areas: Implications for strategies to alleviate nursing shortages in the United States. *The Journal of Rural Health*, 22(2), 151–157. doi:10.1111/j.1748-0361.2006.00024.x

Snavely, T. M. (2016). A brief economic analysis of the looming nursing shortage in the United States. *Nursing Economic$*, 34(2), 98–100.

U.S. Department of Agriculture, Economic Research Service. (2016). Population and migration. Retrieved from http://www.ers.usda.gov/topics/rural-economy -population/population-migration.aspx

Achieving Congruence Between Rural Nursing Practice and Theory: The Synergy Model for Patient Care

Sheila Ray Montgomery and Judith M. Paré

DISCUSSION QUESTIONS

- A rural nurse meets a patient in clinic who has cancelled several appointments. This is very serious because she has a history of an aortic dissection and needs to maintain her blood pressure regimen. The patient states she lives 60 miles from clinic and has been busy at work. The patient states she feels fine, and states that you "just want her money." Her blood pressure at clinic is 190/114. Knowing what you do about rural patients and their view of health, explain to this patient the importance of follow-up care. What characteristics would a nurse need to develop to communicate with this patient?
- Healthcare is changing, and rural clinics are scarce. The doctor has prescribed home healthcare for an infected wound. Explain how you would develop a plan of care for an elderly patient living over 100 miles from clinic. How would you establish resources? What characteristics would the nurse need? What could the nurse expect this patient to express during home visits?
- Using the rural nursing theory as a guide, develop a case study for a rural patient living in an area in your state or country. How would providing care for this patient be different than caring for a patient in an urban area? Match the nurse's characteristics to the patient's attributes.
- How would rural nursing theory help a new nurse from an urban area integrate successfully into a rural community? What nursing characteristics would an urban nurse have that rural nurses would not deem necessary?

Use of the Synergy Model of Patient Care (Synergy Model) creates an environment that allows for assessment of the patient and the nurse; it defines the relationship in such a dynamic manner that it can be applied universally in all types of patient care settings. Working in congruence with the rural nursing theory, the Synergy Model illustrates the true value of patient-centered care and the achievement of optimal health status. Rural nursing theory will be utilized as described using the three concepts established by Long and Weinert in 1989. The three concepts are definition of health, self-reliance, and lack of anonymity of the rural nurse (Long & Weinert, 1989). Although there has been much work to evolve the rural nursing theory, this chapter uses the rural nursing theory base as a touchpoint to begin the discussion of application to nursing practice. This chapter investigates the rural nursing theory and the Synergy Model, and their relationship to the nursing metaparadigm and the utility for application within rural environments and rural nursing practice.

ANALYZING RURAL THEORY

Rural nursing theory development was first introduced in the 1970s (Yura & Torres, 1975). Although there are articles attempting to expand rural nursing theory, the theory-building process continues (Biegel, 1983; Fawcett, 1984; Lee, 1991; Lee & MacDonagh, 2013; Long & Weinert, 1989; Molinari & Guo, 2013). For this chapter, determining a clear definition of what was referred to as "rural nursing theory" was paramount. Rural nursing theory has evolved from multiple studies (Bales, Winters, & Lee, 2013; Courtney, Tong, & Walsh, 2000; Knudtson, 2000; Long & Weinert, 1989; Magilvy & Congdon, 2000; Pierce, 2001; Roberto & Reynolds, 2001). Shannon (1989) described the need for a rural conceptual base and framework for nursing practice. While the process of defining and expanding the rural nursing theory continues, a nursing practice application was clearly expressed in the work present by Long and Weinert (1989) and is used as a base for this application of rural nursing theory to clinical practice.

THE SYNERGY MODEL

Rural Theory and Synergy Model Through the Lens of the Metaparadigm

The nursing metaparadigm is necessary as a starting place for all nursing theory applications because the four elements are the center focus for patient care. The concepts of environment, human beings, nursing, and health are identified as the major nursing concepts for providing humanistic care (Fawcett & DeSanto-Madey, 2013). The rural nursing theory identifies the rural resident as a patient with unique needs, whereas the Synergy Model allows for a clinical interpretation of skills matching the patient and the nurse.

The Synergy Model provides a unique basis for providing individualized care to the patients in rural healthcare environments. Developed by the American Association of Critical-Care Nurses (AACN, n.d.), the basic tenets of the Synergy Model work well with the concepts of rural nursing theory identifying both patient attributes and nurse competencies working together. The Synergy Model includes eight characteristics that allow for numerous nursing competencies to be embedded into daily nursing practices. These nursing characteristics are clinical judgement, clinical inquiry, facilitation of learning, collaboration, systems thinking, advocacy and moral agency, caring practices, and response to diversity. Patient attributes identified by the Synergy Model include resiliency, vulnerability, stability, complexity, resource availability, participation in care, participation in decision making, and predictability. Synergy occurs when the nursing competencies are in harmony with the patient needs. Working together, the Synergy Model and the rural nursing theory provide a basis for patient care in rural settings. The Synergy Model provides a base for utilization in rural nursing and can be adapted to work in congruence with the rural nursing theory concepts (Lee & Mcdonagh, 2013).

There are four major concepts of the nursing metaparadigm that are described within the Synergy Model. Fawcett and DeSanto-Madeya (2013) identify these concepts as human beings, health, environment, and nursing. Articulating the central focus of rural nursing, rural nurses can communicate their similarities and differences to their urban counterparts. By communicating how their practice is the same and how it is different from their urban counterparts, rural nurses will gain an understanding that may decrease a feeling of isolation from their urban counterparts. The commonality that both groups of nurses experience is their commitment to positive patient care outcomes.

Human Beings

"Human beings" are defined as those receiving care and are holistic beings, constantly changing. The human experience includes mind, body, and spirit (Hardin & Kaplow, 2005). The self-reliance of a rural patient creates a unique human experience. For example, availability of resources in rural communities can create a unique challenge for both the patient and the nurse. These challenges can include socioeconomic and geographical challenges that are unique to rural areas, isolation from specialty services needed to treat chronic illnesses, and opportunities for specialty education to enhance nursing practice and the delivery of evidence-based care (Haven, Warshawsky, & Vasey, 2012).

The Synergy Model allows for a unique interpretation of the patients' needs and the needs of the nurse. The rural nurse must often have advanced clinical inquiry skills and be able to match those to the predictability of the patient's physical, mental, and spiritual needs. Rural patients value their self-reliance and the rural nurse must also be able to assess the patient's ability to actively participate in decision making, while preserving the dignity of the individual patient and the cultural mores of that individual and his or her family.

When providing care for older individuals, rural nurses must acknowledge that rural elders may have different expectations than elders residing in urban settings. Elders residing in rural areas typically reside with family in one household and traditionally, caring for elders becomes a community priority (Borowiak, Kostka, & Kostka, 2015). Disenfranchisement from family and community residents may be misinterpreted as noncompliance to a treatment regime when an elder is forced to relocate in order to receive specialty care that cannot be accessed in a rural setting. This is just one example of how rural nurses have to be in tune to the specific needs of their rural patients. Caring for individuals within a rural community can be challenging. Recognizing the complexities of rural communities and prioritizing needs of unique rural individuals require nursing skills or competencies that can be identified/improved through the Synergy Model.

Health

The Synergy Model states,

> A goal of nursing is to restore a patient to an optimal level of wellness as defined by the patient. Death can be an acceptable outcome, in which the goal of nursing is to move a patient towards a peaceful death. (AACN, 2016, p. 1)

The meaning of "health" within the Synergy Model is what the patient says it is. Rural residents define health as being able to be productive within their communities (Lee & McDonagh, 2013). Rural residents achieve health when they have established balance in their lives. Completing activities and being useful have been established as definitions of health for older residents (Shreffler-Grant, Nichols, Weinert & Ide, 2013). The Synergy Model establishes that the goal of health is defined and incorporated into care as defined by the patient (AACN, 2016). The fostering of rural cultural beliefs about health fits into the Synergy Model without conflict, as health is defined by the patient's own definition.

Environment

The "environment" defined by the Synergy Model encompasses the family, patient, and community (AACN, 2016). The patient remains the center of care driving his or her own healthcare delivery. The systems thinking competency within the Synergy Model explores environmental aspects of care. Three outcomes are described: system level, unit level, and patient level. Nursing interventions are continually adjusted to meet the needs or characteristics of the patients and their families within their prospective environments. Within the Synergy Model, care can be delivered through differing systems of healthcare.

The diversity of the model allows for construction of care within even the most rural healthcare systems.

Nursing

The definition of "nursing" by Fawcett and DeSanto-Madeya (2013) is "the nursing actions or processes that are beneficial to human beings" (p. 6). The nursing role, as defined in the Synergy Model, lists competencies that can be adjusted and achieved within the context of the nurse's environment, scope of practice, and expertise level. The nurses' competencies within the Synergy Model are listed from beginner to expert in each characteristic. The beginner to expert level within the Synergy Model allows the nurse to excel in some areas developing strengths while identifying and improving weaknesses. The Synergy Model allows the nurse to grow and develop competencies necessary to care for a wide range of patient specialties. Within rural communities, such versatility is very important. Rural nurses deal with a wide range of illnesses and disabilities often stretching their capabilities.

APPLICATION OF THE SYNERGY MODEL OF CARE TO CURRENT RURAL NURSING PRACTICE

"Rural" has many definitions, many designed to support one research or another. Everyone will agree that rural means being alone at one time or another. Being rural means that there are fewer people around within the community; meaning at one time or another, decisions are made independently. Rural nurses are no different, finding themselves in situations where their resourcefulness shines and patient solutions are creatively discovered. Rural nursing practice is unique in that isolation is not unique, while anonymity is rare. Rural nursing practice means that many have difficulties defining their practice and intersect often with respiratory therapy, medicine, and pharmacy disciplines (Scharff, 2013). When a patient in a rural community begins to have an emergency, often it is the nearest nurse that gets notified. The patient's family might respond saying it will take the ambulance over an hour to arrive when the nurse can be there in minutes. Rural nurses know their communities and their environments—and the communities know them. Being a rural nurse means that everyone knows when a life is saved, everyone knows. Being a rural nurse means when a life is lost, everyone knows. Finally, being a rural nurse means the nurse may be all they have, may be all the nurse's family has. RNs within rural areas have to be able to comfortably practice in a smaller community, which may create a diffuse patient–nurse boundary. In contrast, rural nurses must also be able to deal with critical patient situations and know their boundaries (Hurme, 2009; Institute of Medicine [IOM], 2005). Rural nursing practice needs a care delivery model that will be flexible enough to meet the unique challenges of rural practice. The Synergy Model presents with a growing body of knowledge creating a scheme for clinical nursing practice.

The Mobility and Flexibility of the Synergy Model

The Synergy Model can be utilized as a care delivery model for rural nursing practice. The dynamic nature of the Synergy Model supports nursing practice in acute, chronic care and ambulatory settings. Providing a foundation for many different nursing practice areas, the Synergy Model is being expanded (Carter & Burnette, 2011; Debourgh, 2012; Gralton & Brett, 2012; Smith & Larew, 2013; Swickard, Swickard, Reimer, Lindell, Winkelman, 2014). Magnet hospitals like Baylor and University of Alabama at Birmingham (UAB) have utilized the Synergy Model to guide nursing practice throughout the facility. Collins and Strother (2008) further expanded the model into educational components of hospital nursing competencies, stating "a clinical nurse specialist (CNS) and nurse educator intervene on the individual patient–family level, the nurse–nurse level and systems level to improve outcomes" (p. 1672). The model centers on the needs of the patient as the center of care (Figure 13.1).

Institutions of higher education are utilizing the Synergy Model to create better student outcomes. At Duquesne University, Pittsburgh, Pennsylvania, the student replaces the patient as the center of care. This unique application to an educational model worked, and Duquesne University adopted the Synergy Model as the basic framework for nursing education. Synergy was created between the university, educators, and students, rather than the hospital, patient, and nurse (Duquesne University, School of Nursing, 2008). The usability and resilience of the Synergy Model allows its application to both nursing practice and education. Collins and Strother (2008) developed a competency tool for clinical competency that utilizes and highlights the versatility of the Synergy Model, creating an environment that allows the patient to be central to care delivery. The Synergy Model defines the patient/nurse

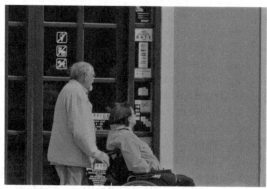

FIGURE 13.1. Disabled elderly person in wheelchair accompanied by caregiver.
Courtesy of Pixabay, https://pixabay.com/en/wheelchair-care-disabled-people-908343/.

relationship in a dynamic format that can be utilized universally in all types of patient care settings.

The Relationship Between Rural Nursing Practice and the Nurse Generalist Identified by the Synergy Model

The Synergy Model recognizes that all patients have similar needs and experience these needs in varied continuums from health to illness (AACN, n.d.). In clinical practice, the rural nurse works within many differing environments requiring competencies that are varied throughout the care spectrum. The concepts of rural nursing theory work in congruence with the Synergy Model to illustrate the impact of nursing care. Shannon (1998) identified a need for a basis of nursing practice that recognized the patients receiving care in rural areas were different from those living in urban environments. No definitive competencies have been developed to define rural nursing practice. This may be because of the generalist nature of rural nursing which is congruent to the Synergy Model's eight nursing competencies (clinical judgement, clinical inquiry, facilitation of learning, collaboration, systems thinking, advocacy and moral agency, caring practices, and response to diversity). The rural nursing theory and the nursing competencies built within the Synergy Model create a relationship that is worthy of further exploration and research.

CRITIQUE OF THE SYNERGY MODEL AS A THEORETICAL FOUNDATION FOR RURAL THEORY AND PRACTICE

The definition of health that expressed rural residents and their lived experiences are related to individuals' ability to be contributors within their communities (Lee & McDonagh, 2013). Rural persons identify health as the ability to participate in the activities in their lives, as the ability to function particularly in rural areas that are dependent on industries in the area. Older residents may define health as relating directly to their ability to work or be useful (Shreffler-Grant et al., 2013). The goal of the Synergy Model is to "restore a patient to an optimal level of wellness as defined by the patient" (AACN, n.d., p. 1). Acknowledging that different patient populations view health differently, the Synergy Model easily incorporates the rural residents' views of health and or wellness.

Bales, Winters, and Lee conducted a qualitative, descriptive study examining health perceptions of rural residents (2013). Six major themes emerged from the research: self-reliance, hardiness, conscientious consumer, informed risk, community support, and inadequate insurance (2013). The study participants included new and old comers to rural communities. Most of the participants attempted to partake in self-care behaviors before seeking medical care, and the degree of self-reliance varied based on how long they lived in a rural area. One couple participating in the study lived rurally only for a short period before retiring. They accessed formal healthcare more quickly than longtime rural residents, and stated the influence included quality healthcare, the diagnosis of chronic health condition, and ease of access before moving to Montana City. In contrast, another participant admitted planning a surgery when ease of travel presented. An older resident cared for her terminally ill husband after undergoing shoulder surgery, demonstrating the endurance rural residents exhibit in the presence of disease burdens. The woman was informed it would cost $118 a day for her husband's care. She abandoned the health recommendations for herself and solicited help from her family to care for her spouse. Despite risks to themselves and warnings from their physicians, these rural residents understood the risk with limited access to emergent healthcare. Wishing to stay within their rural environments, the residents unwaveringly returned to their rural residences. One participant commented, "Those of us that have been here for years, we just try to take care of ourselves without having to get medical attention. Sometimes that is okay. We realize the risk we are taking" (Bales et al., 2013, p. 73). The above provides an example of the harmony that exists between rural nursing theory and the Synergy Model. The attributes of these patients are expressed in the Synergy Model as resiliency, predictability, resource availability, and participation in decision making. The rural nursing theory identifies that rural residents are self-reliant and define health differently than their urban counterparts. Working together between the Synergy Model and the rural nursing theory, a picture of the patient being cared for emerges.

People living in rural communities travel outside their home counties for physician services because of high physician fees, inadequate local services, or an inability of local physicians to meet the needs of the community members (Gamm, Castillo, & Pittman, 2010). Access to healthcare in rural communities is both relative and allegorical. At present, the state of primary healthcare is uncertain. Congress passed the Health Professions Educational Assistance Act of 1976 (HPEA) and the Affordable Care Act (ACA) of 2010. The hope is that one of these legislations helps increase primary care physicians in the rural areas. The Synergy Model allows the nurse to address the concerns of access in healthcare. Of the nursing competencies listed for the nurse systems thinking, collaboration, along with patient advocacy and moral agency, most certainly will be utilized treating rural residents within isolated areas.

Rural residents make decisions to seek care for disease depending on their ideas of the seriousness of their present health condition and their perceptions of the available resources. Rural inhabitants tend to be very independent. The exceptions to seeking medical care are seen in the care sought for children. Rural dwellers will more quickly take children to medical care than themselves (Rasmussen, O'Lynn, & Winters, 2013). As discussed earlier, the eight patient characteristics of the Synergy Model intrinsically recognize the patient's resource availability and participation in care. The Synergy Model patient characteristics support the rural resident in choosing when to seek care, and the nurse competencies allow the nurse to define and develop clinical skills. The nurse can define and develop competencies within the Synergy Model that match the needs of the rural patients and the surrounding community. Different patients develop different ways of operating within the context of their communities. While the rural nursing theory yields the basis for care within rural communities, congruence with the Synergy Model expands the nurse's ability to meet the needs of the individual rural patient. The persons, their direct support system, and their kinship reinforce the foundation of the nurse–patient relationship within the Synergy Model (AACN, n.d.).

Rural nurses experience greater role diffusion to fulfill the requirements of treating patients in underserved and isolated areas. "Health care providers, in rural areas, must deal with a lack of anonymity and much greater role diffusion" (Long and Weinert, 1989, p. 120). While in urban areas nurses may remain distanced from their patients, in rural areas the nurse may have been known to the community for years and most certainly is known as a healthcare provider within the area. The greater role diffusion can be found within the Synergy Model competencies caring practices, response to diversity, and collaboration. The nursing competencies identify and define nurses who are capable and competent to deliver care in rural areas.

FUTURE DIRECTION FOR NURSING RESEARCH

Nurse researchers must examine the utility of integrating the Synergy Model and rural nursing theory for the development of a tool that would aid in the transfer of patients from a rural setting to an urban setting when patient care needs cannot be met locally. The research could be a continuation of the foundational work of Swickard et al. (2014) on the development of a tool using the Synergy Model for patient transfers. The ideal would be an instrument that addresses the unique cultural needs of a rural resident who will now be isolated from home, family, and social supports. The development of this resource would emphasize nurse competencies as identified in the Synergy Model. These competencies would ideally be foundational to the creation of a rural nursing certification specialty.

The need to recognize and support rural nurses is directly linked to retention and recruitment efforts. Future research and exploration into formalizing a rural nurse certification examination are foundational to enhancing rural practice. Although there have been decades of discussion related to rural certification, there is a gap in the literature regarding standardization of this process. Future symposiums highlighting the relationship between rural nursing theory and the Synergy Model hold promise of opening future collaborations across a variety of rural settings and disciplines.

CONCLUSION

Evidence-based practice supports the utility of the Synergy Model for application within rural environments and populations. Although the Synergy Model was originally designed for the critical care environments, it has been expanded into other practice and educational areas. The rural nursing theory foundation can be utilized with the Synergy Model and applied to rural clinical nursing practice. The patient characteristics and the nurse competencies allow for synergy in patient care. The adaptation of nursing competencies into rural clinical practice may have an effect on maximizing resources and creating optimal patient-centered care outcomes. The utility of these theories must be demonstrated by ongoing nursing research. Position papers supported by professional nursing organizations and enhanced lobbying efforts to support legislation that will illuminate the unique needs of rural nursing are essential to support the unique needs of rural nurses and the influence that the application of theory can have on patient care outcomes.

REFERENCES

American Association of Critical-Care Nurses. (n.d.). Synergy model. Retrieved from https://www.aacn.org/nursing-excellence/aacn-standards/synergy-model

American Association of Critical Care-Nurses. (2016). The AACN synergy model for patient care. Retrieved from http://www.aacn.org/wd/certifications/content/synmodel.pcms?menu=certification#Nurse

Bales, R. L., Winters, C. A., & Lee, H. J. (2013). Health needs and perceptions of rural persons. In C. A. Winters (Ed.), *Rural nursing concepts, theory, and practice* (4th ed., pp. 65–78). New York, NY: Springer Publishing.

Biegel, A. (1983). Toward a definition of rural nursing. *Home Health Care Nursing, 1*, 45–46.

Borowiak, E., Kostka, J., & Kostka, T. (2015). Comparative analysis of the expected demands for nursing care services among older people from urban, rural, and institutional environments. *Clinical Interventions in Aging, 10*, 405–412.

Carter, K. C., & Burnette, H. D. (2011). Creating patient-nurse synergy on a medical surgical unit. *Medsurg Nursing Journal, 20*(5), 249–254.

Collins, A. S., & Strothers, D. (2008). Synergy and competence: Tools of the trade. *Journal for Nurses Staff Development, 24*(4), E1–E8. doi:10.1097/01.NND.0000320672.58200.8d

Courtney, M., Tong, S., & Walsh, A. (2000). Older patients in the acute care setting: Rural and metropolitan nurses' knowledge, attitudes and practices. *Australian Journal of Rural Health, 8*, 94–102.

Debourgh, G. (2012). Synergy for patient safety and quality: Academic and service partnerships to promote effective nurse education and clinical practice. *Journal of Professional Nursing, 28*(1), 48–61. doi:10.1016/j.profnurs.2011.06.003

Duquesne University, School of Nursing. (2008). NLN designates Duquesne a center for nursing excellence in education. Retrieved from http://www.duq.edu/news/nln-designates-duquesne-a-center-of-excellence-in-nursing-education

Fawcett, J. (1984). *Analysis and evaluation of conceptual models of nursing.* Philadelphia, PA: F. A. Davis.

Fawcett, J., & DeSanto-Madeya, S. (2013). *Contemporary nursing knowledge: Analysis and evaluation of nursing models and theories* (3rd ed.). Philadelphia, PA: F. A. Davis.

Gamm, L., Castillo, G., & Pittman, S. (2010). Access to quality health services in rural areas—primary care. In L. D. Gamm, L. L. Hutchison, B. J. Dabney, & A. M. Dorsey (Eds.), Rural healthy people 2010: A companion document to Healthy People 2010 (Vol. 2, pp. 17–36), Retrieved from https://srhrc.tamhsc.edu/docs/rhp-2010-volume2.pdf

Gralton, K. S., & Brett, S. A. (2012). Integrating the synergy model for patient care at Children's Hospital of Wisconsin. *Journal of Pediatric Nursing, 27,* 74–81. doi:10.1016/j.pedn.2011.06.007

Hardin, S. R., & Kaplow, R. (2005). *Synergy for clinical excellence: The AACN synergy model for patient care.* Sudbury, MA: Jones & Bartlett.

Haven, D. S., Warshawsky, N., & Vasey, J. (2012). The nursing practice environment in rural hospitals. *Journal of Nursing Administration, 42*(11), 519–525.

Hurme, E. (2009). Competencies for nursing practice in rural critical access hospital. *Online Journal of Rural Nursing and Healthcare, 9*(2), 67–81. Retrieved from http://rnojournal.binghamton.edu/index.php/RNO/article/view/88

Institute of Medicine. (2005). *Quality through collaboration. The future of rural health.* Washington, DC: National Academies Press.

Knudtson, N. (2000). Patient satisfaction with nurse practitioner service in a rural setting. *Journal of American Academy of Nurse Practitioners, 12*(10), 405–412.

Lee, H. J. (1991). Relationship of hardiness and current life events to perceived health and rural adults. *Research in Nursing and Health, 14*(5), 351–359.

Lee, H. J., & McDonagh, M. K. (2013). Updating the rural theory base. In C. A. Winters (Ed.), *Rural nursing: Concepts, theory, and practice* (4th ed., pp 15–34). New York, NY: Springer Publishing.

Long, K. A., & Weinert, C. (1989). Rural nursing: Developing the theory base. *Scholarly Inquiry for Nursing Practice: An International Journal, 3,* 113–127.

Magilvy, J. K., & Congdon, J. G. (2000). The crisis of healthcare transitions for rural older adults. *Public Health Nursing, 17*(5), 336–345.

Molinari, D. L., & Guo, R. (2013). The rural nursing theory: A literature review. In C. A. Winters (Ed.), *Rural nursing: Concepts, theory, and practice* (4th ed., pp. 49–63). New York, NY: Springer Publishing.

Pierce, C. (2001). The impact of culture of rural women's description of health. *Journal of Multicultural Nursing and Health, 7,* 50–53, 56.

Rasmussen, A. D., O'Lynn, C., & Winters, C. A. (2013). Beyond the symptom-action-timeline process: Explicating the health-needs-action process. In C. A. Winters (Ed.), *Rural nursing: Concepts, theory, and practice* (4th ed., pp. 141–157). New York, NY: Springer Publishing.

Roberto, K. A., & Reynolds, S. G. (2001). The meaning of osteoporosis in the lives of rural women. *Healthcare for Women International, 22,* 599–611.

Scharff, J. E. (2013). The distinctive nature and scope of rural nursing practice: Philosophical bases. In C. A. Winters (Ed.), *Rural nursing: Concepts, theory and practice* (4th ed., pp. 241–258). New York, NY: Springer Publishing.

Shannon, A. M. (1998). Developing an educational structure for rural nursing research and theory. In H. J. Lee (Ed.), *Conceptual basis for rural nursing* (pp. 399–407). New York, NY: Springer Publishing.

Shreffler-Grant, J. M., Nichols, E., Weinert, C., & Ide, B. (2013). Complementary therapy and health literacy in rural dwellers. In C. A. Winters (Ed.), *Rural nursing: Concepts, theory, and practice* (4th ed., pp. 469–480). New York, NY: Springer Publishing.

Smith, A. C., & Larew, C. (2013). Strengthening role clarity in acute care nurse case managers application of the synergy model in staff development. *Professional Case Management, 18*(4), 190–198.

Swickard, S., Swickard, W., Reimer, A., Lindell, D., & Winkelman, C. (2014). Adaptation of the AACN synergy model for patient care to critical care transport. *Critical Care Nurse, 34*(1),16–28. doi:10.4037/ccn2014573

Yura, H., & Torres, G. (1975). *Today's conceptual frameworks with baccalaureate nursing programs* (NLN Pub. No. 15–1558, pp. 17–75). New York, NY: National League for Nursing.

CHAPTER 14

Assessing Resilience in Older Frontier Women

Gail M. Wagnild and Linda M. Torma

DISCUSSION QUESTIONS

- Break into small groups and discuss what resilience means to you. How do you see resilience in older women in your own family and friends?
- Identify a group of older women and explore resilience with them. Compare resilience among the groups. How are they alike? How are they different?
- How might nurses work with older women to improve resilience?

Do we help aging adults recognize and perhaps strengthen their resilience? Although there is much written that describes resilience and resilient individuals, there is less information on how one might evaluate individual resilience. Wagnild and Collins (2009) presented a framework for assessing resilience that included the Resilience Scale (RS; Wagnild & Young, 1993) and open-ended questions that provide individuals with opportunities to reflect on and perhaps rediscover their resilience. This strength-based approach encourages individuals to focus on their capabilities and is an important step in helping individuals develop a personal strategy to strengthen resilience. Resilience may facilitate adaptation to changes and challenges that often accompany aging, and this adaptation perhaps will lead to less depression and anxiety, more effective coping, and a more satisfying life. In this chapter, we report on a preliminary study applying this assessment approach with 25 older women.

REVIEW OF LITERATURE

"Resilience" is frequently defined as the ability to adapt or "bounce back" following adversity; it connotes inner strength, competence, optimism, flexibility, and the ability to cope effectively when faced with life's challenges (Hardy, Concato, & Gill, 2004; Wagnild & Young, 1990). Several studies have reported associations between resilience and positive characteristics among aging adults, including forgiveness (Broyles, 2005), morale (March, 2004; Wagnild & Young, 1993), purpose in life, sense of coherence, self-transcendence (Nygren et al., 2005), and self-efficacy (Caltabiano & Caltabiano, 2006). Resilience has also been inversely associated with depression (Torma, 2010; Wagnild, 2009a, 2012; Wagnild & Young, 1993), perceived stress (March, 2004), anxiety (Humphreys, 2003), and fibromyalgia (FM) impact (Torma, 2010).

"Successful" or "healthy aging" has often been defined as physical and mental health that continues into old age, as well as continued social involvement and meaningful activities (Hartman-Stein & Potkanowicz, 2003; Rowe & Kahn, 1997, 1998; Ruuskanen & Ruoppila, 1995; Unger, Johnson, & Marks, 1997). Recently, Harris (2008) has challenged this definition and suggested that rather than striving for successful aging, we should be striving for resilience and resilient responses to life's inevitable difficulties. Aging is a dynamic process, often accompanied by significant adversity, due to the cumulative and synergistic effects of lifestyle behaviors, disease, genetics, and age-related changes (Miller, 2008). The biomedical definition of health as absence of disease inadequately describes the experience of health in persons 65 years of age and older—nearly 90% of Medicare beneficiaries have at least one chronic condition (Hoffman, Rice, & Sung, 1996) and 60% have two or more (Wolff, Starfield, & Anderson, 2002). A person's subjective assessment of his or her ability to function psychologically and physically despite this type of adversity is a much more accurate measure of health in this population (Bryant, Beck, & Fairclough, 2000; Bryant, Corbett, & Kutner, 2001; Wilson & Cleary, 1995).

Aging adults with health problems cannot realistically regain or maintain robust health and independent functioning often associated with a more typical definition of successful aging (Holstein & Minkler, 2003). Many aging adults can strengthen their resilience, however, leading to a meaningful, satisfying, and successful old age, despite declines in health.

BACKGROUND

The percentage of persons more than 65 years of age is expected to grow to an unprecedented 19.6% of the U.S. population by 2030 (Centers for Disease Control and Prevention [CDC], 2003). Currently, older adults constitute approximately 12.2% of the population. In states with substantial frontier populations (six or fewer persons per square mile), the percentage of elders is higher. There are 10 U.S. states in which 30% to 75% of the land area is considered frontier. The proportion of elders in these frontier communities is growing and is projected to double by 2025 (U.S. Census Bureau, 2000). Approximately 15% of the frontier population is 65 years and older; in the three communities reported in this study, 18% to 25% are 65 years and older (Montana County Department of Health and Human Services, 2004).

The majority of elders who survive into old age are women. Approximately 57% of persons 65 years and older are women, and of those 85 years and older, 69% are women. With aging comes a higher incidence of chronic illness and a greater need for healthcare (Wolff et al., 2002). Increasing resilience may help older adults adapt to changes and challenges associated with aging.

Resilience

"Resilience" is the ability to adapt to, learn, and grow stronger from challenges and adversity, leading to lives that are rich, rewarding, and meaningful. Wagnild and Young (1990) identified five interrelated characteristics that constitute resilience and thus enable an individual to adapt and age in a meaningful and satisfying way. These characteristics are:

- *Perseverance*—the act of persistence despite adversity or discouragement
- *Equanimity*—a balanced perspective of life viewed as "sitting loose" and accepting life as it comes
- *Meaningfulness*—recognition of life purpose and a reason for which to live
- *Self-reliance*—belief in one's strengths and capabilities that often comes from experience and wisdom
- *Existential aloneness*—the realization that each life is unique and that while some experiences can be shared, others must be faced alone. Existential aloneness conveys not only a sense of uniqueness but perhaps freedom as well

The process of strengthening resilience in adulthood consists of challenge, support, and success. When confronted with adversity or challenge, a woman who finds a way to meet the challenge and adapt successfully will likely increase her resilience. When she meets subsequent challenges, self-confidence and new problem-solving skills will enable her to adapt successfully again, thus increasing resilience. The process of developing resilience may start early in life with challenges that are successfully met, leading to a greater repertoire of effective problem-solving approaches (Rutter, 1985).

According to Richardson (2002), when individuals are confronted by either planned or unplanned life events, they can choose to reintegrate resiliently, resulting in growth, self-knowledge, and understanding. This leads to an increase in resilience. They can also choose to return to homeostasis, referred to as the "comfort zone." Finally, they can choose to reintegrate with loss, meaning that they may resort to destructive behaviors and substance abuse as a response to life's challenges.

Resilience and Healthy Aging

Resilient women are able to adapt successfully to stress and adversity (Hardy et al., 2004; Wagnild & Young, 1990). Resilience is frequently associated with optimism, flexibility, inner strength, and effective coping. According to Rutter (1985), resilience is not a fixed personality trait. Rather resilience changes as life's demands and circumstances change.

Researchers have focused on resilience and aging only in the last 25 to 30 years with most early research on resilience focusing on children (Garmezy, 1993; Rutter, 1985, 1987, 1993; Werner, 1984, 1992). Wagnild and Young (1990) published one of the first studies on resilience among older women. Their study emphasized strengths and capabilities rather than decline, decrepitude, and disability prevalent in literature up until that time.

The relationship between resilience and healthy aging has been supported in several studies. For instance, resilience is inversely associated with depression (Humphreys, 2003; Wagnild, 2009a, 2009b, 2012; Wagnild & Young, 1993), anxiety (Humphreys, 2003), and perceived stress (March, 2004) and directly related to purpose in life, sense of coherence, self-transcendence, mental health (Nygren et al., 2005; Wells, 2010), morale (March, 2004; Wagnild & Young, 1993), and forgiveness (Broyles, 2005). In several studies with women, resilience is associated with self-reported health status and health-promoting lifestyle practices (Wagnild, 2009a, 2009b; Wells, 2010). In a recent report on 467 urban older women whose average age was 72.3 years (standard deviation [SD] = 7.9), those who were more resilient were significantly more likely to report healthier lifestyles including diet, exercise, stress management, interpersonal support, health responsibility, and self-actualization. More resilient women also reported better overall health and less depression (Wagnild, 2012). This finding was also reported in a recent study that examined resilience as a moderator of the relationship between pain and physical function in older persons who had been living with FM for an average of 23 years (N = 224, average age = 62 years). Levels of resilience were moderately high in this sample despite moderately high levels of pain and functional limitations. Resilience was also positively correlated with age, income, and education, and negatively correlated with depressive symptoms, overall FM impact, and FM pain (Torma, 2010). Resilience did not moderate the effect of pain on physical function as hypothesized, but was instead an independent predictor of physical function in this sample. These findings highlight the important role resilience plays in healthy aging.

RESEARCH METHOD

Design

A descriptive exploratory research design was used for this study. A valid and reliable instrument was used to measure resilience, and open-ended questions specific to the five characteristics of resilience were asked of each participant (Morse, 1991). In addition, each participant was asked about specific challenges she was facing and how she was meeting these challenges. Open-ended questions complemented quantitative measures obtained using the RS (Wagnild & Young, 1993).

Sample

The purposive sample comprised 25 older women who were living independently in their own homes in frontier communities. Inclusion criteria were being 65 years of age or older; being able to read, speak, and write English; and having no known history of cognitive impairment.

Procedures

The study was conducted with the approval of the Institutional Review Board at Montana State University. The researchers invited women to participate who were at Senior Centers, through the Area Agency on Aging, and using a snowball or networking sampling method. The study was explained to women who were interested in participating. Each woman was asked for her consent to participate and to have the assessment audiotaped. The average assessment took 1 hour, with a range of 45 minutes to 2 hours. All were conducted in the women's homes.

Instruments

The RS measured the degree of individual resilience (Wagnild & Young, 1993). The scale covers two factors: personal competence and acceptance of self and life. The RS has been positively correlated with optimism, stress management, self-esteem, and life satisfaction and negatively with depression and helplessness. Items are scored on a 7-point scale from 1 = disagree to 7 = agree. Two subscales derived from factor analysis measure acceptance of self and life (eight items) and personal competence (17 items). Possible scores range from 25 to 175, with higher scores reflecting higher resilience. Scores of 146 to 175 are considered moderate to high, scores from 121 to 145 fall within the midrange, and scores 120 and lower are at the low end of the scale. Cronbach's alpha reliability for the RS in the current study was 0.93.

The health-promoting lifestyle profile (HPLP; Walker, Sechrist, & Pender, 1987) was used to measure health-promoting lifestyles. The HPLP is a 48-item 4-point summated rating scale with "never" coded as 1, "infrequently" coded as 2, "frequently" coded as 3, and "routinely" coded as 4. The HPLP investigates the following six subscales, derived through item analysis: (a) self-actualization, (b) health responsibility, (c) exercise, (d) nutrition, (e) interpersonal support, and (f) stress management. Duffy (1993) reported a Cronbach's alpha internal consistency reliability of 0.92 for the 48-item HPLP with reliability of subscales ranging from 0.65 to 0.85. Cronbach's alpha reliability measures for the HPLP in the current study were 0.91 = total HPLP, 0.91 = self-actualization, 0.87 = health responsibility, 0.65 = exercise, 0.71 = nutrition, 0.80 = interpersonal support, and 0.74 = stress management. These scores are comparable to those reported in previous studies.

Self-reported health status was measured by asking respondents to rate their current health on a 5-point scale as compared to others their age (poor, fair, good, very good, and excellent). This self-report method has been used extensively, corresponds to objective health indicators, and is an acceptable indicator of physical health status (Idler & Benyamini, 1997).

FINDINGS

Demographic Profile

The participants were 25 Caucasian women whose ages ranged from 66 to 85 years (mean age = 75.7 years). Of these, 11 participants were married and living with their spouses and 12 women were widowed; one was divorced and one had never married. Only one participant had fewer than 12 years of education, 11 had completed high school, and 13 had education beyond high school. Nine women reported an annual income of less than $25,000 and eight did not report their income level.

The mean length of time that participants had lived in their community was 45.6 years and ranged from 6 to 73 years. In all, 21 participants reported that they had lived in their communities 25 years or more. Overall, 15 participants resided in a small town, with the remaining 10 participants residing within 2 to 20 miles of the nearest small town. In all, 23 rated their health as good to excellent, with only two reporting their health as fair. All participants reported that they were able to perform activities of daily living without assistance with the exception of one participant who experienced some episodes of urinary incontinence. Most performed instrumental activities of daily living without assistance, with the exception of one participant who needed assistance with housework.

RS and HPLP Scores

The average RS score was 147.1, which is similar to scores obtained on the RS in prior studies with healthy samples of middle-aged and older adults (Broyles, 2005; March, 2004; Nygren et al., 2005; Wagnild, 2003, 2012; Wagnild & Young, 1993) and indicated a moderate-to-high level of resilience. There were nonsignificant relationships between the RS and age, education, and income. The correlation between RS and self-reported health was 0.53 ($p < .02$).

The average score on the HPLP was 142.2. The maximum score possible on the HPLP is 192, suggesting moderate-to-high scores within this sample. There were nonsignificant relationships between the HPLP and age, education, years lived in the community, and income. There were significant relationships between the HPLP and self-reported health status ($r = 0.47, p < .04$). The RS and HPLP were related to each other ($r = 0.52, p < .03$).

Interview Results Within the Resilience Model

Resilience is the ability to adapt successfully to adversity and challenge. Successful adaptation leads to personal growth and self-confidence, which in turn strengthens resilience. According to the model, as resilience develops and strengthens, the probability of adapting successfully to new challenges increases also.

Each participant was asked to describe challenges in her life and responses she used to respond to difficult events. Responses were organized within five essential characteristics of resilience: perseverance, meaningfulness, self-reliance, equanimity, and existential aloneness. Further, each participant was asked to describe how she responded to both minor and major life challenges and the effects of childhood on later adaptation to adversity.

PERSEVERANCE: THE ABILITY TO KEEP GOING DESPITE SETBACKS

Every participant reported that she had been confronted with many challenges; every woman described that meeting challenges required that she put one foot in front of the other and keep going. One woman lost her husband, 45 years of age, to cancer after caring for him throughout his 5-year illness. She admitted that for at least a year after his death, she did not even bother to vacuum or dust because "what was the point?" Gradually she adapted to the loss but it was not easy. She said, "I just made myself make my bed one day, make it the next, and kept on going."

Another participant living with cancer and struggling with the loss of loved ones said, "My sister was murdered two years ago and I've lost two husbands. And that is the hardest. Losing somebody. But my children have seen me get going again. I always get going again. I've been told I have grit!"

A third participant described a friend who was not resilient and aging poorly and said that she stayed in bed with depression most days. She said, "You have to fight all of your life not to be depressed. Sure, I could find a lot to get blue about, too. Because life is kind of depressing. Hard."

MEANINGFULNESS: A SENSE OF PURPOSE IN LIFE

The study participants reported that staying involved in life, having a sense of community, maintaining interests and developing new ones were essential to a healthy old age. Many believed that disengaging from the usual activities of life led to a premature death.

One woman said,

> You have to do something! My husband said that ranchers retired to town and in 3 years they walk themselves to death. They're used to getting up in the morning even if they don't feel good because they have animals to take care of. I think we all have to get up. I think it makes you live longer.

According to the participants, having a purpose in life kept them mentally challenged and permitted them an opportunity to contribute to the well-being of the communities in which they lived. The majority of the women in the study were extensively involved in volunteer work in their communities, which was an important source of productivity for the women and gave them a sense of accomplishment. Many of them had lived in their communities for several decades and were well known.

SELF-RELIANCE: DEPENDING ON ONE'S OWN RESOURCES, JUDGMENT, AND CAPABILITIES

Each woman discussed the process of becoming self-sufficient, or "managing on her own and doing without." There are few if any healthcare resources in many frontier communities, and these women described how they managed nonetheless. In relation to exercising to stay fit, one woman described her resourcefulness while snowbound.

> There's many a trip I've made around the room here. When the walls get to closing in on me, I just make figure eights and walk in my own home. And you can sit in your chair and move your arms and your legs if you have to. There's a lot of things you can make up as you go just to keep moving.

Another woman described how she drove on 1,200 miles of icy roads and frequent blizzard conditions to take her husband to a regional healthcare center for specialized care. She said,

> It was really scary. I thought my husband might die any moment; he was in a lot of pain. And I also knew that we could slide off a mountain pass and never be found. I just kept saying, "one more mile; just one more mile."

But she succeeded and her journey strengthened her self-reliance.

A 76-year-old woman whose husband was terminally ill had to learn to manage their finances for the first time even though her spouse had done so for more than 50 years. She successfully met the challenge.

EQUANIMITY: A BALANCED PERSPECTIVE OF LIFE

Most of the participants were from farming and ranching communities and they had firsthand experience with adversities that many who live in more urban communities do not experience. Because they lived "off the land," drought, hailstorms, early and late frost, poor cattle/grain prices, and the daily uncertainties of farming and ranching led to an attitude of "sitting loose" and "taking what comes." When a crop failed, they learned to start planning for the next season.

Each of the participants reported that a positive attitude was a vital component of health. Many felt that being optimistic, not worrying, focusing on the good parts of life, and having a zest for living were essential to good health. One woman advised, "You don't brood on yourself. You should have a good attitude towards life. Be cheerful. Don't be down in the dumps all the time. Have something to look forward to."

Several participants reported believing that worrying, complaining, and being negative would lead to illness. When asked how they recognized others who were not aging in a healthy way, the most frequent response concerned attitude and outlook on life. One woman expressed it this way:

> You can tell someone is aging well by engaging in a conversation with them. They are outgoing, not gripers and complainers, they are doers. It's more than physical. They may look the age but mentally they are in their 50s.

Another participant, describing someone who responded to life's uncertainties in a positive way, said:

> Their attitude. They'd have a sense of humor; they'd have a smile on their face. They'd have themselves taken care of, you know, not be sloppy, and I guess that's about it. They get out and in amongst people. Do things.

EXISTENTIAL ALONENESS: RECOGNITION OF ONE'S UNIQUE PATH AND THE ACCEPTANCE OF ONE'S LIFE

The women in this study lived in frontier communities, often far from town and even from neighbors. Many were children of early pioneers and homesteaders. Yet they did not complain of loneliness.

One woman had been widowed twice. She lived alone. During our interview together, she looked around her home and described changes she had made to the house. She said, "I've been living the way everyone else wanted me to live and I've finally reached a point where I'm going to do what works for me." Accordingly, her bedroom was open to the living room and she had a walk-in pantry as big as most kitchens because she liked "putting up food." She had gotten rid of her guest room because she did not want houseguests anymore.

Another woman expressed her aloneness this way: "I don't mind being alone. I have so much to do. And I like being able to do exactly what I want, when I want, how I want. No one tells me what to do."

Success and Support

The women's responses to adversity described many creative and successful approaches to relatively minor challenges (e.g., exercising) and to major challenges (e.g., dealing with a spouse's terminal illness). These women were also asked about support in their lives that helped them deal with difficulties. While all identified close family members and friends as sources of support, their sense of community was a source of strength and meaning to each of them as well. Because most had lived in their communities for several decades, they expressed a feeling of connection and affection for their communities. These older women also stated that they continued to contribute to their communities and were recognized by others as a source of valuable information, guidance, and wisdom.

CONTRIBUTION OF EARLY LIFE TO RESILIENCE

When participants were asked to talk about their childhood and how it influenced their current life in terms of health and resilience, each had much to say. These women saw a good start in life as laying the foundation for a lifestyle that helped them to stay resilient throughout their lives. Many reported the importance of having childhood chores and work, which gave them a reason to get up in the morning. Chores also led to self-reliance and "stick-to-itiveness."

One participant said,

Ranch kids have a different outlook on life than the kids that are raised on the asphalt. I mean they have their animals and they have to take care of them. And if you have something in a pen, you gotta feed 'em. When you're a kid, you don't always feel like getting up early in the morning but you just have to keep doing it or the livestock will die. And kids in town, well I say that they don't have that close association with any other living thing. Maybe they got a dog or a cat or a lizard or something, which is good for them, but they don't have that responsibility that kids do that are raised on a ranch.

Each discussed the simplicity of her early life. Most had been raised with very little in terms of material possessions and had learned to be content in their relatively humble circumstances. As farm and ranch kids, they had quickly learned that there were lean and fat years and you "take what comes." This most certainly influenced their equanimity and self-determination to not give up.

Comparison of Quantitative and Qualitative Data

As part of the data analysis, each study participant's individual interview data were compared to her quantitative data; there was consistency between the women's perceptions of health and resilience as described in the interview data and the way they rated themselves on the instruments. A resilient woman continues despite hardship and bounces back from adversity; resilience was a characteristic the participants exemplified. As expected, scores obtained on the RS were moderately high. One would also expect that persons aging well, as these women described themselves, would participate in health-promoting behaviors. Again, scores on the HPLP were moderately high, supporting reports of self-responsibility for health in this sample. Every woman in her interview knew about diet, exercise, stress management, and the need for adequate amounts of sleep. Each had learned from television, reading, and conversations with family and friends. These women were not highly educated and did not have access to specialized healthcare and information. Even so, they were motivated to obtain information that promoted healthy aging.

CONCLUSION

Role Models for Resilient Aging

The elderly frontier women in this study were resilient and healthy, as indicated by their reported independence, moderate-to-high scores in resilience, self-reported health, and health-promoting behaviors. Consistent with Richardson's (2002) position that individuals choose to reintegrate resiliently, return to homeostasis, or reintegrate with loss, these women provided examples within each of the five characteristics of resilience that demonstrated their choices to grow in resilience. They told us that individuals must have a reason to get up in the morning (purposeful life), learn to take what comes (equanimity), never quit trying (perseverance), get comfortable with being alone (existential aloneness), and learn to do what needs to be done (self-reliance). Each woman in this study described the importance of community involvement, identified as a protective factor in older adults' psychological well-being by Greenfield and Marks (2004). These findings are similar to those in a qualitative study by Kinsel (2005), who identified social connectedness and a head-on approach to challenges as factors contributing to resilience.

The women in this study provided many examples of resilient behaviors. Like everyone, they suffered setbacks and losses but they got up again and kept going. More than once was heard the following expression from these ranching and farming women: "When you fall off a horse, you just get back on again." These women knew literally that falling off a horse and getting back on meant not only being able to continue your journey, but also overcoming the fear of getting back on a horse that has thrown you. Ranchers and farmers know that a horse that throws you once may try to throw you again, and this can be intimidating. Dusting yourself off, gathering the reins, and stepping into the stirrup again means facing fear head-on. Achieving success increases resilience.

Future Research and Practice

Research is needed that will develop and test interventions to strengthen resilience among middle-aged and older women. There are many studies that describe the importance of having resilience, but fewer studies describe how to strengthen resilience within this population. Using the resilience model as a guide, a resilience-centered approach would motivate and engage women by focusing on strengths and building personal capacity. This would include working with women to identify what is meaningful in their lives, especially in the midst of loss, illness, and other challenges and encouraging them to give of themselves to others. It means providing support to women who are facing difficulties to develop their self-reliance and encouraging perseverance one step at a time. A resilience-centered intervention would include exploring aloneness or "coming home to yourself" (Northrup, 2006). And finally, strengthening resilience would work toward achieving balance in life and learning to "sit loose" in the saddle of life.

Do early childhood experiences have an effect on later resilience? For instance, Werner, in her 30-year-longitudinal study of 698 infants born in 1955, identified protective factors that strengthened resilience that included strong bonds with adults and involvement in a community group such as a church (1992). The women in this study identified childhood factors they believed had an effect on current resilience such as responsibility resulting in self-reliance and the uncertainty of farming/ranching leading to equanimity and perseverance. They identified their parents as role models and described their involvement in their communities even as children. Their responses and childhood memories were consistent with observations made by Garmezy (1993), Rutter (1985), and Werner (1984) that when children experience a nurturing environment, are given responsibility, experience self-efficacy, and develop a positive outlook in addition to other qualities, they grow into resilient adults.

It is important for healthcare providers to assess risk along with strengths in order to promote health and physical function in older adults. This research was designed to inform the development of methods to assess resilience in older frontier women and to plan interventions designed to strengthen this important protective factor. Increasing resilience will reduce the risk of disability and will promote health and quality of life for a growing number of older adults living in rural and frontier settings.

ACKNOWLEDGMENTS

This research was funded by a grant from Friends Research Institute, Inc, Baltimore, MD, and a block grant from Montana State University College of Nursing, Bozeman, MT. We would like to thank Vonna Koehler, PhD, RN, ARNP, for help in conducting the interviews.

REFERENCES

Broyles, L. C. (2005). *Resilience: Its relationships to forgiveness in older adults* (Unpublished doctoral dissertation). Knoxville: University of Tennessee.

Bryant, L. L., Beck, A., & Fairclough, D. L. (2000). Factors that contribute to positive perceived health in an older population. *Journal of Aging & Health, 12*(2), 169–192.

Bryant, L. L., Corbett, K. K., & Kutner, J. S. (2001). In their own words: A model of healthy aging. *Social Science & Medicine, 53*(7), 927–941.

Caltabiano, M. L., & Caltabiano, N. J. (2006). Resilience and health outcomes in the elderly. In *Proceedings of the 39th Annual Conference of the Australian Association of Gerontology*, November 22–24, 2006. Sydney, NSW, Australia. Retrieved from http://eprints.jcu.edu.au/4271

Centers for Disease Control and Prevention. (2003). Public health and aging: Trends in aging—United States and worldwide. *MMWR. Morbidity & Mortality Weekly Report, 52*(6), 101–106.

Duffy, M. E. (1993). Determinants of health-promoting lifestyles in older persons. *Image: Journal of Nursing Scholarship, 25*(1), 23–28.

Garmezy, N. (1993). Children in poverty: Resilience despite risk. *Psychiatry, 56*(1), 127–136.

Greenfield, E. A., & Marks, N. F. (2004). Formal volunteering as a protective factor for older adults' psychological well-being. *The Journals of Gerontology: Series B, Psychological Sciences and Social Sciences, 59*(5), S258–S264.

Hardy, S. E., Concato, J., & Gill, T. M. (2004). Resilience of community-dwelling older persons. *Journal of the American Geriatrics Society, 52*(2), 257–262.

Harris, P. B. (2008). Another wrinkle in the debate about successful aging: The undervalued concept of resilience and the lived experience of dementia. *International Journal of Aging & Human Development, 67*(1), 43–61.

Hartman-Stein, P. E., & Potkanowicz, E. S. (2003). Behavioral determinants of healthy aging: Good news for the Baby Boomer generation. *Online Journal of Issues in Nursing, 8*(2). Retrieved from http://www.nursingworld.org/MainMenuCategories/ANAMarketplace/ANAPeriodicals/OJIN/TableofContents/Volume82003/No2May2003/BehaviorandHealthyAging.aspx

Hoffman, C., Rice, D., & Sung, H. Y. (1996). Persons with chronic conditions: Their prevalence and costs. *Journal of the American Medical Association, 276*(18), 1473–1479.

Holstein, M. B., & Minkler, M. (2003). Self, society, and the "new gerontology". *Gerontologist, 43*(6), 787–796.

Humphreys, J. (2003). Research in sheltered battered women. *Issues in Mental Health Nursing, 24*, 137–152.

Idler, E. L., & Benyamini, Y. (1997). Self-rated health and mortality: A review of twenty-seven community studies. *Journal of Health and Social Behavior, 38*(1), 21–37.

Kinsel, B. (2005). Resilience as adaptation in older women. *Journal of Women and Aging, 17*(3), 23–39.

March, M. (2004). *Well being of older Australians: The interplay of life adversity and resilience in late life development* (Unpublished doctoral dissertation). Charles Sturt University, Australia.

Miller, C. A. (2008). *Nursing wellness in older adults* (5th ed.). Philadelphia, PA: Lippincott.

Montana Department of Public Health and Human Services. (2004). Montana County health profiles. Retrieved from https://archive.org/details/montana/montanacounty/hea2004mont

Morse, J. M. (1991). Approaches to qualitative–quantitative methodological triangulation. *Nursing Research, 40*(1), 120–123.

Northrup, C. (2006). *The wisdom of menopause.* New York, NY: Bantam Dell.

Nygren, B., Aléx, L., Jonsén, E., Gustafson, Y., Norberg, A., & Lundman, B. (2005). Sense of coherence, purpose in life and self-transcendence in relation to perceived physical and mental health among the oldest old. *Aging and Mental Health, 9*(4), 354–362.

Richardson, G. E. (2002). The metatheory of resilience and resiliency. *Journal of Clinical Psychology, 58*(3), 307–321.

Rowe, J. W., & Kahn, R. L. (1997). Successful aging. *The Gerontologist, 37*(4), 433–440.

Rowe, J. W., & Kahn, R. L. (1998). *Successful aging.* New York, NY: Random House.

Rutter, M. (1985). Resilience in the face of adversity: Protective factors and resistance to psychiatric disorder. *British Journal of Psychiatry, 147,* 598–611.

Rutter, M. (1987). Psychosocial resilience and protective mechanisms. *American Journal of Orthopsychiatry, 57*(3), 316–331.

Rutter, M. (1993). Resilience: Some conceptual considerations. *Journal of Adolescent Health, 14*(8), 626–631, 690–696.

Ruuskanen, J. M., & Ruoppila, I. (1995). Physical activity and psychological well-being among people aged 65 to 84 years. *Age and Ageing, 24*(4), 292–296.

Torma, L. M. (2010). *Fibromyalgia pain and physical function: The influence of resilience* (Doctoral dissertation), Portland: Oregon Health & Science University. Retrieved from http://drl.ohsu.edu/cdm/ref/collection/etd/id/809

Unger, J. B., Johnson, C. A., & Marks, G. (1997). Functional decline in the elderly: Evidence for direct and stress-buffering protective effects of social interactions and physical activity. *Annals of Behavioral Medicine, 19*(2), 152–160.

U.S. Census Bureau. (2000). Index of census 2000/states. Retrieved from https://www.census.gov/main/www/cen2000.html

Wagnild, G. M. (2003). Resilience and successful aging: Comparison among low and high income older adults. *Journal of Gerontological Nursing, 29*(12), 42–49.

Wagnild, G. M. (2009a). A review of the resilience scale. *Journal of Nursing Measurement, 17*(2), 105–113.

Wagnild, G. M. (2009b). *The resilience scale user's guide for the US English version of the resilience scale and the 14-item resilience scale (RS-14).* Worden, MT: The Resilience Center.

Wagnild, G. M. (2012). Resilience and health-promoting behaviors among healthy middle-aged and older adults. Unpublished data.

Wagnild, G. M., & Collins, J. A. (2009). Assessing resilience. *Journal of Psychosocial Nursing and Mental Health Services, 47*(12), 28–33.

Wagnild, G. M., & Young, H. (1990). Resilience among older women. *Image: Journal of Nursing Scholarship, 22,* 252–255.

Wagnild, G. M., & Young, H. M. (1993). Development and psychometric evaluation of the resilience scale. *Journal of Nursing Measurement, 1*(2), 165–178.

Walker, S. N., Sechrist, K. R., & Pender, N. J. (1987). The health-promoting lifestyle profile: Development and psychometric characteristics. *Nursing Research, 36*(2), 76–81.

Wells, M. (2010). Resilience in older adults living in rural, suburban, and urban areas. *Online Journal of Rural Nursing & Health Care, 10.* Retrieved from http://rnojournal .binghamton.edu/index.php/RNO/article/view/55

Werner, E. E. (1984). Resilient children. *Young Child, 40,* 68–72.

Werner, E. E. (1992). The children of Kauai: Resiliency and recovery in adolescence and adulthood. *Journal of Adolescent Health, 13,* 262–268.

Wilson, I. B., & Cleary, P. D. (1995). Linking clinical variables with health-related quality of life. *Journal of the American Medical Association, 273*(1), 59–65.

Wolff, J. L., Starfield, B., & Anderson, G. (2002). Prevalence, expenditures, and complications of multiple chronic conditions in the elderly. *Archives of Internal Medicine, 162*(20), 2269–2276.

Cultural Aspects of Bereavement in Rural Settings

D. "Dale" M. Mayer and Christy Buttler-Nelson

DISCUSSION TOPICS

- Identify three or more ways social determinants of health may affect bereavement.
- Differentiate between primary and secondary losses after death.
- Compare and contrast bereavement support in urban and rural settings.
- Identify what types of bereavement support are available for rural residents in your location.

For life and death are one, even as the river and sea are one.
—Khalil Gibran (1923, p. 84)

Birth and death are irrevocably connected as every person born will someday die and people, who usually experience grief after the death of significant persons in their lives, will enter a period of bereavement. It is important to define the terms "grief" and "bereavement" because common usage makes these terms seem self-explanatory; however, there are differences. Grief may occur in response to conditions other than death, for example, after a divorce, the loss of one's job, an amputation of a limb, even declining health. Based on the work of bereavement researchers Stroebe, Hansson, Stroebe, and Schut (2008), the terms can be differentiated as follows: bereavement is an objective situation that develops after the death of someone significant, whereas grief is the emotional or affective reaction to a loss. For the purposes of this chapter, we focus our attention on bereavement after the death of a person.

Given that humans develop relationships with other people over the course of a lifetime, all individuals will someday be bereaved; thus bereavement is a universal human experience. Death not only leaves a lasting impact on individuals but also on families, friends, and communities. Social customs and cultural rituals frequently influence traditions after a death and these influences may continue into the bereavement experience.

The purpose of this chapter is to describe the cultural aspects of bereavement in rural settings. A case report will be used to illustrate the aspects of one rural family's bereavement experiences. Also included are the perspectives of rural dwellers and healthcare professionals (HCP) who live and work in rural settings. The chapter concludes with evidence-based suggestions for providing bereavement support for rural residents.

HEALTH AND RURAL CULTURE

According to *Healthy People 2020* (Office of Disease Prevention and Health Promotion [ODPHP], 2014, section Topics and Objectives, Overview), "Health starts in our homes, schools, workplaces, neighborhoods, and communities" (para. 1). The social determinants of health are organized around five key areas: economic stability, education, health and healthcare, neighborhood and built environments, and social and community context (ODPHP, 2014). Many people recognize the importance of staying active, eating healthy foods, and avoiding tobacco. Important self-care activities include immunizations, preventative screening examinations, and seeing a doctor during times of illness. Health is also influenced by access to social and economic opportunities, including resources available in the communities where we live, work, and play. It is important to evaluate the safety of the air we breathe, the water we drink, the food we eat, and the safety of our workplaces. Also important are the quality of our relationships and the social interactions we have with family, friends, and neighbors. In summary, where we live impacts our health and living in a rural community has its own unique impact on health.

Bolin and Bellamy (2015) developed *Rural Healthy People 2020* (RHP, 2010) that identifies both challenges and opportunities to promoting health among rural residents. Access to healthcare remains the top priority for rural areas followed by diabetes, mental health, nutrition and weight, and heart disease listed as the top five priorities of *RHP 2020*. Health disparities are present in much of rural America and prevention and care models that build on the strong ties inherent in rural communities are needed to improve the health of rural residents (Bolin & Belamy, 2015). Fahs (2017) reminds us that ". . . being a rural dweller alone does not put your health at risk . . ." (para. 1) but rural residents with limited social and economic resources may experience more negative impacts on their health.

It is important to recognize that rural communities have their own culture. Farmer (2010), a clinical psychologist and syndicated columnist who specialized in rural mental health, posed this question in his newspaper column on urban and rural values, "What makes rural, rural?" (p. 1). Rural residents connect with each other both formally and informally and "everybody knows everybody" (Farmer, 2010, p. 1) allowing rural residents to bond with each other on a deep level due to common ties to the community. Living in a rural community does not necessarily mean rural residents are isolated; in fact, rural residents have frequent social interactions due to long-standing relationships with others in their community. Rural values contribute to feelings of "belonging, emotional support, security and predictability" (Farmer, 2010, p. 1) and rural residents tend to have strong bonds with friends and neighbors. These bonds contribute to a strong sense of community. Rural dwellers are known for their "individualism, hard work, independence, and self-sufficiency (O'Lynn, 2013, pp. 176–177). Rural communities tend to have common gathering places where people meet with their neighbors including the post office, school, grocery store, church, and local taverns or bars.

Rural communities often have an abundance of social capital, for example, when neighbors gather together to assist with a barn raising in a rural county or when rural participants of a cancer support group exchange email messages (Putnam, 2000). Plunkett, Leipert, and Olson (2016) wrote about rural churches, which are often well positioned in their communities, to encourage building on their existing social capital to promote the health of rural residents.

Access to healthcare services is a prerequisite for good health, but rural residents encounter many challenges, including workforce shortages of HCPs and long distances and transportation issues, especially when access to specialty care is needed (Rural Health Information Hub, 2017). Although small rural hospitals may be at increased risk of closure, the critical access hospital (CAH) program in the United States allows communities to transition the local hospital to a CAH. Such hospitals are required to provide short-stay services including emergency, outpatient, primary, and long-term care services, and in turn the CAH then receives increased Medicare reimbursement (Shreffler-Grant & Reimer, 2013). Currently there are 1,339 critical CAHs in the United States (Flex Monitoring Team, 2017) that provide healthcare in rural settings. Rural residents consider CAHs as "not just a safety net for healthcare, [they] also provide a sense of pride for rural communities" (Mayer & Winters, 2016, p. 73).

Case Report—A Family Farm Story

A research study on family bereavement after sudden cardiac death (Mayer, Rosenfeld, & Gilbert, 2013) included interviews with a rural family. Three bereaved family members discussed their bereavement experiences with one of the authors (Dale M. Mayer) and will be used to illuminate cultural aspects of rural bereavement. All names are pseudonyms and an italic font and quotation marks are used to delineate direct quotes. Some details were changed to protect anonymity.

Ron lived with his wife, Marie, on a large farm in a rural area and their two children were attending graduate school and college. Ron was a "very good farmer" and the family had plans for their son to assume responsibility for the farm once he finished college. One morning Marie left for work early and returned home that afternoon to find "nothing had changed, the coffee hadn't been made, [and] everything was just how I left it." Marie found Ron on the floor and she called 911 and told them "you have to send somebody . . . I just need somebody here."

In rural areas, emergency medical services (EMS) are staffed by volunteers who have to leave their activities and travel to the ambulance before proceeding to the location of the 911 call. In Marie's case, it took 30 minutes before a neighbor arrived at the house and 45 minutes before the ambulance arrived. During this time, Marie was connected by phone to a physician (MD) at a CAH located 30 miles away and Marie stated, ". . . she told me to sit down . . . I was [thinking] someone has to come . . . someone has to help me—please Dear Lord and then [the MD] said, sit down . . . are you sitting down? Now I want you to breathe deeply . . ." Marie explained how helpful it was to have someone on the phone with her. Due to the rural nature of the community all EMS providers knew the family; in fact many people in the community had police scanners and were aware that the ambulance was responding to a call. By the time the ambulance arrived, Marie stated, ". . . the whole house just filled up . . . this house was filled . . . by the time the ambulance came, all the neighbors came . . ." Ron's death, due to ventricular fibrillation, "change[d] everything" for this family. After friends and family members from out of town arrived, the funeral was planned. Marie shared that, ". . . there were over 500 [people] at his funeral—it was a big funeral—which is pretty big deal for [name of town]."

Ron's surviving family members talked about the many ways their lives were forever changed after his sudden death. Given that Ron had planted the crop before he died, this family described having to make many decisions, "hard" decisions, immediately after Ron's death, including: Do we keep the farm? Do we sell the farm? Do we lease the farm? With the help of family members and friends, including neighboring farmers, and coupled with the age-old advice of "don't make any major changes for at least a year," they decided to keep the farm. As a family, they continued to operate the farm "with lots and lots of help." Marie's brother arrived to help them harvest the crop the first summer after Ron's death. Other friends and nearby farmers helped reorganize the shop and all the farm implements. Ron's son learned how to operate equipment he had never used before, including the sprayer and air seeder.

Running the farm without Ron was a huge undertaking and this family encountered many stressful situations related to the day-to-day operation of the farm and they were constantly asking themselves: What would Ron do? Examples of decisions included: Where should the new fence go? How much hail insurance should we purchase this year? What variety should we seed and how much fertilizer should we use? Marie shared that, "Things like [fixing farm equipment] are hard for us to do" and her son added, "every time I'm looking for something that I know we have but I don't know where it is, [I'll] think: Oh I'll just run in ask Dad real quick . . ."

This family found it was necessary to make other changes after Ron's death. Marie described having to drive Ron's pickup truck into town a few weeks after his death saying,

I remember that time that I had to take [Ron's truck] . . . into town . . . it must have been within a week or two [after Ron's death] . . . [and] the look on people's face—that was hard and then I knew—we need to get rid of this pick-up because . . . to have the hands go up [to wave] and then just the look on their face—I'm like: Oh God—I can't do this [pause].

Marie also found it helpful to change her job so she could be around more adults. This change allowed her to receive support from others in the community; she shared, "In a small town, life, social life, revolves around the school—so now I go to all the [football and basketball] games . . ." In addition, many people in the community helped Marie and her family after Ron's death. Marie described this saying,

The lawyer, the banker, the [certified public accountant] CPA, people that you knew that were . . . very, very helpful and just being in a small community, all those things that help . . . and small towns are a lot easier to do this in—I suppose if you were in the middle of a big city—I don't know—but I know that [living in a small town] helped . . .

Marie's children mentioned that many people in the community shared stories about Ron with them,

Whenever [my brother] and I go anywhere it seems like somebody pulls us aside and wants to tell us stories . . . Yeah—especially in [name of town]—you go out to a bar on a Friday or Saturday night [and] you get all the old guys sitting in there . . . Are you Ron's daughter?" They'll just pull you over [laughing] . . . for the next 15 minutes you're going to have some stories and part of it is really hard cause then you're just like, Oh God, I miss him so much. But the other part I, Oh wow, I'm so glad that [my dad] had so many friends . . . It's always nice . . .

Marie commented on other changes in her social life after Ron's death, changes that were not easy to accept. She mentioned not fitting in with their couple friends saying, "It's hard, it's hard to be the third wheel. That's what I feel like a lot, in the couples, everybody's couples. They're good, they invite me places, [and] they take me places. I go places, but it's hard . . . I'm the first one to be the single . . . [laughter]." Since Marie lived in a rural community the change in Marie's marital status also impacted her children. Marie mentioned that a girlfriend offered to introduce her to her brother; who was "a really nice guy." Marie felt it was important for her children to hear about this conversation from her and she laughed when they had different responses. Marie's daughter stated, "Mom, I'm not ready for this" and her son commented, "Oh yeah, that's nice . . ." Marie commented that she was not interested in dating yet, although she did leave the door ajar, stating, ". . . So that whole saga [dating] someday may open up but I just said: oh dear God, not right now."

Marie spoke about a local MD, who encouraged them all to get "heart echos and cardiograms and all sorts of [tests] . . ." This MD was described as being ". . . very good about family healthcare and . . . always saying if you need me call me . . ." and also suggested they consider grief therapy. Marie stated, "I went to a therapist down in [name of city 90 miles away]" and Ron's daughter shared, "I go to therapy and I think that's really helpful . . . I can tell—if I skip a week . . ."

This family had a great deal of support from friends and neighbors in the rural farming community, which Marie described saying, ". . . our real close friends—they never left—there was somebody here all the time taking care of stuff." Their lives continued, although at one and a half years after Ron's death, their lives still did not feel "normal." Overall, this family was very proud of their ability to operate the farm and they recognized this as a major accomplishment,

> I think Ron would probably shake his head hilariously at, umm, at how well we've done. I think he'd be proud of us, but at the same time I could just see him going: Oh my God, they're using this, they're using that,—oh my God, they're driving this. Oh, they're going to wreck everything. But we haven't.

Ultimately, they are proud of their successes with the farm and feel that Ron would be proud of them as well.

Cultural Aspects of Rural Bereavement

Bereavement is an experience of such varying intensity that one is rarely prepared to cope with the multiple reactions that accompany the death of an important person in one's life. It is recognized that the causes and circumstances associated with a death influence reactions during bereavement (Parkes, 2011). Certain types of deaths are more challenging for survivors, including suicides, sudden deaths, and deaths occurring out of the expected life sequence (i.e., the death of infants, children, and young adults). Reactions to death are influenced by cultural customs and rural communities have their own culture. Rural residents are proud of their strong sense of community. Not only does "everyone know everyone" (Farmer, 2010, p. 1) but everyone knows about each other's social groups and who have more adversarial relationships.

Most cultures have traditional ways to honor and remember people who have died, which often include some sort of ceremony that may be called by different names, including funeral, celebration of life, or memorial service. Generally, such ceremonies allow family members, friends, and community members to say goodbye in a supportive setting. People may travel great distances to support those bereaved by a death, which allows survivors to be encircled by caring and empathetic friends and relatives. Often people arrive bearing platters of food, a practice which continues for several days. Eventually, supportive friends and extended family members return to their own lives and activities, leaving the bereaved on their own. Although meals may still be delivered to the house, the food may now arrive on a more sporadic schedule. Marie expressed gratitude that not a day passed without someone stopping by or calling to check on her family. This ongoing support was a major aspect of this family's bereavement experiences and allowed the family to continue their lives in spite of a significant loss. One thought as to why it works for this family is the level of support they have in the rural farming community where they live.

In contrast, a person who lives in town, as opposed to a farm, may have a different bereavement experience. The commonality that bridges rural residents, whether they live in a rural agricultural area, or in town, is the social connectedness that allows rural residents to support each other in many ways, including after a death. O'Lynn (2013), in a study of male caregivers in rural settings, provided examples of community support where rural residents look out for and support each other. One participant in O'Lynn's study described his two families as ". . . the 'church family' . . . and the 'bar [tavern] family'" (p. 181). Each of these "families" spends time together, looks out for each other, and provides support in different ways.

Given the lack of anonymity in rural settings when a person in a rural area dies, the whole town knows who died. If the person who died is a prominent member of the community, say a banker, a doctor, or a home health nurse, the death impacts not only immediate friends and family members, but many facets of the community's functioning as well. The bank's employees and customers will be impacted by the death of the banker, but the school board may also be grieving the death of a fellow trustee. The death of the only physician in town will impact both office and hospital staff members, in addition to multitudes of patients and families. Members of a church congregation may profoundly mourn the death of the home health nurse because this person also coached basketball, and was involved with the youth group at church. In rural communities, it is common for the whole community to grieve losses due to death both individually and collectively. This lack of anonymity in rural settings may present challenges for bereaved individuals, including not being able to get a break from grief. For example, a woman may be constantly recognized as the mother whose child died in a farming accident. Every time she stops at the grocery store she is stopped by others offering condolences or sharing their own stories of loss with loss, when all she wanted to do was to get groceries, go home, and make dinner.

When a death occurs, there is a very visible primary loss; in the case report, Marie's primary loss was the death of her husband. However, it is important to recognize that there are less visible secondary losses that also occur (What's Your Grief? 2017). Secondary losses can be described as ripples, similar to throwing a pebble into a lake. The first splash is the primary loss, but the ripples that spread out from that first splash are secondary losses. Marie experienced a primary loss when Ron died, but she had other losses including companionship with her life partner, confidence in her decision making about the farm, and disrupted future plans; all of which are secondary losses. Financial security is commonly a secondary loss, especially when the primary bread winner dies. A surviving spouse may need to seek employment and function in a different capacity that may contribute added stress for surviving family members. Having to relocate due to financial or family issues can be another loss which may also lead to a decline of social support. It is important to recognize secondary losses so that bereaved persons can identify support that will be helpful for them.

In the real-world practice settings of rural communities, one's responsibilities as a professional come ahead of personal emotions. Scharff (2013) describes the nature of rural nursing, writing that ". . . Being rural means that when a nurse walks into the emergency room, it may be her or his spouse or child who needs a nurse, and at that moment being a nurse takes priority over being anyone else . . ." (p. 243). An emergency medicine physician wrote eloquently about the camaraderie of teamwork during a natural disaster, specifically mentioning that death of a patient can affect providers too, stating that as providers they ". . . must nonetheless always put others' feelings first" (Strote, 2014, p. 556). Conversations with HCPs who live and work in rural settings reinforced the concept of putting others first; when an emergency or death occurs in a rural community, HCPs need to control their emotions in order to provide care to others in a professional manner while maintaining confidentiality (J. Shrider-Cobb, personal communication, June 8, 2017).

Given the ubiquitous nature of the Internet, rural residents can use computers to find out who has died, when the service will be, and even post a condolence card to the family on the funeral home website. One social media platform, Facebook (2017), has developed instructions on how to convert a Facebook page into a memorial. Stroebe, van der Houwen, and Schut (2008) critically reviewed the many forms of bereavement support available on the Internet. They concluded that individuals who have Internet access may find bereavement support online; however, they caution that the bereaved, who are in a vulnerable state of mind, must take precautions to ensure they are not taken advantage of online. It is relatively easy to find positive statements about online bereavement support; however, empirical evidence for the effectiveness of online bereavement support is lacking (Stroebe, van der Houwen, et al., 2008).

Bereavement Support for Rural Residents

Social customs and cultural rituals certainly influence the death and bereavement experience and yet little is known on how receptive rural residents are to bereavement support (Blackburn, McGrath, & Bulsara, 2016). Bereavement support may be formal, for example, a grief support group provided by a hospice organization, which is required to offer bereavement support for surviving family members for up to 12 months after a death (Mayer & Winters, 2016). However, not all rural communities have hospice services, thus bereavement support may be provided in other ways. Rural churches are often prominent in their communities and have strong ties to their congregations and local residents; thus a church may invite people going through life transitions, including bereavement, to meet together.

In rural communities, support can be found in many places, including ". . . churches, schools, bridge clubs, civic associations, and even bars" (Putnam, 2017, para. 4). It is important to recognize that bereavement support happens informally too; an example is when people share stories of Ron with his children in the local bar on a Saturday night. Sometimes informal support is unspoken; for example, someone brings a special dessert to a barbeque because the person who usually brings this dessert has died. The significance of this dessert will be recognized by locals, who may share a hug or a knowing smile (J. Shrider-Cobb, personal communication, June 8, 2017) because no words are needed to recognize the absence of an important person. Support in rural communities is bound to be as varied as the rural areas where they live. As with many situations, bereavement support may come from both expected, and unexpected, people. One of the authors received monthly notes from a woman she did not know after a death; the connecting link was the shared experience of the death of a spouse and a friend who knew both their stories.

SUMMARY

Although bereavement is a universal experience and certainly a challenging situation that all will encounter, where we live impacts our experience. There is no one way to grieve and in rural settings bereavement support can be provided by formal and informal networks. What matters is that rural residents find bereavement support in whatever ways that are helpful. Given the cultural impacts associated with life and death, our bereavement experiences will vary, based on not only where we live, but other cultural aspects that contribute to our lives. More research is needed on cultural aspects of bereavement in rural settings, especially on the Internet, although it is clear that bereavement support can be provided in many unique ways.

REFERENCES

Blackburn, P., McGrath, P., & Bulsara, C. (2016). Looking through the lens of receptivity and its role in bereavement support: A review of the literature. *American Journal of Hospice and Palliative Medicine, 33*(10), 989–995. doi:10.1177/1049909115595608

Bolin, J. N., & Bellamy, G. (2015). *Rural healthy people 2020*. Retrieved from https://srhrc .tamhsc.edu/docs/rhp2020.pdf

Facebook. (2017). Memorialized accounts. Retrieved from https://www.facebook.com/ help/1506822589577997

Fahs, P. S. (2017). Social determinants of health and rural nursing. *Online Journal of Rural Nursing and Health Care, 17*(1), 1–2. doi:10.14574/ojrnhc.v17i1.452

Farmer, V. (2010). How urban and rural values differ. Retrieved from http://www .valfarmer.com/article.ec?DocID=1202

Flex Monitoring Team. (2017). *Location of critical access hospitals.* Retrieved from http:// www.flexmonitoring.org/wp-content/uploads/2013/06/CAH_012517.pdf

Gibran, K. (1923). *The prophet.* New York, NY: Vintage Books, Penguin Random House.

Mayer, D., Rosenfeld, A. G., & Gilbert, K. (2013). Lives forever changed: Family bereavement experiences after sudden cardiac death. *Applied Nursing Research, 26,* 168–173. doi:10.1016/j.apnr.2013.06.007

Mayer, D., & Winters, C. (2016). Palliative care in critical access hospitals. *Critical Care Nurse, 36*(1), 72–78. doi:10.4037/ccn2016732

Office of Disease Prevention and Health Promotion. (2014). Social determinants of health. *Healthy People 2020.* Retrieved from https://www.healthypeople.gov/2020/topics-objectives/topic/social-determinants-of-health

O'Lynn, C. (2013). Negotiation of constructed gender among rural male caregivers. In C. A. Winters (Ed.), *Rural nursing: Concepts, theory, and practice* (4th ed., pp. 173–203). New York, NY: Springer Publishing.

Parkes, C. M. (2011). The historical landscape of loss: Development of bereavement studies. In R. A. Niemeyer, D. L. Harris, H. R. Winokuer, & G. F. Thorton (Eds.), *Grief and bereavement in contemporary society: Bridging research and practice* (pp. 1–5). New York, NY: Routledge/Taylor & Francis.

Plunkett, R., Leipert, B., & Olson, J. (2016). Exploring the influence of social determinants, social capital, and health expertise on health and the rural church. *Journal of Holistic Nursing, 34*(3), 236–243. doi:10.1177/0898010115605231

Putnam, R. D. (2000). *Bowling alone: The collapse and revival of American community.* New York, NY: Simon & Schuster.

Putnam, R. D. (2017). Social capital primer. Retrieved from http://bowlingalone .com/?page_id=13

Rural Health Information Hub. (2017). Healthcare access in rural communities. Retrieved from https://www.ruralhealthinfo.org/topics/healthcare-access#barriers

Scharff J. E. (2013). The distinctive nature and scope of rural nursing practice: Philosophical bases. In C. A. Winters (Ed.), *Rural nursing: Concepts, theory, and practice* (4th ed., pp. 241–258). New York, NY: Springer Publishing.

Shreffler-Grant, J. M., & Reimer, M. A. (2013). Implications for education practice and policy. In C. A. Winters (Ed.), *Rural nursing: Concepts, theory, and practice* (4th ed., pp. 439–448). New York, NY: Springer Publishing.

Stroebe, M. S., Hansson, R. O., Schut, H., & Stroebe, W. (2008). *Handbook of bereavement and research: Advances in theory and intervention.* Washington, DC: American Psychological Association.

Stroebe, M. S., van der Houwen, K., & Schut, H. (2008). Bereavement support, intervention, and research on the Internet: A critical review. In M. S. Stroebe, R. O. Hansson, H. Schut, & W. Stroebe (Eds.), *Handbook of bereavement and research: Advances in theory and intervention* (pp. 551–574). Washington, DC: American Psychological Association.

Strote, J. (2014). Enough said. *Annals of Emergency Medicine, 64*(5), 556. doi:10.1016/j .annemergmed.2014.05.026

What's Your Grief? (2017). Secondary loss—One loss isn't enough??!! Retrieved from https://whatsyourgrief.com/secondary-loss-one-loss-isnt-enough

Beyond the Symptom–Action–Timeline Process: Explicating the Health-Needs–Action Process

Andrea Rasmussen, Chad O'Lynn, and Charlene A. Winters

DISCUSSION TOPICS

- Select a subpopulation to:
  - Explore perceptions and responses to health needs
  - Analyze findings and discuss the fit with the Symptom–Action–Timeline (SATL), Symptom Action Process (SAP), and Health-Needs–Action Process (HNAP) models
- Identify responses to health needs in rural men and younger individuals to support the revised HNAP model in these populations.

There is an important study in the first edition of this book by Buehler, Malone, and Majerus (1998) who proposed an initial model detailing how rural dwellers recognize health symptoms and the process rural dwellers go through in relieving those symptoms. As Buehler et al. noted, the significance of such a model is the provision of a framework from which healthcare providers can better assess an individual's interpretation and response to symptoms and then work with them to more accurately interpret symptoms and choose responses that optimize health outcomes. The model also offers healthcare providers a framework to better assess all resources available to individuals (such as self-care or lay resources) that might be tapped to resolve health problems and provide emotional support during illness. The authors recommended additional research to validate the use of their Symptom–Action–Timeline (SATL) process model for rural dwellers.

In 2006, Chad O'Lynn examined the SATL process and made several recommendations that would allow the model to be used in other studies. O'Lynn's literature review supported the SATL process; however, he proposed a revised model titled the Symptom Action Process (SAP). The SAP model was intended to be more inclusive of the various rural subgroups and their health behaviors and holistic health needs. In addition, O'Lynn theorized that findings from studies using the new SAP model would provide health professionals and policymakers a better understanding of how health needs are manifested and interpreted in rural settings.

In this chapter, we report the findings of a literature review designed to examine the level of support for the SATL process (Buehler et al., 1998) and O'Lynn's (2006) SAP model. We specifically address the recommendations proposed by O'Lynn to (a) expand the definition of "symptom" to include psychological symptoms; (b) expand the definition of "symptom" to be more reflective of a health need so that self-care measures to prevent illness or promote health are included; (c) recognize that intentional disregard of a health need is a type of self-care action, especially when mental health needs are involved; (d) embed the model within an environmental context external to the decision tree to account for demographic variables, access to resources, and so on; and (e) design the model to be more circular in nature, allowing for sequential or concurrent health-related actions.

On the basis of the findings from our review of the literature, we recommend the SAP model be expanded and renamed the Health-Needs–Action Process (HNAP) model to incorporate all holistic aspects of the above. We further propose additional studies be conducted with rural populations, both domestically and internationally, to explore support for the revised model.

REVIEW OF THE SATL PROCESS AND THE SAP MODEL

The SATL Process

We present a brief review and graphic depiction of the SATL in this section; however, we refer the reader to Buehler et al. (1998) for more details about the SATL process. The SATL process and SAP model (O'Lynn, 2006) are compared in a graphic description later in the chapter.

The SATL process encompasses four phases: (a) symptom identification, (b) self-care, (c) lay resources, and (d) professional resources (Figure 16.1). The process is preceded by the occurrence of a symptom, defined as an alteration in the usual state of health that requires action. Unless that symptom is recognized by an individual (symptom identification), the SATL process does not continue. It is important to note that "symptom" was defined as a negative entity (Buehler et al., 1998) and the SATL process as one of resolving a problem.

Symptoms are characterized by three general components: (a) physical signs and sensations, (b) degree of interference with the person's usual or desired level of functioning, and (c) intensity and duration of the symptom (Buehler et al., 1998). These three characteristics, coupled with an individual's

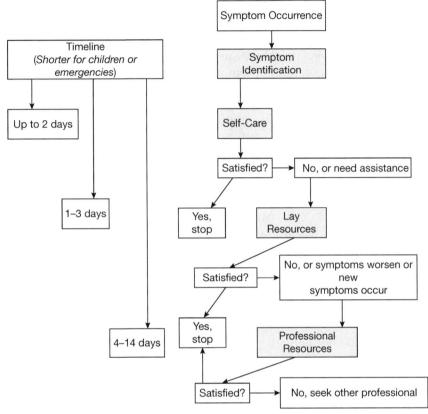

FIGURE 16.1. Symptom–Action–Timeline (SATL) process.
Source: Adapted from Buehler, J., Malone, M., & Majerus, J. (1998). Patterns of responses to symptoms in rural residents: The symptom-action-time-line process. In H. Lee (Ed.), *Conceptual basis for rural nursing* (pp. 153–162). New York, NY: Springer Publishing.

prior experience of and knowledge of the symptom, are used in assigning meaning to the symptom. Based on this meaning, an individual will decide whether to take action. According to Buehler et al. (1998), self-care is the first action taken after identifying a symptom.

"Self-care" refers to the myriad activities initiated by and performed by an individual to relieve a symptom (Buehler et al., 1998). For individuals relying upon others for their health needs (e.g., dependent children and elders), family members or other caretakers would be responsible for initiating activities to address an identified symptom. Self-care activities include applying home remedies, taking over-the-counter medications and herbal preparations, using the Internet and reading reference books to learn more about the symptom and symptom resolution. Self-care activities, as well as all other actions taken in the SATL process, are evaluated by the individual in terms of efficacy, and a decision is made whether to proceed through the SATL process, alter actions, or cease activities.

If self-care activities do not resolve a symptom to the individual's satisfaction, family, friends, and neighbors are consulted. These lay resources are used to provide (a) validation of symptom interpretation, (b) advice and emotional support, and (c) physical care (Buehler et al., 1998). Although not defined by Buehler et al., unlike professional resources, lay resources are not financially reimbursed for their services. If symptoms do not resolve, if symptoms intensify, or additional symptoms occur, professional resources are then sought. If professional resources do not lead to symptom resolution, individuals may seek other professional resources.

The time one takes to navigate the SATL process (Buehler et al., 1998) is influenced by the intensity and duration of a symptom and the degree to which the symptom interferes with usual functioning. Actions are implemented more quickly when a symptom is particularly intense, greatly interferes with usual functioning, or children are involved. If the symptom is interpreted as an emergency, the individual may seek professional care immediately and bypass the early phases of the SATL process. However, if the SATL process is completed in its entirety, the time from symptom identification to self-care can take up to 2 days; from symptom identification to lay resources can take from 1 to 3 days, and from symptom identification to professional resources can take from 4 to 14 days. How individuals progress through the SATL process has great implications for healthcare providers and researchers. It is important to note that a major limitation to the SATL process is the lack of reference to health prevention and health promotion activities utilized by rural dwellers. This is in contrast to both the SAP model proposed by O'Lynn (2006) and the HNAP model proposed by the authors of the present chapter, which accounts for health promotion and illness prevention and incorporates a holistic multitherapeutic approach.

SAP Model

In general, the SAP model supports the SATL process as described by Buehler et al. (1998), but with a few revisions. The authors described a "symptom" as a physical sign or sensation. SATL is focused on problem solving and does not address activities to prevent illness and promote health. O'Lynn (2006) noted that the SATL definition of symptom was quite narrow and proposed that the concept of "symptom" be replaced with "health need." A health need can be a biophysical need, as well as a spiritual, emotional, social, and psychological need. A health need is more holistic than a symptom and would provide a broader perspective of rural dwellers' responses to perceived health and wellness needs (O'Lynn, 2006). The inclusion of psychological symptoms, such as those typically seen in depressive and anxiety disorders, is vital because mental health services are often unavailable or poorly implemented in rural communities (Rural Health Information Hub, 2017; Wilson, Bangs, & Hatting, 2015).

Unlike the linear SATL process, the SAP model includes a circular process that allows for multiple actions—self-care, lay resources, and professional resources—to be incorporated in a sequential *or* concurrent fashion (Figure 16.2). This approach is different from the more linear SATL process, which details the process of resolving a single symptom or health problem, for example, fever or broken bone. The SAP can be used by individuals for multiple symptoms, an important consideration when responding to chronic illnesses. Chronic conditions, such as diabetes or congestive heart failure, are characterized by the recurrence of multiple symptoms with varying degrees of intensity and duration. Using the more circular SAP model, one can readily explain how an individual might use prayer, hot packs, support from friends, prescription drugs, and physical therapy concurrently to manage an illness or injury, and might vary use of these strategies over time as health needs wax and wane.

The SAP model also recognizes the act of ignoring a health need or symptom as a type of self-care action. This is often seen with rural men (Evans, Frank, Oliffe, & Gregory, 2011) and depressed persons seeking treatment for somatic health needs (e.g., fatigue, pain, changes in appetite) while ignoring the depressive symptomatology (lack of interest in usual habits, sadness, etc.) that accompanies the somatic issues. Moreover, some cultural beliefs are rooted in traditions that perceive psychological health needs as conditions resulting from spiritual or magical causes or see the needs as a weakness (Garcia, Gilchrist, Vazquez, Leite, & Raymond, 2011), highlighting the need to consider the context external to the decision-making process to understand rural persons' approaches to health needs. In addition to culture and tradition, gender, race,

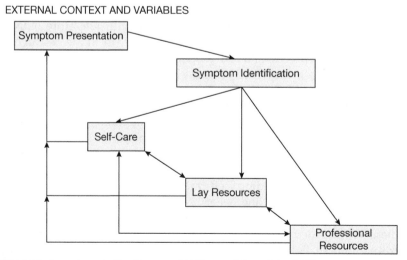

FIGURE 16.2. Symptom–Action Process (SAP): a revision of the SATL process.
Source: Adapted from O'Lynn, C. (2006). Updating the symptom-action-time-line process. In H. Lee & C. A. Winters (Eds.), *Rural nursing: Concepts, theory, and practice* (2nd ed., pp. 138–152). New York, NY: Springer Publishing.

ethnicity, educational achievement, socioeconomic status, family and social role, residential location, and barriers to resources, among others, provide the environment in which decisions are made.

On the basis of our review of the literature, we propose renaming the SAP model as the HNAP model. By replacing the term "symptom" with "health need," we believe that the model more accurately reflects a broader spectrum of rural health demands, including psychological and physiological acute and chronic conditions.

METHOD USED FOR LITERATURE REVIEW

Much of the literature pertaining to rural healthcare focuses on (a) disparities in health for rural dwellers as compared with nonrural dwellers, (b) description of the health of rural dwellers, (c) use of complementary alternative medicine (CAM) and treatments, (d) barriers to accessing healthcare services for rural dwellers, and (e) the experiences and demographics of healthcare providers in rural areas. None of these broad areas of literature directly addresses the SATL process or SAP model in identifying health needs and actions to resolve them, with the possible exception of access barriers. Buehler et al. (1998) touched on access barriers in that additional effort is made to overcome the barriers if children were involved or symptoms were deemed emergent. Access barriers modulate the SATL process rather than serve as foundational antecedents in determining the components of the process itself. O'Lynn (2006) did not include access barriers in his literature review and as a result, barriers to care were not included in this review.

In March 2012, we conducted a search of peer-reviewed resources contained in the Cumulative Index to Nursing and Allied Health Literature (CINAHL), MedLine, Psych Info, PubMed, and Google Scholar, to locate research-based support for the SATL process and SAP model. Resources published from July 2004 through March 2012 were searched using the keyword of "rural" and its associated keywords of "rural health," "rural environment," "rural community," "frontier," and "rural populations." Rural keywords were the primary sorting category to ensure that rural dwellers would be salient in the literature, although use of the SATL process and SAP model may be made in nonrural populations as well. We then combined the rural keywords with other keywords, based on available keyword search options within each database that were suggestive of the SATL process and SAP model, including "self-care," "health needs," "health behaviors," "illness behavior," "attitudes and beliefs for self-care," "decision making," "self-assessment," "alternative therapies," "complementary medicine," and "home remedies." We excluded dissertation abstracts because of the difficulty of obtaining full texts of multiple dissertations. The search yielded a total of 583 journal articles.

From the 583 articles, we excluded review articles, case studies, and anecdotal reports, resulting in a new pool of 87 research-based journal articles. We then excluded all articles reporting studies occurring outside the United States, congruent with O'Lynn's (2006) review. This latter exclusion was reasonable because the study by Buehler et al. (1998) occurred in the United States. These steps resulted in 71 articles available for review.

Following a critical review of the 71 articles, we excluded studies that did not address components relevant to the SATL process or the SAP model and studies that focused only on healthcare providers. The final sample of articles for review included 21 research reports.

FINDINGS FROM THE LITERATURE REVIEW

The 21 studies included in this review were published between July 2004 and March 2012. Participants in these studies represented Arizona, Indiana, Louisiana, Michigan, Montana, New Mexico, North Carolina, North and South Dakota, Pennsylvania, Tennessee, Texas, West Virginia, and Wyoming. All of the studies included rural dwellers, although five studies (24%) included urban participants as a comparison group. The mean age of the rural dwellers in this literature review was 63.12 years. The Buehler et al. (1998) study did not include age ranges; therefore, this study was not included in the current review's mean age calculation. Table 16.1 shows the gender and racial or ethnic characteristics of the participants. Notably absent in the studies were Asian or Pacific Islander participants. Otherwise, non-Hispanic Caucasian, African American, Native American, and Hispanic participants were well represented.

Buehler et al. (1998) and O'Lynn (2006) noted a paucity in the literature of resources that describe the *process* rural individuals undertake in managing

TABLE 16.1 Participants' Demographic Characteristics from the 2012 Literature Review (*N* = 21 Studies)

Characteristic	N	%
Gender		
All female	6	29
Mixed	15	71
All male	0	0
Mean age	63.12 y (*N* = 20)	NA
Race/Ethnicity		
All Non-Hispanic White	3	14
Mixed	13	62
All minority	2	10
Unknown	3	14
U.S. States represented	14	28

symptoms/health needs once they have been identified. We confirmed this paucity in the 2012 literature review. Of the 21 studies reviewed, 13 (62%) minimally supported the tendency of adults to use self-care and lay resources before going to a health professional for nonemergent symptoms (Albert, Musa, Kwoh, Hanlon, & Silverman, 2008; Arcury et al., 2006, 2009; Buehler et al., 1998; Clark et al., 2008; Duran et al., 2005; Garcia et al., 2011; Harju, Wuensch, Kuhl, & Cross, 2006; Ruggiero, Gros, McCauley, De Arellano, & Danielson, 2011; Shreffler-Grant, Weinert, Nichols, & Ide, 2005; Stoller et al., 2011; Vallerand, Fouladbakhsh, & Templin, 2005; Zhang, Jones, Spalding, Young, & Ragain, 2009). However, none of these studies described or tested a comprehensive process of health needs identification and actions.

The majority of the studies we reviewed confirmed the use of self-care strategies to treat symptoms (Albert et al., 2008; Arcury et al., 2006, 2009; Brown & May, 2005; Buehler et al., 1998; Callaghan, 2005; Clark et al., 2008; Duran et al., 2005; Easom & Quinn, 2006; Garcia et al., 2011; Harju et al., 2006; Ruggiero et al., 2011; Shreffler-Grant et al., 2005; Stoller et al., 2011; Vallerand et al., 2005; Winters, Cudney, & Sullivan, 2010; Winters, Cudney, Sullivan, & Thuesen, 2006; Zhang et al., 2009). Many of these studies supported the self-care strategies described by Buehler et al., (1998) and O'Lynn (2006), including taking over-the-counter medications, herbal remedies, CAM, and family remedies; referring to health information sources via the Internet, books, and television; and using physical treatments (e.g., heating pads, stretching, massage, or yoga). A number of authors reported the value of prayer and spirituality as self-care strategies (Arcury et al., 2011; Duran et al., 2005; Easom & Quinn, 2006; Harju et al., 2006; Winters et al., 2010). Buehler et al. (1998) did not discuss these strategies. In some of the studies that compared rural and nonrural dwellers, researchers noted that rural dwellers were more likely than nonrural dwellers to use self-care strategies to treat symptoms (Garcia et al., 2011; Harju et al., 2006; Ruggiero et al., 2011; Winters et al., 2010).

We also found support for the use of lay resources in managing symptoms in the studies reviewed. Primarily, researchers reported the strategies of soliciting the assistance and support of friends and family in managing symptoms and in using formal support groups (Albert et al., 2008; Arcury et al., 2006, 2009, 2011; Buehler et al., 1998; Clark et al., 2008; Duran et al., 2005; Easom & Quinn, 2006; Garcia et al., 2011; Goins, Spencer, & Williams, 2010; Ruggiero et al., 2011; Shreffler-Grant et al., 2005; Stoller et al., 2011; Vallerand et al., 2005; Winters et al., 2006, 2010; Zhang et al., 2009). In addition, in nine (43%) of the studies that we reviewed, the researchers reported the progression to lay resources use after self-care had failed, or the use of lay resources prior to the use of professional resources (Arcury et al., 2006; Brown & May, 2005; Buehler et al., 1998; Clark et al., 2008; Easom & Quinn, 2006; Harju et al., 2006; Shreffler-Grant et al., 2005; Vallerand et al., 2005; Winters et al., 2006).

In terms of gender, women were well represented in the sample of studies we reviewed, including six studies in which women were studied exclusively. In only one study from O'Lynn's review in 2006 (Sellers, Poduska, Propp, & White, 1999) did researchers examine men or men's health exclusively; our literature review did not return any studies that focused exclusively on men. This limitation is significant because Sellers et al. noted that although both men and women may rely on self-care and lay resources before utilizing professional resources, men may interpret symptoms very differently and may delay use of professional resources as long as possible (Levant & Habben, 2003; Sabo & Gordon, 1995; Sellers et al., 1999). Consequently, men may incorporate very different time frames for actions.

Generally, the results of the studies support the finding from Buehler et al., Malone, & Majerus et al. (1998) and O'Lynn (2006) that professional resources are utilized after self-care or lay resources are used. Some of the studies we reviewed included the use of complementary or alternative therapies to manage symptoms (Arcury et al., 2006, 2009, 2011; Buehler et al., 1998; Duran et al., 2005; Easom & Quinn, 2006; Harju et al., 2006; Shreffler-Grant et al., 2005; Winters et al., 2010). Complementary therapies included spiritual interventions, as noted earlier, but also included the use of professional resources such as those provided by a masseuse, acupuncturist, naturopath, chiropractor, and herbalist. Other results supported the finding that professional resources are utilized if symptoms persisted (Arcury et al., 2006; Brown & May, 2005; Buehler et al., 1998; Clark et al., 2008; Easom & Quinn, 2006; Harju et al., 2006; Shreffler-Grant et al., 2005; Vallerand et al., 2005; Winters et al., 2006, 2010).

Consistent with O'Lynn's review (2006), none of the investigators of the studies we reviewed provided specific time frames for utilizing resources as described by Buehler et al. (1998). However, research results did support the timeline tenets within the SATL process, particularly those referring to the use of professional resources. The results found that progression to and direct utilization of professional resources was quicker if (a) symptoms involved children (Buehler et al., 1998), (b) symptoms were perceived as emergent or crisis in nature (Arcury et al., 2006; Brown & May, 2005; Buehler et al., 1998; Clark et al., 2008; Easom & Quinn, 2006; Harju et al., 2006; Shreffler-Grant et al., 2005; Vallerand et al., 2005), (c) the individual perceived a need for a prescription to treat the symptom (Buehler et al., 1998; Harju et al., 2006; Winters et al., 2010), or (d) if the symptom would result in the individual missing work (Buehler et al., 1998; Cudney et al., 2006; Harju et al., 2006).

Buehler et al. (1998) reported that if professional resources were not effective in relieving symptoms, participants continued to work with the professional, sought another professional (particularly a provider of alternative therapy), or accepted the symptom's nonresolution. As noted by O'Lynn (2006), we also found in the studies we reviewed that researchers did not address this specific decision point in the same fashion. However, a number of researchers reported the concurrent use of multiple strategies, including complementary or alternative therapies (Albert et al., 2008; Arcury et al., 2006, 2009, 2011; Brown & May, 2005; Buehler et al., 1998; Duran et al., 2005; Easom & Quinn, 2006; Garcia et al., 2011; Simmons, Huddleston-Casas, & Berry, 2007; Stoller et al., 2011; Vallerand et al., 2005; Winters et al., 2006, 2010). A table of characteristic variables pulled from the literature review is displayed in Table 16.2.

TABLE 16.2 Characteristic Variables Found in the 2012 Literature Review (*N* = 21 Studies)

Characteristic Variables	N	%
Self-care resources utilized	18	86
Lay resources	18	86
Decision-making process	17	81
Rural population only	16	76
Multiple strategies used	15	71
Self and lay care used before professional services	13	62
Health promotion	11	52
Barriers to care	11	52
Lay resources to professional	9	43
Cultural beliefs	8	38
Symptom–action process discussed	7	33
Use of CAM therapies	7	33
Self-efficacy	5	24
Rural vs. nonrural population	5	24
Prayer/Spirituality self-care	4	19
Direct use of professional services when:		
Children are involved	1	5
Prescription is needed	3	14
Possible loss of employment	3	14

CAM, complementary alternative medicine.

DISCUSSION

The literature review provides overall support for aspects of the SATL process and the SAP model used by rural dwellers. Although none of the researchers contradicted the model proposed by Buehler et al. (1998) or O'Lynn (2006), no researcher discussed or tested a comprehensive process for health needs identification and action. It should be noted, however, that the number of studies we reviewed was small. Most of the studies were cross-sectional and descriptive in design, limiting the ability to confirm the use of SATL process or SAP model over time. Similar to O'Lynn's review, most of the research we reviewed had small sample sizes and focused primarily on rural dwellers over 50 years of age (mean age = 63.12 years). To be consistent with the O'Lynn review, we did not include participants residing outside the United States. We recommend studies be conducted with larger samples, younger participants, and with participants from outside of the United States, to further support the proposed change from the SAP to the HNAP model. With the exception of the Asian or Pacific Islander communities, the literature we reviewed represented racial or ethnic diversity. We recommend that studies examining rural Alaskan and Hawaiian communities be conducted to provide additional information about the HNAP model. We concur with O'Lynn (2006) that additional studies of men in rural communities should be conducted to further strengthen the HNAP model. Rural health needs of men differ from those of women and would add great value to this model.

A limitation of the SATL process model by Buehler et al. (1998) is the lack of attention to symptoms that are recognized as problematic but ignored. For example, one may recognize a self-limiting symptom such as a strained muscle, but choose no action to relieve the strain. An interesting finding in our review is that stigma and embarrassment influence health pattern behaviors in rural women diagnosed with depression and other mental health issues (Simmons et al., 2007). Both the SAP and HNAP literature reviews found self-efficacy and health behavior patterns to be similar when comparing rural and nonrural dwellers' compliance with personal health needs management and both SAP and HNAP reviews allow for prevention and management of various health needs, including psychological needs (Garcia et al., 2011; Harju et al., 2006; Simmons et al., 2007; Winters et al., 2010). Additional research is needed to explore how stigma, embarrassment, and other factors such as lack of anonymity, familiarity, and isolation from lay resources influence individuals' recognition and response to health needs.

The emphasis on the timeline aspect of the SATL process model is problematic, in that it suggests a rather linear progression through phases of symptom identification, and actions are taken while previous strategies may be abandoned because of unsatisfactory outcomes. We concur with O'Lynn (2006) that the literature we reviewed did not support this process and that instead, multiple modes of treatment are utilized singularly or concurrently. Our review also supports O'Lynn in that as rural dwellers become more educated and familiar with interpreting and identifying recurring health symptoms, they may bypass self-care and lay care and go directly to professional resources. This is more prevalent in those suffering from chronic conditions (Albert et al., 2008; Buehler et al., 1998; Easom & Quinn, 2006; Stoller et al., 2011; Winters et al., 2006, 2010). A study done by Stoller et al. described the older rural adult who was managing both new symptoms and chronic diseases as a "bricoleur"—a kind of informal professional do-it-yourself person who blends information gathered from multiple sources. Managing the process of chronic symptoms and new health needs is well identified in the proposed HNAP model.

Buehler et al. (1998) and O'Lynn (2006) noted that time frames for action were influenced by whether or not the symptoms were associated with children or with emergent conditions. Our review agrees with this process. In addition, as noted previously, others have suggested that time frames for action are also influenced by whether or not symptoms required a prescription or caused one to miss work (Buehler et al., 1998; Harju et al., 2006; Winters et al., 2006, 2010). It is reasonable to assume that barriers in accessing health resources for rural dwellers, as described widely in the literature, will influence how quickly or slowly one may adopt actions to address health need symptoms. As such, time-frames are descriptive outcomes resulting from the contextual variables.

Perceived barriers such as pain, lack of information, and knowledge were noted in three of the studies we reviewed (Callaghan, 2005; Easom & Quinn, 2006; Vallerand et al., 2005). Lack of information and knowledge (coupled with pain) has been found to be related to health promotion activities (Easom & Quinn, 2006). Adding to that is psychological well-being and the ability of rural dwellers to self-identify their health needs (Callaghan, 2005; Duran et al., 2005; Garcia et al., 2011; Ruggiero et al., 2011; Simmons et al., 2007; Winters et al., 2010). O'Lynn (2006) recognized the importance of including psychological symptoms in the model and noted that mental health services are often unavailable or poorly implemented in rural communities. The HNAP model allows for psychological symptomatology to be identified and treated alongside of physical symptoms (as would be the case in pain management, depression, and/or anxiety with new onset or chronic disease management). Depression in rural women is a growing public health concern, and many of the women underreport their symptoms due to stigma and/or a lack of knowledge regarding their symptoms (Simmons et al., 2007). Oftentimes with depression, anxiety, and other psychological disorders, symptoms present with somatic symptoms as well, making them difficult to identify. Our review validated that multiple strategies are used (as depicted in the HNAP model) to address both psychological and physical health needs in rural populations.

RECOMMENDATIONS FOR THE NEW HNAP MODEL

Figure 16.3 shows a graphic depiction of the HNAP model. The action process of the HNAP is embedded in an external context identical to the SAP model. The two models are similar in all facets of identification, decision-making processes, and actions taken by rural dwellers. The only difference between the SAP and the HNAP model is the replacement of the term "symptom" with "health needs" to include physical and psychological health conditions and states. After health needs are identified in the HNAP model, individuals may incorporate various types of actions: (a) self-care, (b) lay resources, and (c) professional resources in a sequential or concurrent fashion. The contexts will influence which action, or combination of actions, is taken. The sloping nature of the action types reflects the propensity to progress from self-care to lay resources use to professional resources use. The double arrows between action types account for fluid movement among aspects of the model and concurrent use

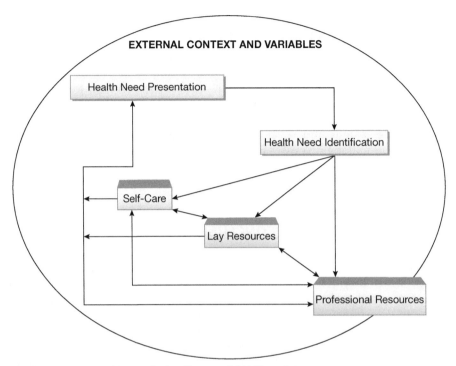

FIGURE 16.3. Health-Needs–Action Process (HNAP) model.
Source: Rasmussen, A.D., O'Lynn, C., & Winters, C.A. (2013). Beyond the symptom-action-timeline process: Explicating the health-needs-action process. In C.A. Winters (Ed.), *Rural nursing: Concepts, theory, and practice* (4th ed., p. 153). New York, NY: Springer Publishing.

of types of actions. More explicit in this model are the arrows leading from the action types back to the symptom occurrence aspect of the model. These arrows close the circle of the process and account for symptoms that might recur, new symptoms that develop, or new actions resulting from new information or previous actions taken by an individual.

Both the SATL process model and HNAP model depict a process in which an individual identifies a problem or health need and takes action(s) to address it. As such, these models may describe the behaviors of all individuals, including nonrural dwellers, although actions taken may differ across populations. To address the limitations of the newly proposed HNAP model, we recommend that further research be conducted to:

1. Evaluate how well the revised HNAP model is empirically supported. If the revised model is well supported, then it may serve as an ideal framework for comparison studies examining health behaviors across participant demographic variables.
2. Identify responses to health needs in rural men and younger individuals to support the revised HNAP model in these populations.

3. Incorporate studies done both internationally and domestically to support rural populations' health need patterns, behaviors, and treatment processes.
4. Address barriers that prevent rural dwellers from health promotion, prevention, and treatment options, including cultural, physical, and psychological impediments that may interfere with the revised HNAP foundation.
5. Provide insight and support regarding cultural practices, beliefs, and decision-making processes in rural dwellers for overall health promotion, illness prevention, and treatment using a holistic interpretation.

CONCLUSION

Buehler et al. (1998) derived the SATL process model from a grounded theory study in which they described the process that a group of rural Montana women used to respond to health symptoms. O'Lynn (2006) completed a literature review to determine the level of support for the SATL process and proposed changes, resulting in a more circular model called SAP. In 2012, a literature review was conducted to determine the level of support for the SATL and SAP models and resulted in the HNAP model. We reviewed 21 research studies located in the CINAHL, MedLine, PsychInfo, PubMed, and Google Scholar databases that focused on the process rural dwellers use to respond to health needs. Those studies provide general support for aspects of the SATL process, the SAP model, and the new HNAP model, although in only seven studies did researchers describe a sequential process of how rural dwellers respond to health symptoms (Albert et al., 2008; Arcury et al., 2009, 2011; Buehler et al., 1998; Stoller et al., 2011; Vallerand et al., 2005; Winters et al., 2010).

We recommend further research with younger participants, rural men, and rural Asian or Pacific Islander participants to determine the support for the revised model. In addition, identifying if cultural, physical, and/or psychological barriers inhibit rural populations (e.g., rural Asian or Pacific Islander) from health promotion, prevention, and treatment would further support the revised SAP model, now renamed HNAP. Finally, we recommend an examination of studies completed outside the continental United States to determine whether the revised model has broad relevance to rural dwellers across the globe.

REFERENCES

Albert, S. M., Musa, D., Kwoh, C. K., Hanlon, J. T., & Silverman, M. (2008). Self-care and professionally guided care in osteoarthritis: Racial differences in a population-based sample. *Journal of Aging and Health*, 20(2), 198–216. doi:10.1177/0898264307310464

Arcury, T. A., Bell, R. A., Snively, B. M., Smith, S. L., Skelly, A. H., Wetmore, L. K., & Quandt, S. A. (2006). Complementary and alternative medicine use as health self-management: Rural older adults with diabetes. *Journal of Gerontology: Social Sciences, 61B*(2), S62–S70.

Arcury, T. A., Grzywacz, J. G., Neiberg, R. H., Lang, W., Nguyen, H. T., Altizer K., … Quandt S. A. (2011). Daily use of complementary and other therapies for symptoms among older adults: Study design and illustrative results. *Journal of Aging and Health, 23*(1), 52–69.

Arcury, T. A., Grzywacz, J. G., Stoller, E. P., Bell, R. A., Altizer, K. P., Chapman, C., Quandt S. A. (2009). Complementary therapy use and health self-management among rural older adults. *Journal of Gerontology: Social Sciences, 64B*(5), 635–643.

Brown, J. W., & May, B. A. (2005). Rural older Appalachian women's formal patterns of care. *Southern Online Journal of Nursing Research, 2*(6), 1–21. Retrieved from http://www.resourcenter.net/images/SNRS/Files/SOJNR_articles/iss02vol06.pdf

Buehler, J., Malone, M., & Majerus, J. (1998). Patterns of responses to symptoms in rural residents: The symptom-action-time-line process. In H. Lee (Ed.), *Conceptual basis for rural nursing* (pp. 153–162). New York, NY: Springer Publishing.

Callaghan, D. (2005). Healthy behaviors, self-efficacy, self-care, and basic conditioning factors in older adults. *Journal of Community Health Nursing, 22*(3), 169–178.

Clark, D. O., Frankel, R. M., Morgan, D. L., Ricketts, G., Bair, M. J., Nyland, K. A., Callahan, C. M. (2008). The meaning and significance of self-management among socioeconomically vulnerable older adults. *Journal of Gerontology: Social Sciences, 63B*(5), S312–S319.

Duran, B., Oetzel, J., Lucero, J., Jiang, Y., Novins, D. K., Manson, Beals, J. (2005). Obstacles for rural American Indians seeking alcohol, drug, or mental health treatment. *Journal of Consulting and Clinical Psychology, 73*(5), 819–829.

Easom, L. R., & Quinn, M. E. (2006). Rural elderly caregivers: Exploring folk home remedy use and health promotion activities. *Online Journal of Rural Nursing and Health Care, 6*(1), 32–46. Retrieved from http://rnojournal.binghamton.edu/index.php/RNO/article/view/164

Evans, J., Frank, B., Oliffe, J. L., & Gregory, D. (2011). Health, illness, men and masculinities (HIMM): A theoretical framework for understanding men and their health. *Journal of Men's Health, 8*(1), 7–15. doi:10.1016/j.jomh.2010.09.227

Garcia, C. M., Gilchrist, L., Vazques, G., Leite, A., & Raymond, N. (2011). Urban and rural immigrant Latino youths and adults' knowledge and beliefs about mental health resources. *Journal of Immigrant Minority Health, 13*, 500–509.

Goins, R. T., Spencer, S. M., & Williams, K. (2010). Lay meanings of health among rural older adults in Appalachia. *The Journal of Rural Health, 27*, 13–20.

Harju, B. L., Wuensch, K. L., Kuhl, E. A., & Cross, N. J. (2006). Comparison of rural and urban residents' implicit and explicit attitudes related to seeking medical care. *National Rural Health Association, 22*(Fall), 359–363.

Levant, R., & Habben, C. (2003). The new psychology of men: Application to rural men. In B. Stamm (Ed.), *Rural behavioral health care: An interdisciplinary guide* (pp. 171–180). Washington, DC: American Psychological Association.

O'Lynn, C. (2006). Updating the symptom-action-time-line process. In H. Lee & C. A. Winters (Eds.), *Rural nursing: Concepts, theory, and practice* (2nd ed., pp. 138–152). New York, NY: Springer Publishing.

Rasmussen, A.D., O'Lynn, C., & Winters, C.A. (2013). Beyond the symptom-action-timeline process: Explicating the health-needs-action process. In C. A. Winters (Ed.), *Rural nursing: Concepts, theory, and practice* (4th ed., pp. 141–157). New York, NY: Springer Publishing.

Ruggiero, K. J., Gros, D. F., McCauley, J., de Arellano, M. A., & Danielson, C. K. (2011). Rural adults' use of health-related information online: Data from a 2006 national online health survey. *Telemedicine and e-Health, 17*(5), 329–334.

Rural Health Information Hub. (2017). Rural mental health. Retrieved from https://www.ruralhealthinfo.org/topics/mental-health

Sabo, D., & Gordon, D. F. (1995). Rethinking men's health and illness. In D. Sabo & D. F. Gordon (Eds.), *Men's health and illness: Gender, power, and the body* (pp. 1–22). Thousand Oaks, CA: Sage.

Sellers, S. C., Poduska, M. D., Propp, L. H., & White, S. I. (1999). The health care meanings, values, and practices of Anglo-American males in the rural Midwest. *Journal of Transcultural Nursing, 10,* 320–330.

Shreffler-Grant, J., Weinert, C., Nicholls, E., & Ide, B. (2005). Complementary therapy use among older rural adults. *Public Health Nursing, 22*(4), 323–331.

Simmons, L. A., Huddleston-Casas, C., & Berry, A. A. (2007). Low-income rural women and depression: Factors associated with self-reporting. *American Journal of Health Behavior, 31*(6), 657–666.

Stoller, E. P., Grzywacz, J. G., Quandt, S. A., Bell, R. A., Chapman, C., Altizer, K. P., … Arcury, T. A. (2011). Calling the doctor: A qualitative study of patient-initiated physician consultation among rural older adults. *Journal of Aging and Health, 23*(5), 782–805.

Vallerand, A. H., Fouladbakhsh, J. M., & Templin, T. (2005). Patients' choices for the self-treatment of pain. *Applied Nursing Research, 18,* 90–96.

Wilson, W., Bangs, A., & Hatting, T. (2015). The future of rural behavioral health. *National Rural Health Association policy brief.* Retrieved from https://www.ruralhealthweb.org/NRHA/media/Emerge_NRHA/Advocacy/Policy%20documents/The-Future-of-Rural-Behavioral-Health_Feb-2015.pdf

Winters, C. A., Cudney, S., & Sullivan, T. (2010). Expressions of depression in rural women with chronic illness. *Rural and Remote Health, 10,* 1–14.

Winters, C. A., Cudney, S., Sullivan, T., & Thuesen, A. (2006). The rural context and women's self-management of chronic health conditions. *Chronic Illness, 2,* 273–289.

Zhang, Y., Jones, B., Spalding, M., Young, R., & Ragain, M. (2009). Use of the Internet for health information among primary care patients in rural West Texas. *Southern Medical Journal, 102*(6), 595–601.

Healthcare Delivery in Rural and Frontier Settings

The focus of this section is the delivery of healthcare in rural and frontier settings. Two chapters appeared in the previous editions of the text; one chapter addresses acceptability as one component of choosing a rural healthcare provider; the second chapter addresses the use of complementary and alternative medicine (CAM). The CAM chapter has been fully updated to include the team's latest work. The remaining five chapters are new and address important challenges facing rural providers including the delivery of palliative care, trauma care, care of veterans and Native Americans, and a healthcare delivery model for critical access hospitals.

CHAPTER 17

Acceptability: One Component in Choice of Healthcare Provider

Jean Shreffler-Grant

DISCUSSION QUESTIONS

- Discuss the aspects of local healthcare that affect the choices that rural dwellers make when deciding whether or not to use local care.
- How can the Acceptability Scale be utilized to improve local rural healthcare?
- Why do you think that the critical access hospital model of care has been implemented so widely across the United States?

Since the early 1980s, access to healthcare has deteriorated in many rural areas in the United States as a result of the closure of rural hospitals and the associated loss of local providers and services that often accompany hospital closure. As one of the major employers in many rural communities, hospital closure can also have a negative economic impact on other local businesses (Balasubramanian & Jones, 2016). In recent years, the rural hospital closure crisis has escalated with 2015 closure rates six times higher than in 2010 (Kaufman et al., 2016; National Rural Health Association [NRHA], 2016). The NRHA (2016) reported that one in three rural hospitals may now be at risk of closure. Much of the blame for closures has long been attributed to factors external to rural communities, such as reduced Medicare reimbursement, a declining rural economy, and provider shortages. In contrast, a substantial volume of evidence has accumulated that indicates that the closures may, in part, be due to influences closer to home. Some rural hospitals are underutilized by local residents, who bypass them to seek care in larger towns and cities (Allen, Davis, Hu, & Owusu-Amankwah, 2015; Amundson, 1993; DeFriese, Wilson, Ricketts, & Whitener, 1992; Escarse & Kapur, 2009; Hall, Marsteller, & Owings, 2010; Liu, Bellamy, Barnet, & Weng, 2008; Liu, Bellamy, & McCormick, 2007; Radcliff, Brasure, Moscovice, &

Stensland, 2003; Weigel, Ullrich, Finegan, & Ward, 2017). As discussed by Lee and McDonagh (2013), "choice" is a new concept that emerged from research about rural persons' health behaviors relevant to the second theoretical statement originally proposed by Long and Weinert (1989). The concept of choice refers to the making of conscious choices by rural dwellers both to live in a rural place and to access healthcare resources. As discussed in this chapter, choice also involves whether or not to access local healthcare resources or alternately, to bypass local care to seek health services in a distant location.

Since the early 1990s, variations of critical access hospitals (CAHs) have been implemented as alternatives to hospitals that are at risk for closure. CAHs must be located in remote rural areas, are limited to short-stay lower-acuity services, and are allowed more flexibility in staffing and other licensure requirements. They are also reimbursed by Medicare on the basis of reasonable cost instead of prospective payment, as compared with traditional rural hospitals. Cost-based Medicare reimbursement is considered advantageous for small hospitals that often serve a high proportion of older patients and are less likely to be able to average risk across large numbers of admissions, as may be necessary under prospective payment (Christianson, Moscovice, Wellever, & Wingert, 1990). Following implementation of the Rural Hospital Flexibility Program, passed into law in 1997, CAHs became a national model and have gained broad support in rural areas across the nation (Shreffler, Capalbo, Flaherty, & Heggam, 1999). By 2006, less than a decade after the CAH model was passed into law, a large majority (80%) of small rural hospitals and more than 60% of all rural hospitals had converted to CAHs (Pink, Holmes, Thompson, & Slifkin, 2007). As of February 2, 2017, there were 1,339 CAHs nationwide (Flex Monitoring Team, 2017). Whether these new CAH models will be any more viable than traditional rural hospitals will likely be tied to how they are viewed and used by the rural residents they are intended to serve.

Improving equity in access to care has been an ongoing concern throughout most of the past half century (Aday, Bagley, Lairson, & Slater, 1993; Patrick & Erickson, 1993), and rural access to care has been a particularly persistent problem (Gamm & Hutchison, 2003). Although equitable access to healthcare in and of itself may be intuitively desirable, it is through presumed links between access to quality health services, appropriate use, and resulting positive health outcomes that access becomes important (Millman, 1993). I conducted a study (1996) to examine rural residents' perspectives on access to healthcare in six communities in Montana with CAHs. The concept of "acceptability" is one dimension of access to care that can be used to explain why people do or do not use local rural healthcare services. As part of the larger study, a scale to measure acceptability was developed and validated. In this chapter, I focus on the Acceptability Scale (see Table 17.1).

TABLE 17.1 Individual Items Included in the "Acceptability Scale"

	Circle One Answer for Each Category					
	Excellent	**Good**	**Average**	**Fair**	**Poor**	
1. How would you rate (facility name) in each of the following categories?						
a. Overall quality of care	5	4	3	2	1	Don't know
b. Medical care	5	4	3	2	1	Don't know
c. Nursing care	5	4	3	2	1	Don't know
d. Staff concern/ compassion	5	4	3	2	1	Don't know
e. "Personal" aspects of care	5	4	3	2	1	Don't know
f. Building cleanliness and condition	5	4	3	2	1	Don't know
g. Acceptability as source of care	5	4	3	2	1	Don't know
2. How would you rate each of the following aspects of overall medical care provided in your community? (Care provided by physicians, nurse practitioners, physician assistants, or other primary care providers at their office or local hospital)						
a. Competence of primary care providers	5	4	3	2	1	Don't know
b. Concern/ compassion for patient	5	4	3	2	1	Don't know
c. "Personal" aspects of care	5	4	3	2	1	Don't know
d. Competence of support staff	5	4	3	2	1	Don't know
e. Acceptability of provider as source of care	5	4	3	2	1	Don't know

Source: Shreffler, M. J. (1996). Rural residents' views on access to care in frontier communities with medical assistance facilities. *Dissertation Abstracts International, 57*, 3131 (No. 9630109).

CONCEPTUAL FRAMEWORK

Access to care was the conceptual framework guiding this study. I conceptualized access to care as having two dimensions. Potential access to care includes properties of the population and healthcare system that affect opportunities to enter into the healthcare system. Actual or realized access to care includes utilization and willingness to use the healthcare system and satisfaction with the care received (Aday & Andersen, 1975; Andersen, McCutcheon, Aday, Chiu, & Bell, 1993).

In several studies published in the 1980s on the relationship between access to care and utilization of care, Penchansky and Thomas (1981; Thomas & Penchansky, 1984) defined access as the fit between clients and the healthcare system. An adequate degree of fit was measured by objective utilization and subjective satisfaction. They identified five components of potential access that are referred to as "the 5 A's":

1. *Availability*—the supply of providers and services relative to clients' needs
2. *Accessibility*—where services are located relative to where clients are
3. *Accommodation*—how services are organized to accept clients
4. *Affordability*—costs of services relative to resources of clients
5. *Acceptability*—the clients' attitudes and opinions about the characteristics of providers and services

Discriminant validity of Penchansky and Thomas's (1981; Thomas & Penchansky, 1984) components of access to care was supported in their studies, and subsets of clients were found to differ significantly in utilization of healthcare, based on how satisfied they were with the components that were salient for them. Although these investigators measured acceptability chiefly by consumers' attitudes and opinions about the physical environment in which care was delivered, they proposed that attitudes about personal and technical practice characteristics of providers and services were also relevant.

METHODS

In the larger study to examine rural residents' perspectives on access to healthcare (Shreffler, 1996), I employed a descriptive survey design. I sent surveys to a random sample of 100 households in each of the six communities with CAHs, and I interviewed a subset of respondents by telephone. I obtained a 63.5% response rate on the mail survey ($N = 381$).

My principal aims in this study were to identify the predictors of use and willingness to use local healthcare, and respondents' satisfaction with care. In interpreting the term "predictors," it should be noted that I sought significant statistical relationships rather than cause and effect relationships. It was not possible to determine from the data whether people used local healthcare because they thought it was acceptable or whether they thought it was acceptable because they had used it.

There were four dependent variables in the analyses to address actual access to care. They were (a) use of the local CAH, (b) use of the local primary care provider, (c) willingness to use the local CAH, and (d) willingness to use the local provider. These use variables were dichotomous yes or no indicators of whether or not the respondents reported actual use of the CAH and the local provider in the recent past. The willingness to use variables were dichotomous yes or no indicators constructed from responses to a question about where respondents would first seek care for a variety of future health concerns. The future health concerns counted as "yes, willing to use" were concerns for which the local CAH and provider(s) offered healthcare services, rather than other services included in the question that were not available locally and for which patients would need to be referred elsewhere.

The major independent variables, or potential predictors, included potential access to care factors. All were measured by respondents' self-report and from their perspectives (vs. from the perspectives of the hospitals or providers). These included characteristics of the population (e.g., age, income, health insurance, and health status) and characteristics of the healthcare system that were operationalized according to "the 5 A's" from Penchansky and Thomas's work (1981; Thomas & Penchansky, 1984), that is, availability, accessibility, accommodation, affordability, and acceptability.

The Acceptability Scale comprised the summed values of responses to twelve 5-point Likert-type rating questions related to the concept of acceptability, included on the mail survey. I based my selection of the questions for inclusion in the scale on Penchansky and Thomas's work (1981; Thomas & Penchansky, 1984). I then validated the questions in telephone interviews from responses to the question: "When you and your household members choose a medical care provider and a hospital to use, can you tell me what factors are important to you?" Responses were related to the technical quality of care, the "art" of care, and the appearance of the facility or office.

The Acceptability Scale items were components of two questions that asked respondents to rate a wide variety of aspects of healthcare in their local communities (see Table 17.1). Response options included excellent, good, average, fair, poor, and do not know. The scale had a possible point range of 12 to 60. The reliability coefficients for the Acceptability Scale were Cronbach's alpha = 0.97 and the Standardized item alpha = 0.97; the inter-item correlations analysis ranged from 0.54 to 0.88.

To identify the predictors of use and willingness to use local healthcare, I built four separate multivariate logistic regression models (one for each dependent variable) in which I first regressed the dependent variable on a set of six community (dummy) variables to control for confounding by community. Then I added independent variables to the model together as a group (not stepwise). Next, I calculated odds ratios and 95% confidence intervals for the independent variables with $p \leq .05$.

I analyzed qualitative comments on several short-answer questions on the mail survey and open-ended questions from the telephone interview regarding access to care by using content analysis methods. I read all qualitative data multiple times and sorted them into similar categories based on the words used in the comments (manifest content) and the apparent meaning of the words (latent content; Catanzaro, 1988). I sought patterns and categories that might add to the understanding of rural residents' views on access to healthcare in their local communities. I then summarized these themes and categories and identified relevant themes using the actual phrases of the respondents.

RESULTS

Table 17.2 shows the descriptive results of the "use of" and "willingness to use" the dependent variables I examined. As can be seen on the table, relatively few respondents ($n = 37, 9.7\%$) reported that anyone in their household had used the local CAH for inpatient care in the prior 2 years, whereas roughly two-thirds of the respondents ($n = 260, 68\%$) reported use of the local provider in the past year. Less than half of the respondents indicated willingness to use the CAH ($n = 162$, 43%) or local providers ($n = 182, 48\%$) for future health concerns.

I computed Acceptability Scale scores for 261 of the total 381 households; I excluded the remaining because of missing values or "don't know" answers. The mean Acceptability Scale score was 46.48 (standard deviation [SD] = 9.87; range = 18–60 points [possible range = 12–60 points]).

On the basis of the logistic regression analysis (summarized in Table 17.3), respondents for households most likely to use the CAH for inpatient care were those who rated their knowledge of local healthcare highly, were older in age, and reported lower incomes. The odds ratio indicates the factor by which the odds of "use" or "willing to use" change when the corresponding variable is changed by one unit. Because in this chapter I focus on the Acceptability Scale,

TABLE 17.2 Frequencies of Dependent Variables "Use of" and "Willingness to Use" Local Healthcare ($N = 381$)

Variable	n	%
"Used the CAHs" for inpatient care in prior 2 years	37	9.7
"Used local provider(s)" in the past year	260	68.0
"Willing to use the CAH" in the future	162	43.0
"Willing to use the local provider(s)" in the future	182	48.0

CAHs, critical access hospitals.

TABLE 17.3 Results of Multivariate Logistic Regression Models to Identify Predictors of "Use of" and "Willingness to Use" Local Healthcare

	β	SE	OR	95% CI
Use of CAHs and				
• Knowledge of local healthcare	0.836*	0.400	2.308	(5.05, 1.06)
• Respondent age	0.035*	0.017	1.036	(1.07, 1.01)
• Household income	−0.533*	0.221	0.587	(0.61, 0.56)
Use of local provider and				
• Acceptability scale score	0.096**	0.024	1.100	(1.15, 1.05)
Willing to use CAHs and				
• Acceptability scale score	0.065**	0.021	1.067	(1.11, 1.02)
• Use local provider	0.936*	0.452	2.549	(6.18, 1.05)
Willing to use local provider and				
• Acceptability scale score	0.088**	0.023	1.092	(1.14, 1.04)
• Used provider in the past	1.879**	0.504	6.546	(17.58, 2.44)
• Community affiliation	1.540**	0.549	4.664	(13.69, 1.59)

CI, 95% confidence interval of the odds ratio; OR, odds ratio; SE, standard error.
Data include significant independent variables only.
*$p \leq .05$.
**$p \leq .01$.

I do not discuss the other results at length, but just as illustration, for every unit increase in the knowledge rating category with an odds ratio of 2.308, the odds of use of the CAH increased by 130%. An odds ratio of 1 is equal odds, so anything significantly over or less than 1 is considered. The Acceptability Scale as well as other variables in this model (distance from CAH, use of local provider, ease of transportation, and community affiliation) were not significant predictors of use of the CAH. I anticipated that few if any covariates would be significant in this model, with only 37 households that had reported use of the CAH.

Households most likely to use the local provider(s) were those that had higher Acceptability Scale scores. For each additional point on the scale, the odds of use of the provider increased by 10%. Other variables in this model (knowledge of local healthcare, distance from CAH, respondent age, income, transportation, and community affiliation) were not significant predictors of use of the local provider.

Households most likely to be willing to use the CAH for future health problems were those with higher Acceptability Scale scores and those that had used the local provider(s) in the past year. Based on the odds ratios for each additional point on the Acceptability Scale, the odds of indicating willingness to use the CAH increased by 7%. Other variables in this model (knowledge, distance from CAH, age, income, transportation, and community affiliation) were not significant predictors of willingness to use the CAH.

Residents most likely to be willing to use the local provider(s) in the future were also those with higher acceptability scores, who used the local provider(s) in the past year, and reported that they were affiliated with the local community. Each point on the Acceptability Scale increased the odds of willingness to use the provider by 9%. Other variables in this model (knowledge, distance from CAH, age, income, and transportation) were not significant predictors of willingness to use the local provider.

Among those who used local healthcare, the Acceptability Scale score was also a significant predictor of satisfaction with care. Because I included only those households that had used both the CAH and local provider(s) in the recent past ($n = 36$) in this analysis, I used Mantel–Haenszel chi-square tests to examine relationships between satisfaction and selected covariates. There was insufficient power to analyze this relationship using multivariate logistic regression models. The Acceptability Scale score was significantly associated with satisfaction with the local CAH, emergency care, local primary care provider(s), and the availability of night or weekend care ($p \leq .01$). Other variables examined were not significantly associated with satisfaction with care.

In the qualitative comments, the rural respondents offered many perspectives related to the relationship between acceptability and use of local healthcare. "He knows what he's doing. He knows my son and my son knows him and that's comforting." "He's a country type doctor. I like that." "The way a hospital is equipped. I want a doctor who is top of the line." "For the doctor—that you have rapport with him, that he gives you accurate information, that you're comfortable that he knows what he's doing." "For the hospital—the nursing care, cleanliness. The doctor—personality. I go to see him the first time—did the medicines help, did the care help the problem?" "They don't have the services, the doctor's not as good, and it's not as good a hospital."

CONCLUSION

In this study, the Acceptability Scale was the most consistent predictor of "use of" and "willingness to use" local rural healthcare, as well as of satisfaction with care. Acceptability is that component of access to care that reflects potential clients' attitudes and opinions about the characteristics of providers and services. Unlike other aspects of access, acceptability reflects making a choice based on an opinion, judgment, and personal preferences on the part of consumers. The current rural reality for obtaining most goods and services including healthcare is that with access to vehicles, modern highways, and health insurance, rural residents are not as affected by distance in choosing healthcare as they once were. This study suggests that those who do not find local healthcare acceptable go elsewhere.

It is interesting to note that a large majority (95%) of the respondents in this study indicated that having local healthcare was very or somewhat important to their household members; "keeping" or maintaining the health services and providers they had was the predominant theme in the qualitative comments—yet only 9.7% of the households had a family member hospitalized in the CAH in the prior 2 years, and only 68.2% had used the local provider(s) in the prior year. A clarification of this discrepancy may be found by considering a second theme that emerged from the data—"just in case," as the following quotes show:

- "You always have certain people who are doubters … but they still want emergency care available in case they need it, even though they don't support it for everyday things."
- "I know that it's not paying its way in taxes but we need it. It's like having an insurance policy. Insurance policies don't pay for themselves either but you need it just in case."

Clearly there was support in these six communities for keeping their local healthcare, as evidenced by the large number of participants who reported that local healthcare was important to their household. The importance of local healthcare, however, was not associated with use of it, while their perception of the acceptability of local healthcare was associated with use.

By improving researchers' understanding of what rural consumers deem acceptable in terms of services and providers, the Acceptability Scale can be used to improve healthcare access for rural residents. In the practice arena, attending to community residents' perceptions of competence, quality, the art of care, and appearance of facilities as well as developing strategies to strengthen and improve these perceptions may reduce out-migration from healthcare that is available locally. In the policy arena, as new models of care are developed or refined, paying substantial attention to features or characteristics that influence acceptability to consumers can make the difference between services that will be used and valued and services that will be bypassed by the residents they are intended to serve. When it comes to rural healthcare, Kinsella's (1982) old baseball adage, "If you build it, [they] will come," does not necessarily hold, unless what is built is acceptable to rural residents.

ACKNOWLEDGMENTS

This research was funded by Health Care Financing Administration Dissertation Grant 30-P-90510/0-01, Hester McLaws Award, Sigma Theta Tau Zeta Upsilon Research Award, and Montana State University College of Nursing.

REFERENCES

Aday, L. A., & Andersen, R. (1975). A framework for the study of access to medical care. In L. A. Aday & R. Andersen (Eds.), *Development of indices of access to medical care* (pp. 1–14). Ann Arbor, MI: Health Administration Press.

Aday, L. A., Bagley, C. E., Lairson, D. R., & Slater, C. H. (1993). *Evaluating the medical care system: Effectiveness, efficiency, and equity.* Ann Arbor, MI: Health Administration Press.

Allen, J. E., Davis, A. F., Hu, W., & Owusu-Amankwah, E. (2015). Residents' willingness-to-pay for attributes of rural healthcare facilities. *The Journal of Rural Health, 31*(1), 7–18. doi:10.1111/jrh.12080

Amundson, B. (1993). Myth and reality in the rural health service crisis: Facing up to community responsibilities. *The Journal of Rural Health, 9,* 176–187. doi:10.1111/j.1748-0361.1993.tb00512.x

Andersen, R. M., McCutcheon, A., Aday, L. A., Chiu, G. Y., & Bell, R. (1993). Exploring dimensions of access to medical care. *Health Services Research, 18*(1), 49–74.

Balasubramanian, S. S., & Jones, E. C. (2016). Hospital closures and the current healthcare climate: The future of rural hospitals in the USA. *Rural and Remote Health, 16,* 1–5. Retrieved from http://www.rrh.org.au/articles/subviewnew.asp?ArticleID=3935

Catanzaro, M. (1988). Using qualitative analytical techniques. In N. F. Woods & M. Catanzaro (Eds.), *Nursing research: Theory and practice* (pp. 437–456). St. Louis, MO: C.V. Mosby.

Christianson, J. B., Moscovice, I. S., Wellever, A. L., & Wingert, T. D. (1990). Institutional alternatives to the rural hospital. *Health Care Financing Review, 11*(3), 87–97.

DeFriese, G. H., Wilson, G., Ricketts, T. C., & Whitener, L. (1992). Consumer choice and the national rural hospital crisis. In W. M. Gesler & T. C. Ricketts (Eds.), *Health in rural North America* (pp. 206–225). New Brunswick, NJ: Rutgers University Press.

Escarse, J. J., & Kapur, K. (2009). Do patients bypass rural hospitals? Determinants of inpatient hospital choice in rural California. *Journal of Health Care for the Poor and Underserved, 20*(3), 625–644. doi:10.1353/hpu.0.0178

Flex Monitoring Team. (2017). Critical access hospital locations. Retrieved from http://www.flexmonitoring.org/data/critical-access-hospital-locations

Gamm, L., & Hutchison, L. (2003). Rural health priorities in America: Where you stand depends on where you sit. *The Journal of Rural Health, 19*(3), 209–213. doi:10.1111/j.1748-0361.2003.tb00563.x

Hall, M. J., Marsteller, J., & Owings, M. (2010). Factors influencing rural residents' utilization of urban hospitals. *National Health Statistical Report, 18*(31), 1–12.

Kaufman, B. G., Thomas, S. R., Randolph, R. K., Perry, J. R., Thompson, K. W., & Pink, G. H. (2016). The rising rate of rural hospital closures. *The Journal of Rural Health, 32*(1), 35–43. doi:10.1111/jrh.12128

Kinsella, W. P. (1982). *Shoeless Joe Jackson comes to Iowa.* New York, NY: Ballantine Books.

Lee, H. J., & McDonagh, M. K. (2013). Updating the rural nursing base. In C. A. Winters (Ed.), *Rural nursing: Concepts, theory, and practice* (4th ed., pp. 15–33). New York, NY: Springer Publishing.

Liu, J. J., Bellamy, G. R., Barnet, B., & Weng, S. (2008). Bypass of local primary care in rural counties: Effect of patient and community characteristics. *Annals of Family Medicine, 6*(2), 124–130. doi:10.1370/afm.794

Liu, J. J., Bellamy, G. R., & McCormick, M. (2007). Patient bypass behavior and critical access hospitals: Implications for patient retention. *The Journal of Rural Health, 23*(1), 17–24. doi:10.1111/j.1748-0361.2006.00063.x

Long, K. A., & Weinert, C. (1989). Rural nursing: Developing the theory base. *Scholarly Inquiry for Nursing Practice: An International Journal, 3*, 113–127.

Millman, M. (Ed.). (1993). *Access to care in America.* Washington, DC: National Academies Press.

National Rural Health Association. (2016). New report indicates 1 in 3 rural hospitals at risk. Retrieved from https://www.ruralhealthweb.org/NRHA/media/Emerge_NRHA/PDFs/02-02-16PI16NRHAreleaseoniVantagestudy.pdf

Patrick, D. L., & Erickson, P. (1993). *Health status and health policy: Quality of life in health evaluation and resource allocation.* New York, NY: Oxford University Press.

Penchansky, R., & Thomas, J. W. (1981). The concept of access: Definition and relationship to consumer satisfaction. *Medical Care, 19*, 127–140. doi:10.1097/00005650-198102000-00001

Pink, G. H., Holmes, G. M., Thompson, R. E., & Slifkin, R. T. (2007). Variations in financial performance among peer groups of Critical Access Hospitals. *The Journal of Rural Health, 23*(4), 299–305. doi:10.1111/j.1748-0361.2007.00107.x

Radcliff, T. A., Brasure, M., Moscovice, I. S., & Stensland, J. T. (2003). Understanding rural hospital bypass behavior. *The Journal of Rural Health, 19*(3), 252–259. doi:10.1111/j.1748-0361.2003.tb00571.x

Rural Assistance Center. (2012). CAH frequently asked questions. Retrieved from http://www.raconline.org/topics/hospitals/cahfaq.php

Shreffler, M. J. (1996). Rural residents views on access to care in frontier communities with medical assistance facilities. *Dissertation Abstracts International, 57*, 3131 (No. 9630109).

Shreffler, M. J., Capalbo, S. M., Flaherty, R. J., & Heggam, C. (1999). Community decision-making about critical access hospitals: Lessons learned from Montana's Medical Assistance Facility program. *The Journal of Rural Health, 15*, 180–188. doi:10.1111/j.1748-0361.1999.tb00738.x

Thomas, J. W., & Penchansky, R. (1984). Relating satisfaction with access and utilization of services. *Medical Care, 22*, 553–568. doi:10.1097/00005650-198406000-00006

Weigel, P. A., Ullrich, F., Finegan, C. N., & Ward, M. M. (2017). Rural bypass for elective surgeries. *The Journal of Rural Health, 33*(2), 135–145 doi:10.1111/jrh.12163

CHAPTER 18

Challenges and Opportunities to Palliative Care for Rural Veterans

Tamara L. Tasseff and Susan S. Tavernier

DISCUSSION TOPICS

Select one rural community to:

- Compare and contrast nonveteran rural populations with rural veteran populations.
- Explore strategies the rural community could implement to provide culturally sensitive care to military veterans.
- Explain how palliative care and hospice care are similar or dissimilar.
- Describe barriers to implementing concurrent palliative care. Identify specific strategies to address those barriers.

Rural veterans are an important subset of both the veteran and the rural population with differing healthcare needs that are sometimes misunderstood. Concurrent palliative care, when delivered as a critical component of comprehensive primary care in rural areas, may offer the best opportunity for rural veterans to remain productive amid the increasing incidence of multiple chronic conditions (MCCs). In this chapter, we describe the rural veteran culture, outline the current research on the barriers to palliative care in the rural setting, and provide direction in the opportunities that exist addressing the concerns of the rural veteran population.

WHO ARE RURAL VETERANS?

Rural veterans are a unique subset of the larger rural-dwelling and veteran population. Approximately 5.2 million veterans live in rural areas (Office of Rural Health, n.d.). They account for nearly 11% of the rural-dwelling population

(Cromartie, 2016), 23% of the veterans living in the United States, and 33% of the veterans enrolled in the Veterans Administration (VA) healthcare system (Office of Rural Health, n.d.). Rural veterans, on average, are older than rural nonveterans (Sibener et al., 2014), and 57% of rural veterans are 65 years of age or older (Office of Rural Health, n.d.).

Of the total number of veterans alive, America's rural veterans represent serving in World War II (4%), the Korean conflict (9%), the Vietnam Era (40%), pre-9/11 (12%), and post-9/11 (11%) (National Center for Veterans Analysis and Statistics, 2016). Although Vietnam Era veterans constitute the largest segment of rural veterans, post-9/11 veterans who served in Iraq and Afghanistan account for 435,000 rural veterans (Office of Rural Health, n.d.). Thirty-six percent of rural veterans, 20% of whom are under 65 years of age, have service-connected disabilities. The majority of rural veterans have multiple, complex, physical and mental health needs that require ongoing care throughout their lives (Farmer, Hosek, & Adamson, 2016).

The Influence of Veteran Culture

Kuehner (2013), a Navy nurse practitioner and a veteran, describes the diverse nature of veterans as individuals who are united by service to a nation who are influenced by a collective military culture. Yet each has a unique story and perspective without any one story revealing the complexity of care needs faced by the veterans after their military service has ended. Similar to Kuehner's assessment of the larger veteran population, rural veterans are diverse and may associate characteristics of both veteran and rural cultural attributes.

Duty, honor, respect, self-sacrifice, integrity, loyalty, and courage are an inseparable part of many rural veterans and the larger veteran population, regardless of the military era or length of their military service (Kuehner, 2013; Meyer, 2015). The military culture is one in which personal privacy is relinquished (Meyer, 2015). Because of this cultural attribute, veterans may distrust healthcare providers based on their experiences with military providers who are compelled to disclose information that may influence the goals of the Department of Defense (Kuehner, 2013).

The military cultural attribute of self-sacrifice for the good of the larger population devalues personal well-being. This leads to a perception that health-seeking behaviors are selfish (Meyer, 2015). This perception is further promoted by the military culture that promotes a "hypermasculine paradigm" (Ashley & Brown, 2015, p. 535) in which help seeking is viewed as weakness. Seeking help for mental health–related issues is often viewed as taboo by many veterans; however, the newest generation of veterans, those who served in Iraq and Afghanistan, may be more open to seeking mental health assistance than older veterans. In a recent survey of 1,501 Iraq and Afghanistan veterans, 58% reported sustaining a mental health injury and 82% reported seeking mental health assistance (Maffucci & Frazier, 2015).

Other studies of veterans reported that rural veterans may utilize emergency departments more than urban veterans to seek mental health treatment rather than seek assistance from available VA or community counseling centers (Johnson et al., 2015). Differences related to the military ethos or war-fighter mentality led to recent changes in the *Diagnostic and Statistical Manual of Mental Disorders* (*DSM*) criteria for posttraumatic stress disorder (PTSD). The original wording in the diagnostic criteria for PTSD used the language related to the patient's endorsement of helplessness, yet military members are trained to confront self-doubt and helplessness as an enemy to be engaged, the opposite of helplessness (Meyer, 2015).

Rural veterans, many of whom joined the military in late adolescence between the ages of 17 and 19 years, internalized the military culture and core values into their personal identities (Kuehner, 2013; Meyer, 2015). Just over 20% of 1,501 veterans of Iraq and Afghanistan believe that civilians understand the sacrifices that veterans have made despite the majority believing they are supported by the public (Maffucci & Frazier, 2015).

Influence of Rural Culture on Rural-Dwelling Veterans

Autonomy, self-reliance, and defining health as the ability to be productive, rather than as the absence of disease (Long & Weinert, 2013), are the attributes of rural culture. Similar to nonveteran rural dwellers, rural veterans frequently encounter transportation challenges, tend to travel farther to receive care, have poorer physical and mental health, poorer quality of life, higher rates of disability, and smaller incomes than urban dwellers and urban veterans; however, rural veterans are more likely than rural nonveterans to have healthcare insurance (National Center for Veterans Analysis and Statistics, 2016). A large majority of Iraq and Afghanistan veterans (71%) surveyed reported service-connected disabilities and chronic pain (64%) and/or PTSD (77%) connected to their military service (Maffucci & Frazier, 2015).

Rural veterans often receive care from local community providers in addition to the VA (Nayar, Apenteng, Yu, Woodbridge, & Fetrick, 2013). Despite access to multiple sources of care, often referred to as "dual care," rural veterans face additional disparities that are different than those encountered by urban veterans and rural dwellers. For example, rural veterans with dementia have a greater likelihood of not receiving timely and effective ambulatory care and were more likely than nonveteran rural dwellers and urban veterans to experience an avoidable hospitalization (Thorpe, Houtven, Sleath, & Thorpe, 2010).

Many health professionals and the public perceive veterans to have abundant access to care from the VA, and within the community through TRICARE (www.tricare.mil) or the Veterans Choice Program (www.va.gov/opa/choiceact). Yet, only active duty military members and veterans who have retired from the military or are Congressional Medal of Honor recipients are eligible for TRICARE, the military equivalent of insurance (Department of Defense, 2016). Not all veterans are eligible for or elect to receive care at VA facilities for a multitude of reasons (Nayar et al., 2013). Many veterans are unfamiliar with the Veterans Choice Program, are uncertain of their eligibility, or do not know how to access it (Maffucci & Frazier, 2015).

Many rural veterans face undue health burdens related to higher rates of chronic disease and disability. Moreover, rural veterans endure challenges of care coordination between the VA, Veterans Choice Program, and local rural healthcare providers, and experienced culturally insensitive care by civilian healthcare teams (Nayar et al., 2013). Gale and Heady (2013) reported a lack of military/veteran cultural competence and understanding of service-connected health issues and behavioral health needs of rural veterans. One-third of Americans under the age of 30, the generation comprising health professionals who will provide care for our rural veterans, are directly related to a military service member (Meyer, 2015). Johnson et al. (2015) noted rural veterans with psychiatric diagnoses, including PTSD, were at higher risk of not receiving appropriate medical services, yet this was not observed in the urban veteran population. Thorpe et al. (2010) examined rural–urban access to ambulatory care for veterans with dementia and found preventable admissions were four times higher for rural veterans than urban veterans. They also found that the association between rurality and preventable hospital admissions was not attributable to overall higher preventable hospital admissions in rural areas. Nayar et al. (2013) found that 74% of rural providers, compared with 59% of urban providers, believed non-VA physicians had enough experience to treat war-related PTSD.

CURRENT RESEARCH ON THE BARRIERS TO PALLIATIVE CARE IN THE RURAL SETTING

Understanding the barriers to palliative care begins with embracing the broad definition of palliative care—improving the quality of life of patients and families facing physical, psychological, or spiritual problems associated with a life-threatening illness through early identification, assessment, and treatment allowing the patient to live as full a life as possible (World Health Organization [WHO], 2015). Despite the broad definition of palliative care and the appropriateness of delivering palliative care at any age and at any stage of a serious illness, 86% of the people who could benefit from palliative care never receive it (WHO, 2015). Basic palliative care can be delivered by primary care providers as a component of comprehensive primary care. Specialized palliative care is often delivered by providers with advanced training in palliative medicine. Palliative care is not hospice care. Hospice care is a special subset of palliative care focused on the end-of-life period. However, the main barrier to offering palliative care may be the misperception that palliative care is synonymous with end-of-life or hospice care (Aslakson et al., 2013; LeBlanc et al., 2015; Meo, Hwang, & Morrison, 2011).

Research related to the perceptions of palliative care held by physicians, nurses, and patients shows these misperceptions exist throughout the world and are not isolated to the United States. Very little published current research exists related to the barriers to palliative care in rural areas. A significant gap exists related to rural veterans' perceptions of palliative care and barriers to rural veterans' experiences of receiving palliative care.

Concurrent palliative care, to improve quality of life, may be offered simultaneously with traditional treatment. Rural veterans suffering from diabetes, heart disease, Parkinson's, Alzheimer's, or other dementias, multiple sclerosis, cancer, kidney disease, and rheumatoid arthritis may be candidates for concurrent palliative care. However, even when physicians and nurses recognize the value of palliative care, they may associate palliative care with a cancer diagnosis and not within the broader context as appropriate to multiple serious chronic conditions (Golla, Galushko, Pfaff, & Voltz, 2014; Kavalieratos et al., 2014). Nurses and physicians more familiar with end-of-life or hospice care may be proponents of palliative care, yet believe that palliative care is appropriate only at the point traditional medical treatments have stopped (Verschuur, Groot, & van der Sande, 2014). This limits a broader application of palliative care to a wide range of serious, chronic illnesses appropriate at any point within the disease trajectory.

Challenges—The Increasing Incidence of Chronic Conditions and the Aging Population

Rural veterans, similar to the aging, rural-dwelling population, are experiencing an increasing incidence of chronic disease that further challenges rural healthcare. Developing chronic conditions increases with aging, and nearly 50% of 45- to 64-year-olds have MCCs and 80% of people older than 65 have MCCs (Gerteis et al., 2014). The rapidly aging population in the United States, increased life expectancy, and the rise in MCCs will increase demands on the U.S. healthcare system, especially in rural areas already burdened by health professional shortages. Increased economic burdens, bothersome symptoms, and stress will likely decrease quality of life for those living with MCCs and their families (Goodman, Posner, Huang, Parekh, & Koh, 2013). This is especially true in rural areas where only 10% of physicians and 16% of nurses practice (Bolin et al., 2015).

Fifty-seven percent of rural veterans are currently over the age of 65 (Office of Rural Health, n.d.) and by 2030, one in five Americans will be 65 or older (Centers for Disease Control and Prevention [CDC], 2013); the vast majority will be living with MCCs. Aging rural veterans and rural nonveterans will be competing for limited healthcare resources, such as available skilled nursing, hospital, and home care in rural areas. Suboptimal symptom management reduces quality of life for rural veterans and rural-dwelling people suffering from serious chronic illnesses or MCCs (CDC, 2013; Institute of Medicine

[IOM], 2015). Aging rural veterans and their families may face additional challenges related to dementia in addition to increases in the incidence of MCCs.

Challenges—Rural Veterans and Early Onset Dementia

Recent studies find rural dwellers and rural veterans who have sustained head trauma, including concussions, have a higher risk of developing dementia or Alzheimer's disease (Alzheimer's Association, 2015). Veterans diagnosed with PTSD, or who have sustained moderate traumatic brain injuries (TBIs), have double the risk of developing Alzheimer's disease and the risk quadruples for rural veterans who have experienced severe TBIs, such as injuries sustained from roadside bomb blasts in Iraq and Afghanistan (Qureshi et al., 2010). Although more research is needed, it is conceivable that rural veterans may develop Alzheimer's years earlier than the traditional Alzheimer's patient (Sibener et al., 2014). An aging rural veteran and rural population, increases in MCCs, and limited availability of skilled nursing beds, healthcare and community support resources, and healthcare professionals require proactive planning now.

Challenges—Confidence and Competence Providing Palliative Care Services

Many physicians and nurses lack experience, confidence, or comfort providing palliative care, especially on an outpatient or ambulatory care basis (Raphael, Waterworth, & Gott, 2014; Schroedl, Yount, Szmuilowicz, Rosenberg, & Kalhan, 2014). Managing referrals (Smith et al., 2013), funding and staffing issues (Raphael et al., 2014; Smith et al., 2013), and difficulties with estimating survival or disease trajectory of nonmalignant diagnoses (Schroedl et al., 2014) remain challenging. Physicians and nurses who practice in rural areas may already experience geographical and professional isolation, and may believe concurrent palliative care should be reserved solely for palliative medicine specialists. Additionally, it is posited that certain professional vulnerabilities may exist for healthcare professionals who believe palliative care is more than end-of-life care when many of their colleagues and patients may perceive that palliative care is solely end-of-life care. Although growing evidence supports the cost-effectiveness of palliative care services (WHO, 2015), convincing rural healthcare administrators and community boards that palliative care is responsible, efficient, and cost-effective care can be challenging and time consuming. However, opportunities exist to proactively screen, explore, and implement alternate healthcare delivery models, and change perceptions through mentoring and education.

Opportunities—Screenings and Creative Alternate Healthcare Delivery Models

Routine screening interventions may assist rural providers with providing higher quality, culturally sensitive care while identifying rural veterans at risk of developing dementia or who may be experiencing a reduced quality of life related to a serious chronic condition and suboptimal symptom management. Less than 40% of non-VA providers screen patients for military service (Meyer, 2015). The VA maintains a website that contains a Military Service Toolkit that provides a screening tool and helpful ideas on how to approach screening patients for military service and questions that may be used to help identify veterans and their specific healthcare needs (VA/U.S. Department of Veterans Affairs, n.d.).

Routine screening of all rural veterans with a history of TBI, depression, and/or PTSD (Qureshi et al., 2010) may help with early identification of veterans who may be most at risk of developing dementia. Early screening and identification provides the opportunity for earlier intervention, including concurrent palliative care, support for the veteran and family, and opportunities for rural community planning and support.

Routine screening of rural veterans with serious chronic conditions may help to identify suboptimal symptom management and reduced quality of life as early in the disease trajectory as possible. The goal of palliative care is to address the stress and symptoms—physical, spiritual, and psychological—of a serious illness at any point within the disease trajectory (WHO, 2015). Routine screening promotes earlier intervention. Many rural healthcare providers have implemented routine depression screening, and this screening is extremely important to rural veterans. Only 6% of Iraq and Afghanistan veterans considered taking their own lives prior to entering military service and the majority, 53% to 73%, reported excellent premilitary health; however, 40% of these same veterans have considered taking their own lives since joining the military and less than 10% reported excellent current overall health (Maffucci & Frazier, 2015). Screening information provides information helpful to considering and designing alternate healthcare delivery models for rural areas.

The VA has shifted focus to community-based clinics and medical home models of care while researching innovative ways to provide care to rural veterans, such as home visits and partnerships with rural community providers (Karlin, Zeiss, & Burris, 2010). The VA has collaborated on several concurrent palliative care research studies, and in 2010, reported providing primary care visits, inclusive of palliative care, to over 21,000 veterans (Shreve, 2010). Current VA research and development efforts are underway to improve access to care for rural veterans through field-based pilot projects in three regions of the United States; VA researchers are pursuing the use of telemedicine/telehealth and virtual consults to provide psychotherapy; interventions for

PTSD, insomnia, Parkinson's disease; and caregiver support to veterans and their caregivers located in rural and remote areas (U.S. Department of Veterans Affairs, 2016). The VA offers multiple continuing education opportunities for community-based non-VA providers and nurses in addition to research collaboration.

Opportunities—Changing Perceptions Through Education and Mentoring

Military culture and palliative care education for health professionals, administrators, and the community are two of the best investments in redesigning rural healthcare delivery models. In 2011, a White House initiative, *Joining Forces*, was launched to promote a greater understanding of the military culture and improve support for veterans. Despite ending in January 2017, over 660 nursing schools in all 50 states (Rossiter, 2015) and more than 100 medical schools across the United States (Association of American Medical Colleges [AAMC], n.d.) committed to greater support of veterans health and culturally sensitive care. Although the vast majority of medical schools reported curriculum on PTSD and TBIs, roughly 25% reported addressing the military culture within their curriculum (Meyer, 2015; Ross, Ravindranath, Clay, & Lypson, 2015).

Physician and nurse perceptions of palliative care likely affect medical and nursing practice. Palliative care perceptions affect when, how, and if palliative care is initiated, impact referral practices, and determine whether concurrent palliative care or only end-of-life care is offered. The IOM (2015) called for better education, communication, policies, payment, and planning related to quality of care through the end of life. The American Association of Colleges of Nursing (AACN) has also studied and adopted 17 updated palliative care competencies for undergraduate nursing students utilizing a panel of palliative care experts and key nursing academic representatives (Ferrell, Malloy, Mazanec, & Virani, 2016).

Although the intent of nursing and medical schools is promising, more educational and palliative care mentoring opportunities are needed to support rural providers and nurses. Mentoring opportunities with health professionals who possess expertise in treating veterans and with palliative medicine specialists are needed and could significantly advance concurrent palliative care availability for rural veterans and rural-dwelling people. Creative solutions and ideas are needed to support and increase the practice of palliative care in rural areas. The potential of telemedicine and virtual consults or e-palliative care, similar to successful e-ICU collaboratives operating in some rural areas, is one idea that may offer specialized support and virtual consults through palliative medicine specialists located in urban centers.

Community education, delivered in collaboration with the VA, veterans, and palliative care experts, is an important step in advancing the understanding of the military culture and the benefits of concurrent palliative care within rural communities. A broadened understanding of the rural veteran culture and concurrent palliative care may allow rural communities to dialogue and discuss proactive solutions to limited healthcare and community resources. Enlisting the help of rural veterans, who may be looking for a renewed purpose and mission, may provide insight into how to partner on rural models of healthcare delivery that incorporate concurrent palliative care and utilize rural veterans to identify and assist other rural veterans in need of concurrent palliative care while providing real-time insight into the rural veteran culture.

Opportunities—Research, Legislative Reform, and Application of the Evidence to Practice

Improving the access and availability of concurrent palliative care for rural veterans is a complex mission in need of a collaborative multifaceted approach. Palliative care, delivered as a complement to primary care for rural veterans with serious chronic conditions, may provide increased quality of life while promoting ethical, efficient, individualized, cost-effective, and resource-conscious care. Controlling symptoms may reduce the stress and symptom burden for both rural veterans and their families. Rural veterans of working age may perceive symptom management related to chronic conditions, or permanent disabling injuries as aligning with rural values such as remaining productive and regaining self-reliance, thus supporting an improved quality of life.

Legislators are also recognizing that palliative care offers affordable, efficient, high-quality care beyond end-of-life care. A bill introduced in the U.S. House of Representatives, H.R. 1676—Palliative Care and Hospice Education and Training Act, is aimed at improving palliative care and hospice education in medical and nursing schools, increasing research, and supporting the development of faculty careers in palliative medicine (Engel, 2017).

More research related to rural veterans, support for faculty, mentors, and education of healthcare professionals in rural communities is needed to promote an understanding of rural veterans and to correct palliative care misperceptions. Research, education, and application of the evidence to improve concurrent palliative care delivery will be needed to improve quality of life for rural veterans and their families living with serious chronic conditions.

CONCLUSION

In a time of healthcare professional shortages, decreasing reimbursements, and limited resources, current healthcare models are insufficient to address the needs of veterans living in rural areas; projections suggest the situation will continue to deteriorate unless healthcare delivery models change. Collaborations between rural providers and the VA not only serve to assist rural veterans, but may also be the best opportunity to develop a national healthcare model that improves the access and availability of concurrent palliative care for rural-dwelling people throughout the United States.

REFERENCES

Alzheimer's Association. (2015). 2015 Alzheimer's disease facts and figures. *Alzheimer's & Dementia, 11*(3), 88. Retrieved from https://www.alz.org/facts/downloads/facts_figures_2015.pdf

Ashley, W., & Brown, J. C. (2015). The impact of combat status on veterans' attitudes toward help seeking: The hierarchy of combat elitism. *Journal of Evidence-Informed Social Work, 12*(5), 534–542. doi:10.1080/15433714.992695

Aslakson, R., Koegler, E., Moldovan, R., Shannon, K., Peters, J., Redstone, L., . . . Pronovost, P. (2013). Intensive care unit nurses and palliative care: Perceptions and recommendations. *Journal of Pain & Symptom Management, 45*(2), 419–420. doi:10.1016/j.jpainsymman.2012.10.123

Association of American Medical Colleges. (n.d.). AAMC supports joining forces. Retrieved from https://www.aamc.org/advocacy/campaigns_and_coalitions/258074/joiningforces.html

Bolin, J. N., Bellamy, G. R., Ferdinand, A. O., Vuong, A. M., Kash, B. A., Schulze, A., & Helduser, J. W. (2015). Rural Healthy People 2020: New decade, same challenges. *The Journal of Rural Health, 31*(3), 326–333. doi:10.1111/jrh.12116

Centers for Disease Control and Prevention. (2013). *The state of aging and health in America 2013* (p. 60). *U.S. Department of Health and Human Services.* Retrieved from http://www.cdc.gov/aging/help/dph-aging/state-aging-health.html

Cromartie, J. (2016). USDA ERS—Population & migration. Retrieved from https://www.ers.usda.gov/topics/rural-economy-population/population-migration/

Department of Defense. (2016). Eligibility. Retrieved from http://www.tricare.mil/Plans/Eligibility

Engel, E. (2017, March 24). Text—H.R.1676—115th Congress (2017-2018): Palliative Care and Hospice Education and Training Act [webpage]. Retrieved from https://www.congress.gov/bill/115th-congress/house-bill/1676/text

Farmer, C. M., Hosek, S. D., & Adamson, D. M. (2016). Balancing demand and supply for veterans' health care: A summary of three RAND assessments conducted under the Veterans Choice Act. *Rand Health Quarterly, 6*(1), 12. Retrieved from https://www.ncbi.nlm.nih.gov/pmc/articles/PMC5158276/

Ferrell, B., Malloy, P., Mazanec, P., & Virani, R. (2016). CARES: AACN's new competencies and recommendations for educating undergraduate nursing students to improve palliative care. *Journal of Professional Nursing, 32*(5), 327–333. doi:10.1016/j.profnurs.2016.07.002

Gale, J., & Heady, H. (2013). Rural vets: Their barriers, problems, needs. *Health Progress, 94*(3), 49–52. Retrieved from http://digitalcommons.usm.maine.edu/insurance/5

Gerteis, J., Izrael, D., Deitz, D., LeRoy, L., Ricciardi, R., Miller, T., & Basu, J. (2014). *Multiple chronic conditions chartbook* (No. AHRQ Q14-0038) (p. 52). Rockville, MD: Agency for Healthcare Research and Quality. Retrieved from http://www.cdc.gov/chronicdisease/overview/

Golla, H., Galushko, M., Pfaff, H., & Voltz, R. (2014). Multiple sclerosis and palliative care: Perceptions of severely affected multiple sclerosis patients and
their health professionals: A qualitative study. *BMC Palliative Care, 13*(1), 1–23.
doi:10.1186/1472-684X-13-11

Goodman, R. A., Posner, S. F., Huang, E. S., Parekh, A. K., & Koh, H. K. (2013). Defining
and measuring chronic conditions: Imperatives for research, policy, program, and
practice. *Preventing Chronic Disease, 10*, E66. doi:10.5888/pcd10.120239

Institute of Medicine. (2015). *Dying in America: Improving quality and honoring individual preferences near the end of life.* Washington, DC: National Academy of Sciences.
Retrieved from http://publications.amsus.org/doi/full/10.7205/MILMED-D-15
-00005

Johnson, C. E., Bush, R. L., Harman, J., Bolin, J., Evans Hudnall, G., & Nguyen, A. M.
(2015). Variation in utilization of health care services for rural VA enrollees
with mental health-related diagnoses. *The Journal of Rural Health, 31*(3), 244–253.
doi:10.1111/jrh.12105

Karlin, B., Zeiss, A., & Burris, J. (2010). Providing care to older adults in the Department
of Veterans Affairs: Lessons for us all. *Generations, 2*, 6–12.

Kavalieratos, D., Mitchell, E. M., Carey, T. S., Dev, S., Biddle, A. K., Reeve, B. B., . . .
Weinberger, M. (2014). "Not the 'Grim Reaper Service'": An assessment of provider
knowledge, attitudes, and perceptions regarding palliative care referral barriers
in heart failure. *Journal of the American Heart Association, 3*(1), 1–11. doi:10.1161/
JAHA.113.000544

Kuehner, C. A. (2013). My military: A navy nurse practitioner's perspective on military
culture and joining forces for veteran health. *Journal of the American Association of
Nurse Practitioners, 25*, 77–83. doi:10.1111/j.1745-7599.2012.00810.x

LeBlanc, T. W., O'Donnell, J. D., Crowley-Matoka, M., Rabow, M. W., Smith, C. B.,
White, D. B., . . . Schenker, Y. (2015). Perceptions of palliative care among hemato-
logic malignancy specialists: A mixed-methods study. *Journal of Oncology Practice,
11*(2), e230–e238.doi:10.1200/JOP.2014.001859

Long, K. A., & Weinert, C. (2013). Rural nursing: Developing the theory. In C. A. Winters
(Ed.), *Rural nursing concepts, theory, and practice* (4th ed., pp. 1–14). New York, NY:
Springer Publishing.

Maffucci, J., & Frazier, C. (2015). *7th annual member survey: The most comprehensive look
into the lives of post-9/11 veterans.* New York, NY: Iraq and Afghanistan Veterans of
America. Retrieved from https://iava.org/wp-content/uploads/2016/05/IAVA_
MemberSurvey_Final_single_pgs.pdf

Meo, N., Hwang, U., & Morrison, R. S. (2011). Resident perceptions of palliative care
training in the emergency department. *Journal of Palliative Medicine, 14*(5), 548–555.
doi:10.1089/jpm.2010.0343

Meyer, E. G. (2015). The importance of understanding military culture. *Academic
Psychiatry, 39*, 416–418. doi:10.1007/s40596-015-0285-1

National Center for Veterans Analysis and Statistics. (2016, August). *Characteristics of rural
veterans: 2014 data from the American Community Survey.* U.S. Department of Veterans
Affairs. Retrieved from https://www.va.gov/vetdata/docs/SpecialReports/Rural_
Veterans_ACS2014_FINAL.pdf

Nayar, P., Apenteng, B., Yu, F., Woodbridge, P., & Fetrick, A. (2013). Rural veterans'
perspectives of dual care. *Journal of Community Health, 38*(1), 70–77. doi:10.1007/
s10900-012-9583-7

Qureshi, S. U., Kimbrell, T., Pyne, J. M., Magruder, K. M., Hudson, T. J., Petersen, N. J., . . . Kunik, M. E. (2010). Greater prevalence and incidence of dementia in older veterans with posttraumatic stress disorder. *Journal of the American Geriatrics Society, 58*(9), 1627–1633. doi:10.1111/j.1532-5415.2010.02977.x

Raphael, D., Waterworth, S., & Gott, M. (2014). The role of practice nurses in providing palliative and end-of-life care to older patients with long-term conditions. *International Journal of Palliative Nursing, 20*(8), 373–379. doi:10.12968/ijpn.2014.20.8.373

Ross, P. T., Ravindranath, D., Clay, M., & Lypson, M. L. (2015). A greater mission: Understanding military culture as a tool for serving those who have served. *Journal of Graduate Medical Education, 7*(4), 519–522. doi:10.4300/JGME-D-14-00568.1

Rossiter, R. (2015, November 10). AACN supports Joining Forces Wellness Week. *Press Release.* American Association of Colleges of Nursing: Washington, DC.

Schroedl, C., Yount, S., Szmuilowicz, E., Rosenberg, S. R., & Kalhan, R. (2014). Outpatient palliative care for chronic obstructive pulmonary disease: A case series. *Journal of Palliative Medicine, 17*(11), 1256–1261. doi:10.1089/jpm.2013.0669

Shreve, S. (2010). Hospice and palliative care by the VA, beyond the VA. *Generations 2,* 49–56.

Sibener, L., Zaganjor, I., Snyder, H. M., Bain, L. J., Egge, R., & Carrillo, M. C. (2014). Alzheimer's disease prevalence, costs, and prevention for military personnel and veterans. *Alzheimer's & Dementia: The Journal of the Alzheimer's Association, 10*(3), S105–S110. doi:10.1016/j.jalz.2014.04.011

Smith, A. K., Thai, J. N., Bakitas, M. A., Meier, D. E., Spragens, L. H., Temel, J. S., . . . Rabow, M. W. (2013). The diverse landscape of palliative care clinics. *Journal of Palliative Medicine, 16*(6), 661–668. doi:10.1089/jpm.2012.0469

Thorpe, J. M., Houtven, C. H., Sleath, V., & Thorpe, C. T. (2010). Rural-urban differences in preventable hospitalizations among community-dwelling veterans with dementia. *Journal of Rural Health, 26*(2), 146–155. doi:10.1111/j.1748-0361.2010.00276.x

U.S. Department of Veterans Affairs. (n.d.). VA Community Provider Toolkit: Serving Veterans through partnership. Retrieved from https://www.mentalhealth.va.gov/communityproviders/screening_howto.asp

U.S. Department of Veterans Affairs. (2016). Health services research & development. Retrieved from https://www.hsrd.research.va.gov/for_researchers/sig/default.cfm#rural

U.S. Department of Veterans Affairs Office of Rural Health. (n.d.). Rural veterans. Retrieved from http://www.ruralhealth.va.gov/aboutus/ruralvets.asp

Verschuur, E. M., Groot, M. M., & van der Sande, R. (2014). Nurses' perceptions of proactive palliative care: A Dutch focus group study. *International Journal of Palliative Nursing, 20*(5), 241–245. doi:10.12968/ijpn.2014.20.5.241

World Health Organization. (2015, July). Palliative care. Retrieved from http://www.who.int/mediacentre/factsheets/fs402/en

CHAPTER 19

The "Golden Hour" in Rural America

Renae Christensen

DISCUSSION QUESTIONS

- What are the three goals of the Institute for Healthcare Improvement "Triple Aim" initiative?
- Discuss the ways a rural emergency department (ED) nurse can positively affect patient outcomes.
- What are the advantages of rapid transfer of an ED patient to a higher level of care from a critical access hospital?
- When should decision for transfer occur?

I work in the flat plains of the Midwest as a nurse in a critical access hospital (CAH) and also as a RN/paramedic answering the ambulance call of the sick and injured who have dialed 911 in a frontier county. According to Nayar, Yu, and Apenteng (2013), "the defining characteristics of frontier areas are geographical isolation and low population density. Section 799A, Health Care in Rural Areas, passed by Congress in 1988, defined 'frontier' as an area with less than 7 persons per square mile" (p. 258). Our CAH is a trauma-receiving hospital, and the next nearest hospital is 45 minutes by ground ambulance and is a Trauma Level 3 facility. According to Coleman, Baker, Gallo, and Slonim (2012),

> CAHs comprise approximately 17% of the nation's hospitals and are defined as rural hospitals with no more than 25 beds that meet government standards for CAH designation, have the capacity to provide acute or emergency care, and are located >35 miles from a large medical center. (p. 7)

Although our situation is defined as "frontier," it is not unique (see Figure 19.1). "In 2007, there were 452 counties that met the frontier definition of fewer than 7 people per square mile" (Nayar et al., 2013, p. 258). The Affordable Care Act provides increased reimbursement to Montana, Nevada, North Dakota, South

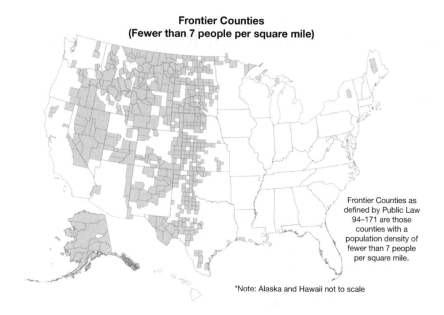

Frontier Counties
(Fewer than 7 people per square mile)

Frontier Counties as
defined by Public Law
94–171 are those
counties with a
population density of
fewer than 7 people
per square mile.

*Note: Alaska and Hawaii not to scale

FIGURE 19.1. Frontier counties United States, 2005 (conventional definition)
Source(s): U.S. Census Bureau, 2010 Decennial Census, Summary File 1

Dakota, and Wyoming because more than half of the counties in the state meet frontier criteria (Rural Health Information Hub, 2017).

A common statement in the care of cardiac patients is "time is muscle" meaning the focus is on the rapid care of patients and the prevention of loss of muscle. Treatment within the first hour has been coined the "Golden Hour." According to Gregory (2007), the standard of care for many medical emergencies requires specialized teams and protocols to provide the most rapid transition from arrival in the emergency department (ED) to definitive treatment. This approach has demonstrated positive patient outcomes for such common conditions as myocardial infarction (heart attack), cardiac arrest, and stroke (p. 1614). Many studies have been done to determine the benefits of rapid treatment. "Patients with delayed admission to the intensive care unit (ICU) had significantly higher ICU and hospital mortality and longer ICU and hospital length of stays compared with non-delayed patients" (Gregory, 2007, p. 1614).

The Golden Hour begins at the onset of symptoms or injury. Delay in recognition and treatment of the symptoms of a heart attack or stroke can result in extended injury and poor health outcomes. A car accident on a rural road that is infrequently traveled and with poor cell phone reception can delay treatment. Because of my unique position as an RN at a CAH and a RN/Paramedic for the ambulance, I recognized that the Golden Hour in rural America might be longer than 60 minutes.

THE CRITICAL ACCESS HOSPITAL

Rural hospitals differ from urban hospitals in availability of resources, staff, specialty services, and diagnostic and interventional modalities. When complex or uncommon clinical problems are encountered, resources can be taxed. At our facility, there are two RNs in the facility at all times and occasionally a patient care technician. A radiology technician and laboratory technician are on call and need to be available within 30 minutes. The on-call medical provider is not required to be in the facility, but must be able to be at the patient bedside within 20 minutes. The on-call provider can be a physician, a physician assistant (PA), or a nurse practitioner (NP). The midlevel provider (PA, NP) must have a physician available for consultation by phone. There are no surgical services available at our facility. If a complex patient is brought in by ambulance, it is not uncommon for the ambulance team to assist in the ED and/or prepare for continued transportation of the patient to another facility once stabilized. Direct communication with an off-site medical specialist is available at the touch of a button via the tele-ED system allowing for enhanced medical expertise, staff support, and the initiation of transfer of a critical patient.

Emergency Medical Treatment and Active Labor Act

Emergency Medical Treatment and Active Labor Act (EMTALA) was signed into law by President Reagan in 1986 as a mandatory set of rules set up for hospitals and physicians governing when a patient must be transferred (Stickler, 2006). If a patient presents for care at a hospital, a qualified medical provider must screen the patient and examine the affected systems with consideration of complications. A standard screening must be performed for each patient who arrives to ensure that problems are identified appropriately. Once the problems have been identified, the hospital resources need to be evaluated to determine if the hospital has sufficient staff and equipment to care for the patient. Appropriate treatment to stabilize the patient before transfer is necessary. The patient or representative must be informed of the risks and benefits of being transferred, and written permission for transfer must be obtained. In addition, the receiving facility must be contacted to determine that it has adequate resources and staffing to care for the patient. All medical records should accompany the patient in transfer to maintain continuity of care. Personnel accompanying the patient must have appropriate skills to care for the patient and have the necessary equipment for sustaining the stability of a patient during the transfer.

THE GOLDEN HOUR AT OUR CAH

According to the Golden Hour, patients treated within the first hour of injury have a mortality rate of 10%, versus a mortality rate of 75% if treatment occurs within 8 hours (Avtgis, Pollack, Martin, & Rossi, 2010, p.p. 282–283). Only 5% to 10% of trauma patients require transfer to a higher level of care (Whedon & Von Recklinghausen, 2013). Nonetheless, a timely decision to transfer is necessary for positive patient outcomes.

In a rural trauma site review, it was noted that our CAH might have delays in identifying the need to transfer patients. Following the review, information was evaluated for a 6-month period and it was determined that trauma patients were spending long periods in the ED before they were being transferred to a higher level of care. The times to transfer ranged from a minimum of 62 minutes to a maximum of 417 minutes with an average of 165 minutes; no trends were identified. Each individual provider's average was within a few minutes of the combined average. With support from the medical staff, and assurances of adequate resources, a plan was designed to improve time to transfer by using a systematic approach to every patient assessment to facilitate early identification of patients who might need to transfer.

The Team

The medical staff was supportive of the project. Quality Management confirmed that the information was valid and agreed with the need for improvement.

> Essential elements of shared leadership are relationships, dialogues, partnerships, and understanding boundaries. The application of shared leadership assumes that a well-educated, highly professional, dedicated workforce is comprised of many leaders. It also assumes that the notion of a single nurse as the wise and heroic leader is unrealistic and that many individuals at various levels in the organization must be responsible for the organization's fate and performance. (Sullivan, 2013, p. 43)

By identifying the team players and drawing from their knowledge, the challenges were identified, and goals were set. The requested resources (*ACLS Reference Manual*, a "Go To" book for stroke and a cardiac "Go To" reference) were placed in the ED to support standard assessments and improve staff confidence during critical patient care. Nursing input was valued as well as physician involvement causing the entire project to be a group vision to improve patient outcomes. Excessive transport times are " . . . characteristic of immature trauma systems" and ". . . total elapsed time to definitive care is often measured in hours rather than minutes" (Whedon & Von Reckling, 2013, p. 260). By focusing on the fact that every minute counts and reducing nonessential tests such as CT scans that are not determining the need for transfer, patients were transferred more rapidly. Sometimes, receiving providers do not accept the patient without additional testing. Delays in transfer because of waiting for radiology results when it is known that the patient is requiring transfer to a higher level of care no matter what the radiology results are should no longer be acceptable.

During a recent trauma review, it was determined that initiation of transfer of a patient should occur within the first 15 minutes of a patient arriving at the ED. In the review of a nearby hospital's goals, it was determined that if a patient needs to be transferred to a higher level of care, its goal is to have the patient out the door within the first hour. The new goal for our hospital is 45 minutes. By focusing on rapid transfers, the staff will be more aware of the fact that every minute counts.

By reviewing the problem and focusing on improved patient satisfaction and having a shared commitment from team members, we believed we could improve patient outcomes. The Emergency Committee and Quality Assurance will review the statistics again to assure that the time to transfer is improving and identify any further stumbling blocks that exist. Sustaining the project to improve transfer times was a team effort.

Rogers' Theory of Diffusion of Innovation

Rogers' theory of knowledge diffusion provides an excellent framework for making change; it consists of five steps (Sullivan, 2013). The framework emphasizes the reversible nature of change and how participants may initially adopt and then later refuse a proposal, or vice versa (p. 58). People do not buy what you do, but instead, they will buy in why it is done. Rogers' theory begins with knowledge—either foundational or acquired. The second step is persuasion—which may be supportive of an idea or not. The third step is a decision to accept or reject the idea. The fourth step is implementation and requires action to put the idea into use. The final step is confirmation, which requires review of the concept of validity or need for changes (see Figure 19.2). These steps make sense when making a process improvement change.

McGrath and Zell (2001) reported an interview with Rogers who said that if one person adopts an idea and shares their enthusiasm for the change, then

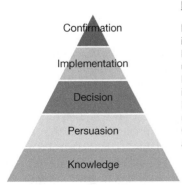

Rogers' Theory

Knowledge - person becomes aware of an innovation and has some idea of how it functions
Persuasion - person forms a favorable or unfavorable attitude toward the innovation
Decision - person chooses to adopt or reject the innovation
Implementation - person puts an innovation into use
Confirmation - person reevaluates the decision and verifies validity.

FIGURE 19.2. Rogers' theory

the next person also will be more likely to adopt the change because of fear of being left out. The power of persuasion can be a large influence on the adoption of a change. Moreover, once an idea is implemented, it is reevaluated to determine that it remains beneficial. Sometimes during the reevaluation process, it is determined that the change has not been accepted and further investigation into the problem needs to occur to maximize the change process. These steps seem reasonable in the medical field because nurses and physicians may implement a treatment followed by reevaluation; therefore, management of healthcare also reasonably follows the same path.

Patient Experience

One example of a typical patient experience is a stroke resulting in a fall at home that causes an injury. The American Heart Association (2017) advises, "The time-sensitive treatment relies on people calling 911 as soon as they notice facial drooping, arm weakness or speech difficulty" (Guidelines urge new approach to treating worst strokes, para. 23). Some patients may be fortunate enough to have someone witness the incident, and activate a call to 911. Other patients may wear a device that can be activated by the push of a button to request assistance. Some unfortunate patients may be discovered by a family member or neighbor hours or even days after the incident before assistance can be requested. The delay in these patients' care can result in additional skin breakdown, dehydration, and numerous other complications. The Golden Hour of treatment of a stroke begins at the onset of symptoms. The American Heart Association (2017) reports, "The mainstay of treatment has long been tissue plasminogen activator, or tPA—a clot-busting drug approved by the Food and Drug Administration in 1996 that must be given intravenously within 4.5 hours to be effective" (Guidelines urge new approach to treating worst strokes, para. 4).

Once the call to 911 has been received, an ambulance will be dispatched. The ambulance will arrive with several trained personnel to assess the patient and equipment to transfer the patient to a gurney. Next, they will carry the patient to the ambulance for further transfer to the nearest facility, which is most often the CAH. During the transport to the CAH, the crew can begin to obtain a history of the patient, complete a physical examination, and treat the patient according to the needs that are identified. By establishing contact with the receiving facility, the ambulance can allow maximum staff available at the receiving facility to treat the patient expediently. Once arriving at the CAH, the medical provider will assess the patient and order labs and radiology as appropriate. The decision to transfer a patient may be immediately evident depending on whether the patient is still within the 4.5-hour window of acceptable administration of tPA, or may be postponed until lab or radiology results are available. Ischemic stroke accounts for approximately 87% of all strokes resulting in 690,000 Americans who have clot-caused strokes each year (American Heart Association, 2017). Identifying if the patient has an ischemic or hemorrhagic stroke is necessary to determine the appropriate care which requires a CT scan. A patient with a hemorrhagic stroke is not a candidate for the thrombolytic, tPA, without causing further damage. Delay in receiving the thrombolytic will result in extending the stroke deficit.

Once it is determined the patient needs a higher level of care, the provider can initiate conversation with the receiving facility. EMTALA rules require that the patient be stabilized before transfer and that the patient be transferred to a facility that has appropriate space and resources to care for the patient (Stickler, 2006). Sometimes a message is left for the accepting facility to have a provider call back, and delays in transfer often have occurred because of the receiving facility requesting further testing before it will accept the patient. Another impediment that can occur when transferring a patient is the receiving facility may request additional imaging before accepting the patient and even more troublesome is when the test is repeated on patient arrival to the receiving facility incurring an additional expense.

The collaboration of care must be done expediently to promote rapid transfer of the patient. The method of transfer could be as simple as private vehicle if the patient is stable enough; ground ambulance transfer with Basic Life Support, Advanced Life Support, or Specialty Care Transport; or air transport via helicopter or fixed wing may be arranged depending on the severity of the patient condition and availability. In South Dakota, many times air transfer is not available due to weather conditions. The risks and benefits of transferring a patient need to be weighed by the provider attending the patient as he or she is responsible for the patient during transfer. Many ambulance services in rural areas are not staffed broadly and several have given up their coverage of a service area due to lack of staffing. The earlier a decision for transfer is made and arrangements for transfer are formulated, the quicker a patient can get to specialty care at a higher level of care.

Process Improvement

Process improvement is the task of reviewing the existing practice and improving the process to meet new standards of quality. According to the Institute for Healthcare Improvement (IHI, 2017), "The U.S. healthcare system is the most costly in the world, accounting for 17% of the gross domestic product with estimates that percentage will grow to nearly 20% by 2020" (IHI Triple Aim Initiative, para 2). The current system of care is created with a volume-based reimbursement and rural providers are not able to sustain the current habits. Despite the largest cost expenditure, the United States fails in prevention of medical errors, timely care, and coordination of care and underperforms in comparison to other countries in efficiency, access, and life outcomes (Faguet, 2013). The IHI's "Triple Aim Initiative" (2017) simultaneously focuses on three dimensions: improving the patient experience of care; improving the health of populations; and reducing the per capita cost of healthcare. New efforts have been made to transition reimbursement to value-based reimbursement where patient satisfaction and outcomes are reflected in payment. Some may think: Why is it so important to focus on rapid transfer and nurses have no influence on the result? The reality is that a nurse is the first point of contact for the patient at a rural hospital. The nurse can expedite the care of the patient by assembling the team rapidly and being prepared to promptly carry out the orders given by the provider. In 1 year, our CAH was able to reduce the time that a patient was at our facility by 30 minutes by focusing on the need for rapid transfer. The goal of our project is to provide better care to the patients, with smarter spending, and have healthier people. Transparency is necessary to continue the process improvement for patient-centered care and eliminate wasteful spending.

CONCLUSION

Rural systems face unique challenges due to their lack of specialty care, but I would argue that rural nursing is a specialty that is not recognized. The Golden Hour for a patient in rural America requires an extraordinary team effort of resources to have the best patient outcomes because the closest trauma center is not the first stop for Emergency Medical Services. As a paramedic who responds to the initial call for help and as a nurse who works in a CAH, I have explored the transitions of care and the consequences of delay in transfer. The increased awareness of the length of stay in the ED for patients transferring to a higher level of care has resulted in the team focusing on ways to decrease these times and improve patient outcomes. Some progress has been gained in shaving off time in the ED at our CAH, but there remains work to be done. Work has begun to initiate a statewide project that would have all CAHs review time to transfer data and evaluate it for further improvement. Rural American patients can be assured that during their Golden Hour the staff will be doing everything within their resources to provide the best outcomes possible.

REFERENCES

American Heart Association. (2017). Guidelines: Acute ischemic stroke. Retrieved from http://www.heart.org

Avtgis, T. A., Polack, E. P., Martin, M. M., & Rossi, D. (2010). Improve the communication, decrease the distance: The investigation into problematic communication and delays in inter-hospital transfer of rural trauma patients. *Communication Education*, 59(3), 282–293. doi:10.1080/03634521003606194

Coleman, N. E., Baker, D., Gallo, J., & Slonim, A. D. (2012). Critical outcomes: Clinical and team performance across acute illness scenarios in emergency departments of critical access hospitals. *Journal for Healthcare Quality: Official Publication of the National Association for Healthcare Quality*, 34(3), 7–15. doi:10.1111/j.1945-1474.2011.00141.x

Faguet, G. (2013). *Affordable care act: A missed opportunity, a better way forward*. New York, NY: Algora.

Gregory, C. J. (2007). Golden hours wasted: The human cost of intensive care unit and emergency department inefficiency. *Critical Care Medicine, 35*(6), 1614–1615.

Institute for Healthcare Improvement. (2017). IHI Triple Aim initiative. Retrieved from http://www.ihi.org/engage/initiatives/TripleAim/Pages/default.aspx

McGrath, C., & Zell, D. (2001). The future of innovation diffusion research and its implications for management: A conversation with Everett Rogers. *Journal of Management Inquiry, 10*(4), 386–391. Retrieved from http://search.proquest.com/docview/203315226?accountid=35812

Nayar, P., Yu, F., & Apenteng, B. A. (2013). Frontier America's health system challenges and population health outcomes. *The Journal of Rural Health, 29*(3), 258–265. doi:10.1111/j.1748-0361.2012.00451.x

Rural Health Information Hub. (2017). Health and healthcare in frontier areas. Retrieved from https://www.ruralhealthinfo.org/topics/frontier#definition

Stickler, J. (2006). EMTALA: The basics. *JONA's Healthcare Law, Ethics, and Regulation, 8*(3), 77–81.

Sullivan, E. J. (2013). *Effective leadership and management in nursing* (8th ed.). Boston, MA: Pearson/Prentice Hall.

Whedon, J., & Von Recklinghausen, F. (2013). An exploratory analysis of transfer times in a rural trauma system. *Journal of Emergencies, Trauma and Shock, 6*(4), 259–263. doi:10.4103/0974-2700.120368

CHAPTER 20

Palliative Care for Rural Chronically Ill Adults

Jane A. Schantz

DISCUSSION QUESTIONS

- Many rural healthcare centers are staffed by generalists who do a wide variety of types of care in their daily work. Given this, what do you think is the best way for generalists to provide high-quality palliative care (PC) to their patients?
- Describe the differences and similarities between PC and hospice.
- Interdisciplinary teams (IDTs) typically consist of doctors, nurses, social workers, and chaplains. Why do you think this is important in PC? Where do these roles differ or overlap?

Palliative care (PC; also known as palliative medicine) is coming into its own as a medical specialty, primarily for adults with serious, life-threatening, and/or chronic illness. For many years, PC has been thought to be synonymous with end-of-life (EOL) care and hospice. But in the past decade, national organizations such as the Center to Advance Palliative Care (CAPC), the National Hospice and Palliative Care Organization, Hospice and Palliative Nurses Association, and American Academy of Hospice and Palliative Care have worked hard to distinguish and define palliative medicine in its own right, and to promote its establishment within the larger healthcare system. Although there remains a fair amount of misunderstanding among the general public and even the medical community as to what it is, "PC" is now a phrase with which many American adults are at least familiar, as it is a topic that is currently popular in the media. Typically, PC is described as being an umbrella specialty, within which EOL care and hospice reside. Both PC and hospice emphasize a palliative approach to symptom management and an interprofessional, team-based, holistic model of individualized care that focuses both on the patient and his or her loved ones. But increasingly there is an effort to separate the terms "PC" and "hospice," as PC matures as a field of medicine. This comes in part to dispel the common misunderstanding that "PC" is simply coded language for EOL care.

PC IN RURAL SETTINGS

The purpose of this chapter is to report on the state of PC in rural settings, comparing it to what is assumed to be the standard, PC in urban/suburban settings. A case study will illustrate the need for home-based PC services for chronically but not yet terminally ill patients. We look at the most commonly identified challenges for rural PC, as well as strengths and recommendations for future programs.

In the United States, hospice services are regulated by Medicare, which defines eligibility as requiring a terminal diagnosis with a life expectancy of 6 months or fewer if the illness runs its expected course (Centers for Medicare & Medicaid Services [CMS], 2015, p. 3). In order to receive hospice, the patient must agree to forgo all curative treatment for the hospice diagnosis and any secondary diagnoses contributing to the patient's terminal prognosis. Conversely, PC is offered regardless of prognosis and often along with curative treatment. CAPC (n.d.) defines PC as:

Specialized medical care for people living with serious illness. It focuses on providing relief from the symptoms and stress of a serious illness. The goal is to improve quality of life for both the patient and the family.

Palliative care is provided by a team of palliative care doctors, nurses, social workers and others who work together with a patient's other doctors to provide an extra layer of support. It is appropriate at any age and at any stage in a serious illness and can be provided along with curative treatment. (Definition of Palliative Care, para. 1)

PC is of special interest to nurses. Nurses have always played a key role in PC, as the patient-centered, holistic model is essentially the nursing model itself, and nurses are central providers of hospice care.

Hospital-Based PC

Whether in urban, suburban, or rural settings, PC is most commonly practiced in the inpatient, acute care environment. Inpatient PC consultation is frequently sought amid an acute-on-chronic health crisis and usually focuses on one or more of the following: emotional support, symptom management, discussion of prognosis and goals of care, healthcare literacy and decision making, advance directives, patient and family communication and coping, resource utilization, spiritual concerns, care coordination across levels of care, and/or EOL care and bereavement (Manfredi et al., 2000; Quill, 2015). These interventions have been repeatedly shown to increase patient and family satisfaction and well-being. They have also been shown to decrease healthcare costs at the EOL through improved symptom management, clarified goals of care, and shortened length of stay, as well as fewer hospital readmissions, emergency department (ED) visits, and emergent hospitalizations (Armstrong, Jenigiri, Hutson, Wachs, & Lambe, 2013; McGrath, Foote, Frith, & Hall, 2013; Meier & Sieger, 2015; Wachterman et al., 2016). One landmark study showed cost savings of as much as $1,700 per admission for those who survived to discharge and $4,900 per admission for those who died inpatient (Morrison et al., 2008). These benefits have been demonstrated in both urban and rural hospitals.

At its 2015 national conference, CAPC declared, "Mission accomplished!" in reference to inpatient PC service penetration in hospitals across the United States. Indeed, between 2009 and 2015, the availability of hospital-based PC services increased by 78% nationally. In 2015, 4.8% of all hospital admissions involved PC (Rogers & Dumanovsky, 2017). For rural hospitals, however, this declaration appears to be premature.

Approximately 51 million people live in the rural United States and depend on their community hospitals (American Hospital Association, 2015). In their state-by-state report card for 2015, CAPC reported that in sole community provider (SCP) hospitals with 50 or more beds, only 45% reported PC programs. There are little data on hospitals with fewer than 50 beds. The availability of PC varied widely by state and by region. Three states had no PC programs in any SCPs (Mississippi, Arkansas, and Alaska). New England had the highest penetration at 89%, which is not surprising given the proximity to multiple major hospitals and academic medical centers. The central southern region had the poorest penetration in SCPs, at 19% (Morrison & Meier, 2015). Critical access hospitals have fewer than 25 beds and a very small census mean of just over four patients per day. In these hospitals, which number more than 1,300 in the United States, PC programs are rare (Mayer & Winters, 2016).

In one study to assess rural PC needs, researchers surveyed 236 hospitals in seven Rocky Mountain states (Fink, Oman, Youngwerth, & Bryant, 2013). The authors found significant barriers to providing PC, including lack of access to PC resources, lack of administrative support, lack of training and mentorship, and lack of basic knowledge about PC practice. They also found confusion as to the difference between PC and hospice. Although there was interest in professional development, distance, lack of time, and lack of coverage were all identified as additional barriers. These themes were repeated in studies of outpatient PC programs (Bakitas et al., 2015; Evans, Stone, & Elwyn, 2003; Keim-Malpass, Mitchell, Blackhall, & DeGuzman, 2015; Leadbeater & Staton, 2014; Robinson et al., 2009; Robinson, Pesut, & Bottorff, 2010).

Outpatient and Home-Based PC

Although successes in increased PC utilization in hospitals deserve celebration, many clinicians recognize that inpatient PC consultation, which is still too often employed only for EOL concerns, is akin to closing the barn door after the horses have escaped. Earlier intervention through outpatient and home-based PC services may prevent acute hospitalization. And for those patients who do receive early PC referral, the benefits of inpatient consultation may be amplified by ongoing outpatient support and home-based services to maintain effective symptom and chronic illness management, and to prevent unnecessary rehospitalization. The focus of national PC leaders now turns to applying the PC model to management of chronic illness through outpatient and home-based PC services.

Rogers and Dumanovsky (2017) found that the majority of PC inpatients fell into one of four top diagnosis groups: 8% had neurologic disease, 12% had pulmonary disease, 13% had cardiac disease, and 26% had cancer. These categories represent diseases that often have a high degree of symptom burden over a prolonged period, well before the last 6 months of life. Pain, dyspnea, fatigue, weakness, dehydration, nausea, constipation, and other symptoms are common and can be disabling in advanced illness. Patient and family functional status can be significantly impaired without proper treatment and support. Outpatient and home-based PC services are aimed at effectively monitoring and treating patients with advanced chronic illness, reducing acute symptoms and exacerbations, supporting patient and family coping, facilitating access to resources, and smoothing transitions between care settings (Brumley, 2007; CAPC, n.d.; Davis, Temel, Balboni, & Glare, 2015; Twaddle & McCormick, 2016). The following case study illustrates the need for home-based PC services.

CASE STUDY

Horace (85) and Ida (83) Gregson (not their real names) had been married 65 years. He was a veteran and had worked in banking until his retirement and they had traveled the world together. They lived in their own modest split-level home. They had two adult children, both of whom lived several states away. Horace was admitted to hospice after an acute hospitalization for congestive heart failure (CHF). He had secondary diagnoses of cardiovascular disease with intermittent angina, chronic asthma, and macular degeneration, which had left him legally blind and unable to drive. Ida was able to care for him despite her moderately severe arthritis and her mild dementia. Horace was a

(continued)

(*continued*)

proud man who did not like to be dependent on anyone, did not want to use oxygen, and insisted on continuing with certain routines such as fetching the mail and shoveling snow. He and Ida were resistant to home hospice at first, but grew to be very fond of their hospice nurse, their home health aide, and the volunteer who drove the Gregsons to get groceries and to the library for audiobooks.

The hospice nurse assessed Horace during weekly visits and worked with his physician to adjust medications for anginal pain, edema, hypertension, dyspnea, and a recurrent cellulitis on Horace's leg. The home health aide spent an hour a day 5 days a week to assist Horace with showering and do some light housekeeping. Over time, Horace's symptoms of CHF stabilized and it became increasingly clear he was not going to continue to qualify for hospice services. But Ida's dementia was worsening and her ability to care for Horace was inconsistent. The hospice team did not feel it was safe to discharge Horace from hospice services. Working within Medicare regulations, they found a way to recertify him for another benefit period, but at the end of that period, he had to be discharged. Horace and Ida hired some help with housecleaning twice a week but were unwilling to hire strangers for home healthcare. Within 6 weeks of discharge, Horace was taken to the ED after a fall at home. Following his hospital admission where he was given intravenous fluids, he was again referred to hospice in acute heart failure. Horace's hospice nurse found that he had been taking too much diuretic, as he could not see the labels on his pill bottles and Ida's dementia now made it difficult for her to manage his medications. Over the following 18 months, Horace was discharged from hospice, hospitalized, and readmitted to hospice two more times. In the 2 years since his initial hospice admission, the longest he went without hospice services was 2 months. By the time Horace died, Ivy's dementia was so severe, she was unable to care for him. Fortunately, Horace *was* on hospice during his last 3 months of life, and the hospice team assisted the family in making plans for Ivy's care.

The issues represented in this case are all too common. Patients living with advanced chronic illness tend to be older, have multiple comorbidities, and may have family members who also carry a chronic disease burden. Medicare regulations stringently dictate that patients must be demonstrating a steady decline to continue to qualify for hospice; yet, this is not the usual illness trajectory for advanced cardiac or lung disease. Both of these illnesses are known for periods of fragile stability that may be prolonged but are easily disrupted by something like an overly salty meal or a common upper respiratory infection, which can quickly imperil these patients with symptoms such as severe dyspnea that require rapid, skilled intervention. Without access to PC services, these patients end up repeatedly hospitalized for acute symptoms that could often be managed at home with nursing support. Mr. Gregson was on and off hospice services for 2 years because there was no alternative care service available. He clearly deteriorated whenever services were removed, and he and his wife both suffered. Home-based PC is the solution to this problem.

Community- or Home-Based PC

In a systematic review, Kirby et al. (2016) compared the needs of patients with life-limiting illness, and their families and caregivers, in rural versus urban settings. They found that rural EOL residents had higher rates of severe CHF, cancer, renal failure, and emphysema, with poorer symptom management, fewer physician visits, and poorer access to home care services, including PC. Patients and caregivers lacked information about PC and EOL care, and caregivers lacked support for practical skills that would allow patients to stay home longer (p. 291). Rural cancer patients were less likely to understand their prognosis, or to know that treatment intent was palliative rather than curative (p. 292). However, they also found that rural residents had resilience, greater acceptance of death, and good community support networks.

Ideally, community- or home-based PC (CHBPC) is modeled on the interprofessional team used in both inpatient PC programs and home hospice services, represented by a physician and/or nurse practitioner, RN, social worker, and chaplain; however, these services are not all reimbursable by Medicare and other forms of insurance (Meier, Bowman, Collins, Dahlin, & Twohig, n.d.). Therefore, various program structures are being trialed around the country. The rural context brings additional barriers to reaching this ideal. There is still a lack of research on true PC in rural settings in the United States (Bakitas et al., 2015; Kirby et al., 2016; Robinson et al., 2009). The literature on PC for patients at the EOL is somewhat more robust, if research from other countries is included, as much of it originates in Canada and Australia. With the exception of financial analysis, much of this EOL research can be applied to the assessment of CHBPC, as the practice issues are closely related.

Certain themes stand out across the literature. There is wide general agreement that rural disparities in availability of PC services, compared to urban and suburban communities, are common. Most also agree that outpatient and CHBPC programs in rural areas cannot be generically designed but must be tailored to the needs of the community being served (Bakitas et al., 2015; Kirby et al., 2016; Murphy, 2010; Pesut et al., 2013; Robinson et al., 2010; Temkin-Greener, Zheng, & Mukamel, 2012). Issues related to geographical distance and "windshield time," lack of PC specialists, staff recruitment and retention, limited access to resources such as durable medical equipment and pharmacies, and financial constraints are common. Millions of people reside more than

60 minutes from a hospice agency, and many areas lack residential/inpatient hospice facilities as well as 24-hour (crisis) support. The idea of implementing telehealth technologies is frequently mentioned, with mixed reports on its feasibility and efficacy (Bakitas et al., 2015; Charlton, Schlichting, Chioreso, Ward, & Vikas, 2015; Evans et al., 2003; Holland et al., 2014; Lynch, 2012; Robinson et al., 2010).

In looking at program development, additional topics unique to rural settings are being discussed and debated, including generalist versus specialist practice, rural–urban partnerships, and the role of the interdisciplinary team (IDT). Building capacity in communities was another strong theme. These aspects of PC practice encompass those areas that most urgently need to be tailored to fit the needs of the community being served. Across all models, nursing care is integral to PC and education for nurses and other providers is another major area of discussion.

Many rural and remote settings rely on generalists to cover the wide variety of healthcare needs for these communities. Any model of CHBPC necessarily relies on these local providers, whether for direct treatment or referral, and building and maintaining good relationships with them is crucial. In fact, utilizing existing professionals is repeatedly reported as an element of program successes. Because PC is only a small portion of what they do, however, it is more difficult for these professionals to obtain and maintain sufficient training and skills to meet the variety of needs presenting within PC. Various solutions to this challenge are being tried, many focusing on specialist support being made available to the generalists.

Hospice organizations are one source of specialist support. Traveling teams of PC specialists may visit patients directly or be available via tele- or videoconferencing. Mobile health clinics are another potential solution (Bakitas et al., 2015; Lynch, 2012; Robinson et al., 2009; Spice, Paul, & Biondo, 2012). Howell et al. (2011) report on a shared care model that involves primary care patients in need of PC, an advanced practice nurse who acted as care coordinator, input on symptom assessment and management by an IDT, and involvement of home care services. The results were improved patient quality of life and reduction of symptoms. Mitchell et al. (2016) evaluated another pilot program that also involved a specialist nurse practitioner coordinating care with support of the patient's generalist primary care provider and a one-time IDT case conference for each patient. The results included prompt initiation of treatment with good follow-up and coordinated, integrated care. Patients reported being satisfied with the service. Financial viability was not established.

Telephone and videoconferencing may seem like an obvious answer to the geographical challenges of rural care. In some programs, these have been successfully utilized whereas in others results were more mixed. Watanabe et al. (2013) describe a virtual clinic where patients traveled to a facility, received an in-person assessment by a nurse including physical assessment and completion of a variety of assessment tools, and then participated in an IDT videoconference that resulted in recommendations for care. The nurse provided follow-up. Although this method was determined to be feasible and patients reported satisfaction, problems identified included patient travel time and increased time needed for scheduling, and limited awareness of the clinic despite promotional efforts. Leadbeater and Staton (2014) found that often the necessary technology was not available in rural areas. After-hours telephone support, on the other hand, has been shown to increase a sense of security and reduce feelings of isolation experienced by families caring for a PC patient (Wilkes, Mohan, White, & Smith, 2004).

Ceronsky, Shearer, Weng, Hopkins, and McKinley (2013) studied the effects of the Minnesota Rural Palliative Care Initiative, which sought to build PC capacity over 18 months using 10 community teams in a variety of service areas ranging in population from 9,000 to 200,000. All communities had existing hospice programs and four participating hospitals were critical access hospitals. The teams involved the collaboration of a wide variety of existing agencies and institutions, comprising an interdisciplinary approach. Only one community had a previously existing PC program. Based on their analysis, the authors proposed five recommendations:

> First, external resources and support are necessary to support community development of palliative care services. Second, ongoing networking is critical to sustainability and continued progress. Third, defining community-based metrics is essential to quantify the impact on cost, quality, readmissions, and patient and family satisfaction. Fourth, reimbursement for palliative care services as a covered benefit would make a significant difference to the sustainability of programs in rural communities. Fifth, development of palliative care programs and services must align with other efforts to redesign care delivery to maximize efficiency for rural providers. (p. 312)

More research such as this is needed to guide PC program development in rural areas.

CONCLUSION

As our nation's population ages in the next two decades, there will be mounting pressure to find effective ways to care for burgeoning numbers of chronically ill adults. Palliative medicine offers a sound solution by providing holistic patient- and family-centered care with an emphasis on quality of life. Much work needs to be done to develop models of home-based care that are tailored to the communities they serve and covered by Medicare and other insurers. Nurses will undoubtedly play key roles in delivering this specialized care, and are well suited to do so.

REFERENCES

American Hospital Association. (2015). Rural and small hospitals fact sheet. Retrieved from http://www.aha.org/content/13/fs-rural-small.pdf

Armstrong, B., Jenigiri, B., Hutson, S. P., Wachs, P. M., & Lambe, C. E. (2013). The impact of a palliative care program in a rural Appalachian community hospital. *American Journal of Hospice and Palliative Medicine, 30*(4), 380–387. doi:10.1177/1049909112458720

Bakitas, M. A., Elk, R., Astin, M., Ceronsky, L., Clifford, K. N., Dionne-Odom, N., . . . Smith, T. (2015). Systematic review of palliative care in the rural setting. *Cancer Control, 22*(4), 450–464.

Brumley, R. (2007). Increased satisfaction with care and lower costs: Results of a randomized trial of in-home palliative care. *Journal of the American Geriatrics Society, 55*(7), 993–1000. doi:10.1111/j.1532-5415.2007.01234.x

Center to Advance Palliative Care. (n.d.). About palliative care. Retrieved from https://www.capc.org/about/palliative-care

Centers for Medicare & Medicaid Services. (2015). *Medicare benefit policy manual.* Retrieved from https://www.cms.gov/Regulations-and-Guidance/Guidance/Manuals/downloads/bp102c09.pdf

Ceronsky, L., Shearer, J., Weng, K., Hopkins, M., McKinley, D. (2013). Minnesota rural palliative care initiative: Building palliative care capacity in rural Minnesota. *Journal of Palliative Medicine, 16*(3), 310–313. doi:10.1089/jpm.2012.0324

Charlton, M., Schlichting, J., Chioreso, C., Ward, M., & Vikas, P. (2015). Challenges of rural cancer care in the United States. *Oncology (Williston Park, N.Y.), 29*(9), 633–640. Retrieved from http://www.ncbi.nlm.nih.gov/pubmed/26384798

Davis, M., Temel, J., Balboni, T., Glare, P. (2015). A review of the trials which examine early integration of outpatient and home palliative care for patients with serious illnesses. *Annals of Palliative Medicine, 4*(3). doi:10.3978/j.issn.2224-5820.2015.04.04

Evans, R., Stone, D., & Elwyn, G. (2003). Organizing palliative care for rural populations: A systematic review of the evidence. *Family Practice, 20*(3), 304–310. doi:10.1093/fampra/cmg312

Fink, R. M., Oman, K. S., Youngwerth, J., & Bryant, L. L. (2013). A palliative care needs assessment of rural hospitals. *Journal of Palliative Medicine, 16*(6), 638–644. doi:10.1089/jpm.2012.0574

Holland, D. E., Vanderboom, C. E., Ingram, C. J., Dose, A. M., Borkenhagen, L. S., Skadahl, P., . . . Bowles, K. H. (2014). The feasibility of using technology to enhance the transition of palliative care for rural patients. *CIN: Computers, Informatics, Nursing, 32*(6), 257–266. doi:10.1097/CIN.0000000000000066

Howell, D., Marshall, D., Brazil, K., Taniguchi, A., Howard, M., Foster, G., & Thabane, L. (2011). A shared care model pilot for palliative home care in a rural area: Impact on symptoms, distress, and place of death. *Journal of Pain and Symptom Management, 42*(1), 60–75. doi:10.1016/j.jpainsymman.2010.09.022

Keim-Malpass, J., Mitchell, E. M., Blackhall, L., & DeGuzman, P. B. (2015). Evaluating stakeholder-identified barriers in accessing palliative care at an NCI-designated cancer center with a rural catchment area. *Journal of Palliative Medicine, 18*(7), 634–637. doi:10.1089/jpm.2015.0032

Kirby, S., Barlow, V., Saurman, E., Lyle, D., Passey, M., & Currow, D. (2016). Are rural and remote patients, families and caregivers needs in life-limiting illness different from those of urban dwellers? A narrative synthesis of the evidence. *Australian Journal of Rural Health, 24*(5), 289–299. doi:10.1111/ajr.12312

Leadbeater, M., & Staton, W. (2014). The role and organisation of community palliative specialist nursing teams in rural England. *British Journal of Community Nursing, 19*(11), 551–555. doi:10.12968/bjcn.2014.19.11.551

Lynch, S. (2012). Hospice and palliative care access issues in rural areas. *American Journal of Hospice and Palliative Medicine, 30*(2), 172–177. doi:10.1177/1049909112444592

Manfredi, P. L., Morrison, R. S., Morris, J., Goldhirsch, S. L., Carter, J. M., & Meier, D. E. (2000). Palliative care consultations: How do they impact the care of hospitalized patients? *Journal of Pain and Symptom Management, 20*(3), 166–173. Retrieved from http://www.ncbi.nlm.nih.gov/pubmed/11018334

Mayer, D. D. M., & Winters, C. A. (2016). Palliative care in critical access hospitals. *Critical Care Nurse, 36*(1), 72–78. doi:10.4037/ccn2016732

McGrath, L. S., Foote, D. G., Frith, K. H., & Hall, W. M. (2013). Cost effectiveness of a palliative care program in a rural community hospital. *Nursing Economic$, 31*(4), 176–183. Retrieved from http://www.ncbi.nlm.nih.gov/pubmed/24069717

Meier, D. E., Bowman, B., Collins, K. B., Dahlin, C., & Twohig, J. S. (n.d.). *Palliative Care in the Home: A guide to program design.* New York, NY: Center to Advance Palliative Care.

Meier, D. E., & Sieger, C. E. (2015). *A guide to building a hospital-based palliative care program.* New York, NY: Center to Advance Palliative Care.

Mitchell, G. K., Senior, H. E., Bibo, M. P., Makoni, B., Young, S. N., Rosenberg, J. P., & Yates, P. (2016). Evaluation of a pilot of nurse practitioner led, GP supported rural palliative care provision. *BMC Palliative Care, 15*(1), 93. doi:10.1186/s12904-016-0163-y

Morrison, R. S., & Meier, D. E. (2015). *America's care of serious illness: 2015 state-by-state report card on access to palliative care in our nation's hospitals.* New York, NY: Center to Advance Palliative Care.

Morrison, R. S., Penrod, J. D., Cassel, J. B., Caust-Ellenbogen, M., Litke, A., Spragens, L., & Meier, D. E. (2008). Cost savings associated with U.S. hospital palliative care consultation programs. *Archives of Internal Medicine, 168*(16), 1783–1790. doi:10.1001/archinte.168.16.1783

Murphy, S. (2010). Territory palliative care: A model for remote area palliative care provision. *Progress in Palliative Care, 18*(1), 27–30. doi:10.1179/096992610X12624290276304

Pesut, B., Hooper, B., Sawatsky, R., Robinson, C. A., Bottorf, J. L., & Dalhuisen, M. (2013). Program assessment framework for a rural palliative supportive service. *Palliative Care: Research and Treatment, 7,* 7–17. doi:10.4137/pcrt.s11908

Quill, T. (2015). The initial interview in palliative care consultation. In R. M. Arnold (Ed.), *UpToDate.* Retrieved from https://www-uptodate-com

Robinson, C. A., Pesut, B., & Bottorff, J. L. (2010). Issues in rural palliative care: Views from the countryside. *Journal of Rural Health, 26,* 78–84. doi:10.1111/j.1748-0361.2009.00268.x

Robinson, C. A., Pesut, B., Bottorff, J. L., Mowry, A., Broughton, S., & Fyles, G. (2009). Rural palliative care: A comprehensive review. *Journal of Palliative Medicine, 12*(3), 253–258. doi:10.1089/jpm.2008.0228

Rogers, M., & Dumanovsky, T. (2017). *How we work.* New York, NY: Center to Advance Palliative Care.

Spice, R., Paul, L. R., & Biondo, P. D. (2012). Development of a rural palliative care program in the Calgary Zone of Alberta Health Services. *Journal of Pain and Symptom Management, 43*(5), 911–924. doi:10.1016/j.jpainsymman.2011.05.019

Temkin-Greener, H., Zheng, N. T., & Mukamel, D. B. (2012). Rural-urban differences in end-of-life nursing home care: Facility and environmental factors. *Gerontologist, 52*(3), 335–344. doi:10.1093/geront/gnr143

Twaddle, M. L., & McCormick, E. (2016). Palliative care delivery in the home. In C. Ritchie & M. Silveira (Eds.), *UpToDate*. Retrieved from https://www.uptodate.com/contents/palliative-care-delivery-in-the-home

Wachterman, M. W., Pilver, C., Smith, D., Ersek, M., Lipsitz, S. R., & Keating, N. L. (2016). Quality of end-of-life care provided to patients with different serious illnesses. *JAMA Internal Medicine, 176*(8), 1095–1102. doi:10.1001/jamainternmed.2016.1200

Watanabe, S., Fairchild, A., Pituskin, E., Borgersen, P., Hanson, J., & Fassbender, K. (2013). Improving access to specialist multidisciplinary palliative care consultation for rural cancer patients by videoconferencing: Report of a pilot project. *Supportive Care in Cancer, 21*(4), 1201–1207. doi:10.1007/s00520-012-1649-7

Wilkes, L., Mohan, S., White, K., & Smith, H. (2004). Evaluation of an after-hours telephone support service for rural palliative care patients and their families: A pilot study. *Australian Journal of Rural Health, 12*(3), 95–98. doi:10.1111/j.1440-1854.2004.00568.x

CHAPTER 21

Healthcare Delivery Model for Critical Access Hospitals

Susan Wallace Raph and Rayn Ginnaty

DISCUSSION QUESTIONS

- What factors influence nurse staffing in the rural or frontier critical access hospital (CAH) setting? Can the national nursing productivity benchmarks be applied to this setting?
- The rural nurse is described by Scharff as the expert generalist. What strategies are available to help rural nursing staff develop and maintain the practice competencies necessary for quality safe patient care?
- Using the Centers for Medicaid & Medicare Services (CMS) definitions, identify CAH facilities in your area. What challenges might they experience in recruiting and retaining qualified nurses?
- The *Management of Outcomes for Rural Efficiency (MORE)* Contract supports nursing functions that are considered nonproductive. How would you advocate to CAH administration for the resources needed to secure this contract?

The financial viability of healthcare agencies is dependent upon an effective level of nurse staffing that balances the demands for quality and safety. Despite adjusted cost reimbursement models, critical access hospitals (CAHs) are challenged to achieve financial success due in part to nurse staffing variables that are impacted by the highly variable and extremely low patient census unique to the rural setting. Designing a productivity model within a framework that accounts for rural and frontier staffing variables provides an opportunity to effectively manage nurse staffing and patient outcomes for the CAH setting.

CRITICAL ACCESS HOSPITALS

In an effort to reduce the financial vulnerability of rural hospitals and improve access to healthcare, the Balanced Budget Act of 1997 created the CAH designation. Eligible facilities receive 101% cost-based reimbursement from Medicare rather than the standard prospective payment system. The CAH must have 25 or fewer acute care inpatient or swing beds; be located more than 15 miles from another hospital or CAH in an area with mountainous terrain or only secondary roads; maintain an annual length of stay of 96 hours or less for acute care patients; and provide 24/7 emergency care services (Centers for Medicaid & Medicare Services [CMS], 2016a). A CAH serving a population of less than 2,500 people more than an hour away from an urban healthcare facility faces unique challenges that directly influence the financial viability of the organization.

Nurse Staffing

In an analysis of state staffing laws, Douglas (2010) called for solutions that balance safety, quality, and cost. The author identified 36 variables that contribute to the highly complex and dynamic decision-making process used by rural nurse executives to determine appropriate nurse staffing, and hypothesized that trust, effective communication, and collaboration between nurse executives, finance personnel, and the bedside staff are foundational to the process. The variables are further delineated in Table 21.1 into factors influenced or mediated by the patient, organization, and nursing infrastructure.

Each of the variables requires constant assessment and attention and reflects the dynamic healthcare environment. CAH facilities in the rural and frontier areas face unique factors that further complicate nurse-staffing decision making.

Rurality

Many communities are served by a CAH in what is considered a frontier and remote (FAR) part of our nation, a designation characterized by four levels of combined low population size and a high degree of geographical remoteness as noted on Box 21.1 (U.S. Department of Agriculture [USDA], 2015). The most remote areas (Level 4) are measured by their distance and travel time of 15 minutes or more from an urban area of 2,500 to 9,999 people. States with the highest shares of frontier areas include Wyoming, Montana, North Dakota, South Dakota, Nevada, and Alaska.

Rural and frontier healthcare in general and rural nurse staffing is impeded by multiple factors associated with the setting. Cramer, Jones, and Hertzog (2011) cite low patient acuity, rapidly fluctuating patient volumes, and greater rates of nurse shortages as compelling factors that influence nurse staffing issues in the rural setting. Newhouse (2005) conducted focused interviews with rural nurse executives and identified three major forces that distinctly influence

TABLE 21.1 Nurse Staffing Variables

Patient	Organizational	Nursing Infrastructure
Experience of staff	Educational requirements	Safety
Cultural influence	Treatment requirements	Quality/performance benchmarks
Intensity of situation	Observation/intervention requirements	Fatigue considerations
Severity of illness	Number of registered nurses (RNs)	Patient satisfaction
Family/situation needs	Number and mix of staff	Nurse satisfaction
Special credential requirements	Setting/environment	Continuity of care
	Physical plant	Role and skill competence
	Ancillary/support staff availability	Legislative/regulatory requirements
	Physician preferences	Admission, discharges, and transfers
	Variations in technology	Quality considerations
	Number of patients	Budget considerations
	Range of conditions	Working conditions
		Team dynamics
		Individual nurse (staff dynamics)
		Policies and procedures requirements
		Safety considerations

rural nursing: the external environment, organizational factors, and nursing infrastructure. The external environment provides not only physical isolation, but also little to no control over the type of population served, services offered, and regulatory mandates. Internal organizational factors such as patient acuity, technology, financial margins, leadership, culture, and resources, shape and mold policy and decisions. The nursing infrastructure reflects the unique variables managed by the rural nurse executive, a position often held by a novice administrator. Lower salaries, provider–RN conflict, continuity of care, competency, culture, politics, and leadership issues compound the complex setting. The group identified solutions that reflect an overarching theme of regulatory changes to support the rural context of care. MacKinnon (2012) conducted institutional ethnography to elicit general themes regarding rural nurse staffing.

BOX 21.1 USDA, Economic Research Service, Criteria for Defining Four FAR Area Levels, 2017

- **Level 1**—FAR areas consist of rural areas and urban areas up to 50,000 people who are 60 minutes or more from an urban area of 50,000 or more people.
- **Level 2**—FAR areas consist of rural areas and urban areas up to 25,000 people who are 45 minutes or more from an urban area of 25,000 to 49,999 people; and 60 minutes or more from an urban area of 50,000 or more people.
- **Level 3**—FAR areas consist of rural areas and urban areas up to 10,000 people who are 30 minutes or more from an urban area of 10,000 to 24,999; 45 minutes or more from an urban area of 25,000 to 49,999 people; and 60 minutes or more from an urban area of 50,000 or more people.
- **Level 4**—FAR areas consist of rural areas that are 15 minutes or more from an urban area of 2,500 to 9,999 people; 30 minutes or more from an urban area of 10,000 to 24,999 people; 45 minutes or more from an urban area of 25,000 to 49,999 people; and 60 minutes or more from an urban area of 50,000 or more people.

FAR, frontier and remote; USDA, U.S. Department of Agriculture.

Recommendations include the need for staff competency, safety standards, and flexibility in the decision-making process of nurse staffing. Scharff (2013) described the rural nurse as an expert generalist who moves easily from one role to another depending on the circumstances. Ruberg (2015) acknowledged the lack of publicly reported data for CAHs to support benchmarking for safe nurse staffing and captured the challenges in applying mandated nurse–patient ratio legislation to the CAH setting, and identifies seven nurse staffing best practices for the CAH setting:

- Effective communication between hospital management and nursing staff
- Formal information sharing
- Effective nursing leadership
- Open and collaborative discussion on patient acuity and case mix
- Educational opportunities for nurses
- Creation of data collection and decision-making tool
- Establishment of a comprehensive nurse-staffing plan

Ruberg (2015) suggested the comprehensive nurse-staffing plan include position control through accurate documentation of total RN full-time equivalents (FTEs) required to staff a CAH, short- and long-term position control analysis, monitoring of patient volumes, and flexing up core staffing levels through an additional staffing request document completed by the charge RN in the unit.

Evaluation of the comprehensive nurse-staffing plan includes the measurement and tracking of three metrics. The total overtime worked by RNs during each pay period and totaled quarterly is compared to the same quarter from the previous year to account for seasonal trends. This metric is also compared as a percentage total regular RN hours worked and adjusted for the average daily census in the emergency department (ED) and inpatient units. Additionally, nurse turnover ratios are followed to assess changes made to affect nurse satisfaction and the total expenses related to nurse recruitment are tracked.

Ultimately, nurse staffing is based on patient census and the services offered by the CAH. Patient census can vary dramatically from day to day, a phenomenon not uncommon to most healthcare agencies. However, a consistently low and highly variable census presents unique challenges for a CAH to maintain a competent minimum staffing that is safe and cost-effective. By definition, the CAH must staff a minimum of one RN, clinical nurse specialist, or licensed practical nurse on-site 24/7 whenever the CAH has one or more patients (CMS, 2016b). When additional services are offered, the requirements for nurse staffing increase. With an eye on required professional staffing for perinatal units, the rural CAH settings have witnessed a decline in births. Simpson (2011) reported 14% of hospitals with less than 100 births in 2008 discontinued birthing services in 2010 due in part to lack of provider coverage and costs. An analysis of the birth distributions found 7.9% of hospitals in the United States had less than 100 births, and that 72.3% of these hospitals continued to meet the minimum staffing guidelines of two in-house obstetrician (OB)-skilled nurses established by the Association of Women's Health Obstetric and Neonatal Nurses.

Healthcare Productivity

In today's healthcare environment it is essential for hospitals to determine adequate staffing levels to ensure high-quality care while remaining financially viable. This challenge becomes even greater in the CAH setting. Many CAHs find it challenging to meet budget through a strong nursing model and increased focus on implementing a system to monitor nursing productivity. There is inherent difficulty in the evaluation of nurse staffing. The outcomes of nursing have generally been measured within a structural variable of staff mix or nursing hours per case or patient day, the results of which have been regarded as inconsistent due to narrow conceptual models and inadequate research tools (Jones & Yoder, 2010; Sidani, Doran, & Mitchell, 2004). The cost of a single unit of nursing care has not been captured and as such is generally not itemized or reimbursed. Instead, nursing care is bundled into a room charge that is insufficient in capturing the predictive precision necessary for determining safe and effective staffing plans or efficiency and effectiveness of transitional care approaches. This imperfect financial approach diminishes the visibility and the value of nursing. The current prospective payment system of healthcare creates a ceiling for the price of nursing care and limits incentive to increase its provision (Wendel, O'Donohue, & Serratt, 2014). Identifying valid and reliable empirical indicators of efficient and cost-effective nursing care is therefore necessary.

As a social science concerned with decision making, economic theory reflects the accuracy of predicting the choices made regarding resource allocation (Jones & Yoder, 2010). The authors identify the economic concepts of scarcity, utility, cost, supply, demand, price, and marginal analysis as relevant to nursing administration. Ultimately, a cost–benefit analysis reveals the benefits of selecting one option over another. A positive net benefit reflects both the profit and the utility or happiness for the agency. Nursing is currently a scarce commodity measured in the time needed for individual nursing activities and associated variable costs. Administrative nursing decisions regarding models of nurse staffing and transitional care are influenced by two key variables: volume and quality care. Nursing managers incorporate the use of marginal analysis to determine the amount of additional resources needed to reach maximum efficiency for the volume of nursing care produced (Jones & Yoder, 2010). This is commonly referred to as a "nurse-staffing matrix." Variables that may enhance efficiency include technology, skill mix changes that facilitate delegation, physical design of the unit, patient acuity, available support staff, and policy and procedural changes that eliminate waste and nonvalue added activities (Jones & Yoder, 2010). Conversely, if the demand for nursing resources outweighs the supply, negative consequences such as missed nursing care, overtime, and decreased quality occur.

The concept behind nursing productivity is basic to understanding the workload needed to provide patient care at the bedside. In its simplest definition, productivity is defined as the measurement of the efficiency and amount of labor required to provide elements of nursing care. However, the consistency of productivity outcomes depends on the variables and setting in which it is used. Holcomb, Hoffart, and Fox (2002) cite that the differences often applied to the productivity calculation can be grouped into four categories: human resources, material resources, patient quality, and types of services provided. The variables in nurse staffing fall mainly into the human resources category. In order for nursing productivity to be an effective measurement, key definitions of direct patient care and indirect patient care requirements need to be determined (Holcomb et al., 2002). One method used to determine nursing productivity is by calculating nursing hours per patient day (NHPPD), typically derived from a benchmark provided by a national company. NHPPD is the total number of nursing staff providing patient care compared to the number of patients. The hours reflect the amount of time in a 24-hour period where a nurse is providing direct care to the patient at the bedside. The NHPPD become part of a unit-based matrix or tool used to determine staffing levels given a preidentified number of patients. A matrix is developed based on key variables including patient volume, acuity, known admissions, discharges, and transfers. Often the matrix is set to meet key financial metrics while giving nursing leadership the ability to balance staff schedules based on average daily patient volume (Donovan, 2004). A facility with lower patient volumes and little variation to the average daily census requires a minimal staffing level. In most cases, minimal staffing can be two nurses or one nurse and certified nursing assistant. Greater variation in the average daily census requires more flexibility in the nurse staffing model.

The staffing variables, Douglas (2010) recognizes, are impacted differently in the critical access or frontier setting. For example, most CAHs cannot afford ancillary support staff so the primary nurse or the nurse executive, who may not be accounted for in the NHPPD matrix development, completes these important patient care functions. The ability to ensure and measure positive patient outcomes based on these variables can be extremely costly for a CAH as it requires additional resources. Many of these variables fall into the fixed or nonproductive hours not considered to be direct hands-on patient care. However, the work contained in the nonproductive hours often leads to innovative, evidence-based practice changes, and quality care improvement (Altman & Rosa, 2016). CAHs often find it difficult to staff additional nursing resources in various roles to ensure key performance metrics are analyzed, regulatory requirements have been met, and identified staff competency and trainings have been completed.

PLAN AND RECOMMENDATIONS

Development and staffing of the necessary services that support the competency, quality, and safety measures for effective nurse staffing can be not only difficult to staff but also costly for a CAH. The use of dedicated staff for transitional care, infection prevention, quality monitoring, and evidence-based practice education are core foundational services for an organization, but provision of these services is often the last priority for a nurse executive who is challenged with recruitment and retention of qualified nurse staff for direct patient care. These tasks are generally added to the nurse executive's already full portfolio of organizational oversight. Taking a collaborative approach in sharing such resources with other CAH facilities or contracting with regional urban healthcare agencies offers a cost-effective and more efficient avenue for ensuring adequate nurse staffing and the necessary support resources. Depending on the size of the CAH, monthly or quarterly outcome management consultation and services are provided to assess, plan, implement, and evaluate the educational needs of nurses staffing, monitor and report quality and safety indicators, and assist in making improvements in care that are evidence based. Establishing collaborative and contractual relationships with referral healthcare organizations and other outlying CAH facilities enhances the communication necessary for efficient transitional care practices and improved patient outcomes.

CAH Healthcare Delivery Model

Management of Outcomes for Rural Efficiency (*MORE*) is presented as a model for rural and frontier CAHs to tap existing evidence-based quality, safety, transitional care, and educational resources from regional urban healthcare systems to support the nursing productivity infrastructure. The *MORE* model, presented in Figure 21.1, represents the core of patient-centered rural nurse staffing that is surrounded by multiple staffing variables that affect productivity, quality care, and patient safety. The infusion of contracted outcome management (*MORE*) services and consultation serves to control the variables through a cost-effective nursing productivity and support framework.

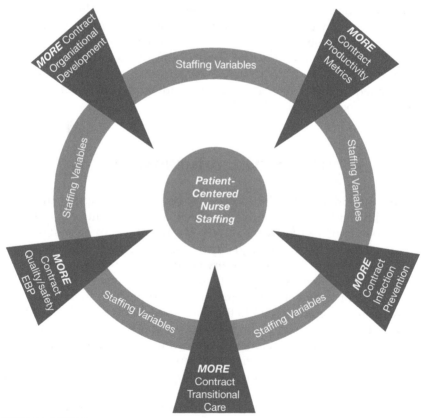

FIGURE 21.1. MORE model.
EBP, evidence-based practice; MORE, Management of Outcomes for Rural Efficiency

CONCLUSION

The rural and frontier CAH setting uniquely affects the provision of quality safe nurse staffing. Nurse executives in this setting are challenged with balancing the financial demands of the organization, a low volume–highly variable patient census, staffing of an expert generalist nursing staff, and provision of core nurse functions that ensure quality patient care. Contracting for evidence-based urban outcome management services to enhance and support core nursing functions offers the CAH setting an opportunity for fiscally responsible nurse staffing.

REFERENCES

Altman, M., & Rosa, W. (2016). Redefining "time" to meet nursing's evolving demands. *Nursing Management, 46*(3), 60–63. doi:10.1097/01.NURSE.0000476236.55728.47

Centers for Medicare & Medicaid Services. (2016a). Critical access hospital. *Rural Health Series.* Retrieved from https://www.cms.gov/Outreach-and-Education/Medicare-Learning-Network-MLN/MLNProducts/downloads/critaccesshospfctsht.pdf

Centers for Medicare & Medicaid Services. (2016b). State operations manual: Appendix W—Survey protocol, regulations and interpretive guidelines for critical access hospitals (CAHs) and swing-beds in CAHs. Retrieved from https://www.cms.gov/Regulations-and-Guidance/Guidance/Manuals/Downloads/som107ap_w_cah.pdf

Cramer, M. E., Jones, K. J., & Hertzog, M. (2011). Nurse staffing in critical access hospitals: Structural factors linked to quality care. *Journal of Nursing Care and Quality, 26*(4), 335–343. doi:10.1097/NCQ.0bo13e318210d30a

Donovan, L. (2004). Mapping a staffing blueprint to match competencies. *Nursing Management, 35*(Suppl. 5), 14. doi:10.1097/00006247-200410005-00005

Douglas, K. (2010). Ratios: If only it were that easy. *Nursing Economic$, 28*(2), 119–125.

Holcomb, B., Hoffart, N., & Fox, M. (2002). Defining and measuring nursing productivity: A concept analysis and pilot study. *Journal of Advanced Nursing, 38*(4), 378–386. doi:10.1046/j.1365-2648.2002.02200.x

Jones, T. L., & Yoder, L. H. (2010). Economic theory and nursing administration research: Is this a good combination? *Nursing Forum, 45*(1), 40–53. doi:10.1111/j.1744-6198.2009.00160.x

MacKinnon, K. (2012). We cannot staff for "what ifs": The social organization of rural nurses' safeguarding work. *Nursing Inquiry, 19*(3), 259–269. doi:10.1111/j/1440-1800.2011.00574.x

Newhouse, R. P. (2005). Exploring nursing issues in rural hospitals. *Journal of Nursing Administration, 35*(7), 350–358.

Ruberg, G. G. (2015). *Best practices for nurse staffing in critical access hospitals* (Master's thesis). Available from UMI Dissertation Publishing. (UMI No. 1592033)

Scharff, J. E. (2013). The distinctive nature and scope of rural nursing practice: Philosophical bases. In C. A. Winters (Ed.), *Rural nursing: Concepts, theory, and practice* (4th ed., pp. 241–258). New York, NY: Springer Publishing.

Sidani, S., Doran, D. M., & Mitchell, P. H. (2004). A theory-driven approach to evaluating quality of nursing care. *Journal of Nursing Scholarship, 36*(1), 60–65. doi:10.1111/j.1547-5059.2004.04014.x

Simpson, K. R. (2011). An overview of distribution of births in United States hospitals in 2008 with implications for small volume perinatal units in rural hospitals. *Journal of Gynecologic and Neonatal Nursing, 40,* 432–439. doi:10.1111/j.1552-6909.2011.01262.x

U.S. Department of Agriculture (2015). 2010 Frontier and remote (FAR) area codes. Retrieved from http://www.ers.usda.gov/data-products/frontier-and-remote-area-codes/documentation.aspx

Wendel, J., O'Donohue, W., & Serratt T. D. (2014). *Understanding healthcare economics: Managing your career in an evolving healthcare system.* Boca Raton, FL: CRC Press.

CHAPTER 22

Tribal Nations

Jenifer Show and Elizabeth Kinion

DISCUSSION TOPICS

- Go to the National Congress of American Indians website (www.ncai .org). Select one current news article from the site to discuss during class.
- Provide examples of structural, cognitive, and financial barriers that you have experienced when dealing with a healthcare system. If you have not personally experienced a healthcare barrier, share your personal experience that prevented/eliminated one of the three healthcare barriers.
- Identify a research question you would like to explore regarding AI access to healthcare.

American Indian (AI) or Alaska Native (AN) refers to "persons having origins in any of the original peoples of North, South, and Central America, who maintain tribal affiliation or community attachment" (U.S. Office of Management and Budget, 1997, para. 104). Once considered a forgotten and dwindling population, the American and AN populace has grown at rates twice as fast as the overall U.S. population (U.S. Census Bureau, 2010). According to the 2010 census, 5.2 million people in the United States self-identified as being either AI or AN; this is a 9.7% increase from the 2000 census, when 4.1 million people self-identified. However, AIs and ANs account for only 1.7% of the total U.S. population (U.S. Census Bureau, 2010). In the United States, many AI populations reside on reservations or other trust lands (Office of Minority Health, 2015). AIs who live on federal reservations face a number of social and economic challenges that are comparable to third world countries (Native American Aid, 2015).

"There are over 560 federally recognized Indian Nations that are sovereign nations within the United States" (National Congress of American Indians

[NCAI], n.d.). As sovereign nations, tribes have the natural authority to govern all affairs involving their people (NCAI, n.d.).

> Sovereignty is a legal word for the authority to self-govern. Tribal sovereignty means that each tribe has the inherent legal and political authority to govern itself. Currently, 566 sovereign tribal nations (variously called tribes, nations, bands, pueblos, communities, and Native villages) have a formal nation-to-nation relationship with the U.S. government. Tribal governments exercise jurisdiction over lands that would make Indian Country the fourth largest state in the nation, and are an important and unique member of the American family of governments, which includes tribal governments, the U.S. federal government, and the U.S. states. The U.S. Constitution recognizes that tribal nations are sovereign governments. As members of tribes, American Indian and Alaska Native people have both an ethnic and political status. Tribes are governments that have distinct legal and political authority to represent their citizens and to regulate all activities occurring on their lands, including research. Similar to federal and state governments, tribes have sovereign power over their lands, citizens, and related affairs. Researchers are required to follow the laws of each tribe, including the tribe's research regulation policies and any tribal laws pertaining to research being conducted with tribal citizens and on tribal lands (NCAI Policy Research Center, 2012, p. 4).

HEALTHCARE

Technically, a number of AIs have access to free healthcare through the Indian Health Service. However, funding for the Indian Health Service is often so severely below the actual need that the healthcare services are not readily available. Consequently, healthcare quality and access become a fleeting reality. The principal reason for the funding challenges experienced by the Indian Health Service is rooted in the discordant relationship between AIs and the U.S. government.

Over the past 10 years, Indian Health Service has made progress in closing the gap in health outcomes. Of critical importance is the need to build on recent increases in funding (Sequist, Cullen, & Acton, 2011).

Indian Health Service

The Indian healthcare system represents a model for many rural health programs through respect for cultural beliefs, blending of traditional practices with the modern medical model, and an emphasis on public health and community outreach activities (Indian Health Service [IHS], n.d.-c). As with many bureaucratic federal agencies, the Indian Health Service is not without challenges.

In exchange for land and natural resources, the U.S. government established the Indian Health Service as an agency within the Department of Health and Human Services to provide federal health services to AIs and ANs (U.S. Department of Health and Human Services [USDHHS], 2011). The Indian Health Service is the result of a long history of treaties and legislation, establishing a trust responsibility on behalf of the U.S. government. This trust responsibility of the federal government was to guarantee adequate healthcare for AIs. However, this obligation is not being properly fulfilled (Warne, 2006).

The provision of health services to members of federally recognized tribes grew out of the special government-to-government relationship between the federal government and Indian tribes. This relationship, established in 1787, is based on Article I, Section 8 of the Constitution, and has been given form and substance by numerous treaties, laws, Supreme Court decisions, and Executive Orders. The Indian Health Service is the principal federal healthcare provider and health advocate for Indian people and its goal is to raise their health status to the highest possible level. The Indian Health Service provides a comprehensive health service delivery system for approximately 2.2 million American Indians and Alaska Natives who belong to federally recognized tribes in 36 states. (IHS, n.d.-a, para. 1)

The Indian Health Service has 12 areas across the United States. The areas are "Alaska, Albuquerque, Bemidji, Billings, California, Great Plains, Nashville, Navajo, Oklahoma, Phoenix, Portland, and Tucson. Each of these areas has a unique group of Tribes that they work with on a day to day basis" (IHS, n.d.-e). Indian tribes and organizations interact with the Indian Health Service and make budget recommendations. Not unlike other agencies who report to the U.S. government, the Indian Health Service budget process is rather lengthy.

The budget formulation process begins at the Area level, where two tribal representatives serve as Area representatives on the Indian Health Service Budget Formulation Work Group. This group convenes twice annually for a National Work Session and Evaluation Planning meeting. Prior to finalization, the Indian Health Service budget is reviewed by several U.S. government agencies such as the United States House of Representatives and the Senate Committees on Appropriations, Subcommittee on Interior, Environment and Related Agencies and the Senate Committee on Indian Affairs." (IHS, n.d.-b)

The Indian Health Service budget is a discretionary budget. Discretionary budgets are described as optional funding determined by the number of qualified recipients. The discretionary status of the Indian Health Service budget signifies that the U.S. Congress has the authority to determine whether they are obligated to fund discretionary programs (Westmoreland & Watson, 2006). As discretionary budgets, funding may increase, stay stagnant, or decrease annually. The Indian Health Service budget has remained relatively stagnant over the past few decades, barely rising with the increased cost of healthcare. When compared to other governmental budgets, the Indian Health Service budget is considerably less than other federal programs with mandatory budgets. Due to fluctuations in federal funding and the uncertain annual budget processes, many tribes have experienced challenges in meeting the basic healthcare needs of their citizens (NCAI, 2016).

In contrast to discretionary budgets, mandatory budgets are not subject to budgetary cycles and are guaranteed. Additionally, mandatory budgets may increase annually based on inflation. This accounts for increased cost of care and the potential cost of an increase in the number of eligible users (Malerba, 2013). Three examples of agencies with mandatory budgets include Medicare, Medicaid, and the Department of Veterans Affairs. Mandatory funding has increased substantially over the years, whereas the Indian Health Service budget has increased at a much slower rate (Westmoreland & Watson, 2006). It is interesting to note that AIs, the sole population group in the nation born with the inherent right to healthcare, has gated access based on discretionary funding.

Health Disparities

AI and AN populations experience more significant health-related disparities than any other population in the United States. Specific health diseases such as diabetes, alcoholism, unintentional injuries, and suicide are just a few of the top health concerns that adversely affect AI/AN populations at far higher rates than any other race (Warne, 2006). The overwhelming majority of these disparities is preventable and is influenced by behavior and lifestyle choices (IHS, 2017).

Not unlike other rural communities, the survival and prosperity of tribal communities depend on the safety, health, and wellness of the citizens. Unfortunately, AIs suffer disproportionately from unmet health needs. For example, the life expectancy of AIs is 4.2 years less than the average for all U.S. populations (NCAI, 2015). Additionally, the Indian healthcare delivery system faces significant funding disparities, notably in per capita expenditures for health. In 2013, the Indian Health Service per capita expenditures for patient health services were $2,849, compared to $7,717 per person for healthcare spending nationally (NCAI, 2015).

Decades of research have traced two ominous but very real characteristics regarding the direction of our nation's healthcare system. The first is that the United States has the worst rankings in terms of mortality and health status when compared to other developed nations (Davis, Stemikis,

Squires, & Schoen, 2014). The second, and possibly the most distressing characteristic, is that individuals who occupy the lower ranks of our socioeconomic hierarchy are typically the ones who experience the worst health outcomes and have the highest levels of morbidity and mortality (Palloni & Yonker, 2015). The latter is an extremely unfortunate circumstance since, in the United States, many racial and ethnic minorities disproportionately occupy the lower rungs of our nation's socioeconomic ladder, making up over 50% of the economically disadvantaged (USDHHS, 2011).

Of the 46.5 million people living in poverty in the United States, racial and ethnic minorities make up the bulk of this figure. They include African Americans, AIs or ANs, Hispanics or Latinos, Asian Americans, Native Hawaiians, and other Pacific Islanders. Out of all minorities surveyed in the U.S. Census for 2010, those who self-identified as AI or AN had the highest national poverty rate of any race at 27% (U.S. Census Bureau, 2010).

AIs who live on federal reservations face a number of social and economic challenges that are comparable to third world countries (Native American Aid, 2015). For example, isolation and lack of economic opportunity on or near reservation lands leads to a drastic increase in unemployment that is not seen anywhere else in the United States. Unemployment rates on AI reservations can be astronomically high, ranging anywhere from 40% to 80%. For instance, one reservation within the Northern Great Plains region had one of the highest unemployment rates at 77% (Unemployment on Indian Reservation, 2010).

Housing is typically substandard as well; some houses lack necessities such as sewer, running water, electricity, heating, or cooling. About 40% of on-reservation housing is considered to be, by definition, inadequate (U.S. Commission on Civil Rights, 2004). Overcrowding further complicates the housing issue; it is not uncommon for three or more generations to occupy one dwelling at a time.

Educational attainment is also severely lacking. Only 17% of AIs have a bachelor's degree and a meager 6% have a graduate degree. This pales in comparison to the non-Hispanic White population where the bachelor degree attainment rate is 33% and the graduate degree attainment rate is 12% (Office of Minority Health, 2015). The combination of socioeconomic factors illustrated here creates a perfect storm for health inequity in AI/AN communities.

The circumstances that surround the health status of all people, especially AIs, are shaped by three interrelated but controllable factors: the distribution of money, power, and resources (World Health Organization [WHO], 2015). Regrettably, each of these is in significantly short supply for AIs. The underfunding of the Indian Health Service is a prime example of a resource limitation facing many AIs and ANs.

To appreciate the complexities of access to healthcare in AI populations, one must consider the multitude of factors that influence their access to care. Socioeconomic status, facility staffing, geography, culture, and funding issues are just a few of the many problems that shape healthcare across Indian Country (Artiga, Arguello, & Duckett, 2013). "Concerns about the quality of care provided to American Indians/Alaska Natives in Indian Health Service facilities has been identified recently by federal officials and tribal members" (U.S. Government Accountability Office [GAO], 2017) . . .

> Recognizing the challenges Indian Health Service faces with overseeing and providing quality healthcare in its facilities, it finalized the development of a quality framework in November 2016 that outlines, at a high level, the Indian Health Service's plan to develop, implement, and sustain a quality program intended to improve patient experience and ensure delivery of reliably high quality healthcare. (GAO, 2017, para. 3)

Healthcare Access Barriers

The Healthcare Access Barriers (HCAB) model provides a practical framework for taking into account a triad of categorically modifiable barriers associated with access to care (Carrillo et al., 2011). The triad includes financial, structural, and cognitive barriers. These interrelated barriers are associated with distinct healthcare characteristics: decreased screenings, late presentation for care, and lack of treatment (Carrillo et al., 2011). The combination of these factors ultimately contributes to poor health outcomes and health disparities.

According to the HCAB model, financial, structural, and cognitive barriers intermingle, resulting in healthcare deficits. Each of the barriers encompasses a number of specific circumstances that can influence healthcare access (Carrillo et al., 2011). One of the first barriers mentioned by the HCAB model is financial, and consists of two distinct dynamics: the cost of care and the health insurance status of the population (Carrillo et al., 2011). In AI populations, the funding of already minimally available healthcare services is a constant concern and an ever-present issue. While healthcare costs have soared over the past few decades, the federally appointed budget of the Indian Health Service has not kept pace with inflation, nor has it increased to support the demographic growth of Indian Tribes (Malerba, 2013). In fact, while other federally funded programs such as Medicare, Medicaid, and the Department of Veterans Affairs have seen their budgets increase to account for inflation and the increased number of people eligible for their services, the Indian Health Service budget has remained relatively stagnant (Westmoreland & Watson, 2006). Furthermore, since the start of the sequestration, a number of federal budgets have been cut, and the Indian Health Service has suffered even greater financial losses. In fact, sequestration of the Indian Health Service budget resulted in a 5% reduction in funds that the Indian Health Service has never managed to recover (Malerba, 2013). Presently, it is estimated that the Indian Health Service functions at only 59% or less of the total actual need (National Tribal Budget Formulation Workgroup, 2013).

When the already historically troubled budget of the Indian Health Service is faced with more budgetary cuts and does not increase over time to cover rising healthcare costs, a couple of problems occur. First, decreased availability of funds forces the Indian Health Service to ration the amount of services it provides and second, the Indian Health Service has to limit the per capita amount spent on its beneficiaries (National Tribal Budget Formulation Workgroup, 2013).

In addition to healthcare access deficits caused by financial challenges, structural barriers originating within the medical institution or organization also impede entry to care (Carrillo et al., 2011). Structural barriers are numerous and may include availability of a healthcare home, waiting time for appointments, facility hours of operation, transportation to healthcare facilities, inconsistent healthcare providers, limited telephone access to providers, and retention and recruitment of providers.

A number of the aforementioned structural barriers often affect AI populations. Two primary structural barriers affecting health in AI populations include unfilled vacancies in the healthcare workforce and geographical isolation of Indian reservations. Recruitment and retention of medical providers by the Indian Health Service is often difficult and remains a large challenge for the organization (Sequist et al., 2011). The lack of healthcare providers is extremely prevalent across Indian Country. Vacancy rates for key health disciplines remain high within the Indian Health Service ranging anywhere from 6.6% to 25% (IHS, n.d.-d). With a lack of qualified medical personnel available, many medical professionals who take the challenge to work for the Indian Health Service often find themselves getting frustrated with the inability to provide high-quality care, and eventually leaving the organization thus creating high turnover rates (U.S. Commission on Civil Rights, 2004). Not surprisingly, high turnover rates leave gaps in the already undermanned Indian Healthcare System, greatly disrupting continuity of care and compromising quality of service and leading to provider burnout (U.S. Commission on Civil Rights, 2004).

Adding to the difficulty of recruiting and retaining healthcare providers are the isolated locations of many of the hospitals and clinics within the Indian Health Service. Most Indian Health Service facilities are located in what can be considered rural or frontier areas such as Montana, North/South Dakota, or Alaska. Healthcare professionals are often unwilling to move to these geographically remote tribal communities where everyday conveniences are lacking, as are job opportunities for spouses, community activities for their children, adequate educational systems, and sufficient housing (U.S. Commission on Civil Rights, 2004).

Compounding the many financial and structural barriers to healthcare access in AI populations are cognitive barriers. Cognitive barriers are more abstract in nature and typically encompass issues such as the patient's beliefs, the complex patient–provider relationship, and the knowledge about disease processes (Carrillo et al., 2011). One of the major cognitive barriers to healthcare for many AIs is the inherent mistrust of healthcare providers, as well as the federal organization charged with providing them care (Guadagnolo et al., 2009).

The mistrust AIs experience toward the Indian Health Service and its subsequent providers is deeply rooted in their historically rocky relationship with the federal government and the dominant White culture. Actions of the federal government caused AIs to endure generations of ". . . disenfranchisement; extermination of tradition, language and land rights; broken treaties; sterilization of Native American women; placement of Indian children in Indian boarding schools; and other experiences of oppression . . ." (U.S. Commission of Civil Rights, 2004, p. 29).

The combined maltreatments of AI people throughout history have resulted in deeply rooted feelings of unresolved anger, grief, and distrust that have managed to transfer across into today's generations (Sotero, 2006). Feelings of distrust, especially toward healthcare systems and providers, may negatively affect a person's willingness to access healthcare services (Armstrong et al., 2006). While there are limited studies examining this phenomenon in AI populations, one of the few studies available on this topic found that low trust/ confidence in healthcare providers was a significantly reported barrier to AI patients seeking general medical care (Guadagnolo et al., 2009).

Steps Forward

Although a number of compounding factors presently affect the health of AIs, Tribes and the Indian Health Service have taken steps to alleviate some of the many barriers. For instance, in an attempt to reduce staff shortages, the Indian Health Service has implemented a series of special pay, bonuses, and allowances for qualified healthcare professionals who opt to work within their organization (U.S. Commission of Civil Rights, 2004). Additionally, the Indian Health Service offers the Health Professions Scholarship Program and loan repayment program, both of which allow for financial assistance either during completion of school or after completion of school in exchange for a time in service commitment (U.S. Commission of Civil Rights, 2004; IHS, n.d.-f).

> Tribal Colleges and Universities located on or near Indian Reservations are unique public institutions of higher education founded and charted by AI/AN Tribal governments . . . Tribal colleges and universities provide a social and cultural foundation for engaging AI/ANs in college access and completion through community-based research, wrap-around support, and social entrepreneurship for Nation building. Tribal colleges and universities work closely with tribes, communities and schools to provide education career pathways. (American Indian Higher Education Consortium [AIHEC], 2017, p. 3).

In recent years, an increasing number of Tribal Colleges and Universities are offering courses in nursing and other healthcare fields.

The mission and function of the Tribal College and Universities is to "help expand educational opportunities and improve educational outcomes for all AI/AN students including opportunities to learn their Native languages, cultures, and histories and receive complete and competitive educations that prepare them for college, careers and productive satisfying lives" (The White House, 2011, para. 11).

Grant-funded programs to support nurse education are also available to select universities. The purpose of grant-funded programs is to ". . . increase the number of nurses, nurse midwives, nurse anesthetists, and nurse practitioners who will deliver healthcare services to Native American Indian and Alaska Native communities" (IHS, n.d.-f, para. 2). The primary objectives of grant-funded programs authorized under section 112 of the Indian Health Service Care Improvement Act are to (a) recruit and retain AI/AN individuals to become nurses, (b) provide scholarships to AI/AN individuals enrolled in nursing schools, (c) provide a program that encourages AI/AN nurses (graduate and undergraduate) to provide or continue to provide healthcare services in AI/AN healthcare programs, and (d) provide a program that increases the skills of, and provides continuing education to, AI/AN nurses (IHS, n.d.-f, para. 3).

CONCLUSION

AIs experience some of the most significant health disparities more than any other race. This is despite the fact that AIs/ANs are the only group of people who are legally guaranteed, through a number of government-to-government treaties, the right to healthcare. Although facing a number of financial, structural, and cognitive challenges, greater numbers of AIs are seeking education as nurses or other healthcare providers through programs offered at Tribal Colleges and Universities. This, coupled with the educational support provided through Indian Health Service, offers a glimmer of hope for improved healthcare on the reservations one person at a time.

REFERENCES

American Indian Higher Education Consortium. (2017). *Tribal colleges & universities: Educating, engaging, innovating, sustaining, honoring.* Retrieved from http://www.aihec.org/who-we-are/docs/AIHECbrochure2017.pdf

Armstrong, K., Rose, A., Peters, N., Long, J. A., McMurphy, S., & Shea, J. A. (2006). Distrust of the health care system and self-reported health in the United States. *Journal of General Internal Medicine, 21*(4), 292–297. doi:10.1016/j.healthplace.2012.01.007

Artiga, S., Arguello, R., & Duckett, P. (2013). Health coverage and care for American Indians and Alaska Natives. *The Henry J. Kaiser Family Foundation.* Retrieved from http://kff.org/report-section/health-coverage-and-care-for-american-indians-and-alaska-natives-issue-brief/

Carrillo, J. E., Carrillo, V. A., Perez, H. R., Salas-Lopez, D., Natale-Pereira, A., & Byron, A. T. (2011). Defining and targeting health care access barriers. *Journal of Health Care for the Poor and Underserved, 22,* 562–575. doi:10.1353/hpu.2011.0037

Davis, K., Stremikis, K., Squires, D., & Schoen, C. (2014, June 1). Mirror, mirror on the wall, 2014 update: How the U.S. Health Care System compares internationally. *The Commonwealth Fund.* Retrieved from http://www.commonwealth.org

Guadagnolo, B. A., Cina, K., Helbig, P., Molloy, K., Reiner, M., Cook, E. F., & Petereit, D. G. (2009). Medical mistrust and less satisfaction with health care among Native Americans presenting for cancer treatment. *Journal of Health Care for the Poor and Underserved, 20*(1), 210–226.

Indian Health Service. (n.d.-a). Agency overview. Retrieved from https://www.ihs.gov/aboutihs/overview

Indian Health Service. (n.d.-b). Annual budget. Retrieved from https://www.ihs.gov/aboutihs/index.cfm/annualbudget

Indian Health Service. (n.d.-c). For providers. Retrieved from https://www.ihs.gov/forproviders

Indian Health Service. (n.d.-d). IHS recruitment. Retrieved from https://www.ihs.gov/dhps/index.cfm/programperformancedata/recruitment

Indian Health Service. (n.d.-e). Locations. Retrieved from https://www.ihs.gov/locations

Indian Health Service. (n.d.-f). Student opportunities. Retrieved from https://www.ihs.gov/nursing/studentops

Indian Health Service (IHS). (2017). Indian health disparities. Retrieved from https://www.ihs.gov/newsroom/factsheets/disparities/

Malerba, M. (2013). The effects of sequestration on Indian health. *Hastings Center Report, 43*(6), 17–21.

National Congress of American Indians. (n.d.). Tribal Nations & the United States: An introduction. Retrieved from http://www.ncai.org/about-tribes

National Congress of American Indians. (2015). *Fiscal year 2016 Indian Country Budget Request: Promoting self-determination, modernizing the trust relationship.* Washington, DC: Author.

National Congress of American Indians. (2016, February). A quiet crisis: Federal funding and unmet needs in Indian country, 2016 update. Retrieved from http://www.ncai.org/resources/testimony/a-quiet-crisis-federal-funding-and-unmet-needs-in-indian-country-2016-update

National Tribal Budget Formulation Workgroup. (2013). *Creating a legacy of honor and trust: Striving for health parity for all American Indians and Alaska Natives.* Retrieved from http://www.nihb.org/docs/07112013/FY%202015%20IHS%20budget%20full%20report_FINAL.pdf

Native American Aid. (2015). Living conditions. Retrieved from http://www.nrcprograms.org/site/PageServer?pagename=naa_livingconditions

NCAI Policy Research Center and MSU Center for Native Health Partnerships. (2012). *"Walk softly and listen carefully": Building research relationships with tribal communities* (p. 4). Washington, DC, and Bozeman, MT: Author.

Office of Minority Health. (2015). Profile: American Indian and Alaska Native. Retrieved from http://minorityhealth.hhs.gov/omh/browse.aspx?lvl=3&lvlid=62

Palloni, A., & Yonker, J. (2015). A search for answers to continuing health and mortality disparities in the United States. *Journal of American Society on Aging, 38*(4), 12–18.

Sequist, T., Cullen, T., & Acton, K. (2011). Indian health service innovations have helped reduce health disparities affecting American Indian and Alaska Native people. *Health Affairs, 30*(Suppl. 4), 3–10.

Sotero, M. (2006). A conceptual model of historical trauma: Implications for public health practice and research. *Journal of Health Disparities Research and Practice, 1*(1), 93–108.

Unemployment on Indian Reservations at 50 Percent: The Urgent Need to Create Jobs in Indian Country: Hearing before the Committee on Indian Affairs, Senate 111th Cong. 1 (2010) (testimony of Byron Dorgan).

U.S. Census Bureau. (2010, January). *The American Indian and Alaska Native populations: 2010.* Retrieved from http://www.census.gov/prod/cen2010/briefs/c2010br-10.pdf

U.S. Commission on Civil Rights. (2004, September). *Broken promises: Evaluating the Native American health care system.* Washington, DC: Author.

U.S. Department of Health and Human Services. (2011). Indian Health Service, U.S. Department of Health and Human Services-IHS. Retrieved from healthfinder.gov/FindServices/Organizations/Organization.aspx?code=HR0079

U.S. Government Accountability Office. (2017, January). *Indian Health Service: Actions needed to improve oversight of quality of care.* Retrieved from https://www.gao.gov/assets/690/681952.pdf

U.S. Office of Management and Budget. (1997). The 1997 revisions to the standards for the classification of federal data on race and ethnicity. Retrieved from http://www.whitehouse.gov/omb/fedreg_1997standards

Warne, D. (2006). Research and educational approaches to reducing health disparities among American Indian and Alaska Natives. *Journal of Transcultural Nursing, 17*(3), 266–271.

Westmoreland, T. M., & Watson, K. R. (2006). Redeeming hallow promises: The case for mandatory spending on health care for American Indians and Alaska Natives. *American Journal of Public Health, 96*(4), 600–605.

The White House. (2011). Executive order 13592—Improving American Indian and Alaska Native educational opportunities and strengthening tribal colleges and universities. Retrieved from https://obamawhitehouse.archives.gov/the-press-office/2011/12/02/executive-order-13592-improving-american-indian-and-alaska-native-educat

World Health Organization. (2015). Social determinants of health: Key concepts. Retrieved from http://www.who.int/social_determinants/thecommission/finalreport/key_concepts/en/

Improving Health Literacy About Complementary and Alternative Therapy Among Rural Dwellers

Jean Shreffler-Grant, Elizabeth Nichols, and Clarann Weinert

DISCUSSION QUESTIONS

- Discuss how the findings of each study included in this chapter led to the subsequent studies.
- Do you think that rural dwellers' tendency to be self-reliant and seek advice from informal sources contributes to the use of complementary and alternative medicine (CAM) as part of their health-seeking behaviors?
- How can the intervention discussed in the Healthcare Choices: Be Safe and Be Wise section of this chapter affect the healthcare choices made by older rural adults?
- How can nurses use the results of the studies discussed in this chapter to benefit the health of their rural clients/patients?

Adequate health literacy is necessary in today's healthcare marketplace so that consumers are able to understand and evaluate information regarding conventional or allopathic healthcare (Institute of Medicine [IOM], 2004). Health literacy is defined in *Healthy People 2010* as "the degree to which individuals have the capacity to obtain, process, and understand basic health information and services needed to make appropriate health decisions" (U.S. Department of Health and Human Services, 2000, Section 11–12).

Health literacy is even more important for evaluating complementary and alternative medicine (CAM). Healthcare consumers usually have some assistance from providers to interpret information about allopathic care and often receive instructions and advice to guide healthcare decision making and action taking. This is less likely with CAM. These therapies are often self-prescribed or self-directed in nature and are less regulated or controlled by governmental agencies or allopathic providers. Further studies have found that often there is limited communication between consumers and allopathic providers about consumers' use or potential use of CAM (Eisenberg et al., 1993, 1998; Vallerand, Fouladbakhsh, & Templin, 2003).

During the past several decades, the use of CAM in the United States has grown significantly (Barnes, Bloom, & Nahin, 2008; Eisenberg et al., 1993, 1998; IOM, 2005). CAM has become an important component of the U.S. healthcare system as consumers, including those living in rural areas, increasingly use CAM as an adjunct to or substitute for conventional healthcare (Arcury, Preisser, Gesler, & Sherman, 2004; Astin, 1998; Eisenberg et al., 1998; Harron & Glasser, 2003; McFarland, Bigelow, Zani, Newson, & Kaplan, 2002). Some people use CAM instead of allopathic care because of the lower cost of CAM, which is particularly evident during downturns in the economy (Tanner, 2009). The National Center for Complementary and Integrative Health (NCCIH) defines CAM as a group of diverse healthcare systems, practices, and products that were developed outside of mainstream Western, conventional, or allopathic medicine (NCCIH, 2017). The CAM therapies and products are not considered part of allopathic care in part because there is insufficient evidence that they are safe and effective. Types of CAM range from therapies provided by practitioners such as naturopathic physicians and acupuncturists to self-care practices, such as herbs and magnets.

Approximately 40% of adults in the United States report having used some form of CAM in the past 12 months (Barnes et al., 2008; Barnes, Pewell-Griner, McFann, & Nahin, 2004). In addition, roughly one in nine (11.8%) children used CAM in the past 12 months (Barnes et al., 2008). Not surprisingly, use among children whose parents used CAM was significantly higher (23.9%) than among children whose parents did not use CAM (5.1%). When cost concerns cause a delay in seeking allopathic care, CAM is more likely to be used by both adults and children than when cost is not a concern (Barnes et al., 2004). Despite the widespread use and acceptance of CAM in the general population, consumers are reluctant to inform allopathic providers that they used CAM (Eisenberg et al., 1993, 1998).

On the basis of the literature, the demographics of those in the general U.S. population who use CAM vary; but in general, CAM is used more often for chronic than acute health conditions and use is more common among women than men, younger adults than older, those with higher incomes and more education, and those living in the West than in other parts of the country (Astin, 1998; Astin, Pelletier, Marie, & Haskell, 2000; Cherniack, Senzel, & Pan, 2001; Eisenberg et al., 1998). Studies have found that individuals with chronic illness have a variety of reasons for using CAM, including (a) symptom relief, (b) ineffectiveness of allopathic treatments, (c) side effects of allopathic treatments, (d) dissatisfaction with allopathic care, (e) concerns about adverse effects of allopathic care, (f) desire for control, and (g) the ready availability of CAM (Johnson, 1999; Montbraind & Laing, 1991; Rao et al., 1999; Vincent & Furnham, 1996).

Despite extensive literature searches, no empirical studies on health literacy specifically about CAM could be located at the time when this research team began its work. There is also very limited evidence in general about how much CAM users know about the products and treatments they use, what sources of information they use, or how they evaluate and use the information they have or acquire (IOM, 2005). Evidence is also lacking about how consumers in the United States decide when and how to use CAM and whether or not they comply with instructions from CAM providers or product labels. One study found that while 80% of older study participants reported using two or more CAM therapies, their self-rated knowledge about most of the therapies was very low (King & Pettigrew, 2004). The IOM cited three primary sources of information that consumers use about CAM: word of mouth, the Internet, and health food stores. The few studies evaluating the quality of information available from these sources suggested that quality may be a concern.

The purpose of this chapter is to present a summary of a series of research studies conducted by a team of investigators at the Colleges of Nursing at Montana State University (MSU) and the University of North Dakota on the use of CAM by older rural dwellers. The results of these projects raised a number of researchable questions regarding the health literacy levels about CAM among older rural adults, particularly rural adults with chronic illnesses. The results are relevant to the second rural nursing theoretical statement identified by Long and Weinert (1989) and further discussed and updated by Lee and McDonagh (2013). Self-reliance and use of informal networks for advice and care are the characteristics of rural residents that influence their health-seeking behaviors. These characteristics can also affect the choices that rural adults make when deciding about the use of complementary or alternative therapies.

HEALTHCARE CHOICES: A STUDY OF COMPLEMENTARY THERAPY USE AMONG OLDER RURAL DWELLERS

At the time this study was conducted, a number of well-known studies had demonstrated that use of CAM was growing among the general population in the United States, but little was known about use of these therapies among rural residents. Most of the national studies did not report where study participants lived and some used only urban participants. To address this gap in the literature, the Healthcare Choices study was conducted with older adults living in sparsely populated rural areas in Montana and North Dakota (Shreffler-Grant,

Weinert, Nichols, & Ide, 2005). The purpose of the study was to explore use of, cost of, and satisfaction with the quality and effectiveness of CAM from the perspectives of the older rural adult participants. The study was conducted during 2000 to 2003 and funded by NCCAM (R15AT09501). A descriptive survey design was used to generate data from a random sample of older adults in 19 rural communities in Montana and North Dakota. An interview instrument was developed to elicit data addressing the specific aims; it was piloted prior to use. Telephone interviews were conducted with 325 older adults. Participants ranged in age from 60 to 98 years ($m = 71.7$). Most of the participants (67.7%, $n = 202$) reported having one or more chronic illnesses. Only 17.5% ($n = 57$) reported using CAM providers, whereas 35.7% ($n = 116$) used self-prescribed CAM practices. When these two categories of use were combined, a total of 45.2% of the participants used some form of CAM, or used CAM providers, self-prescribed CAM practices, or both. This finding demonstrated that these older rural residents were using as much or more CAM than participants in national studies (36%–40%) that included all adult age groups.

Relevant to the issue of health literacy about CAM, the participants in this study most often learned about the CAM therapies by word of mouth from relatives or friends, consumer marketing, or reading, rather than from healthcare professionals (Shreffler-Grant et al., 2005). Much of the CAM used by participants of this study was self-prescribed, raising questions about whether the participants had sufficient knowledge and information for safe and effective use of the CAM products. In addition, a majority (64.6%, $n = 210$) of the participants reported that they had at least one significant acute or chronic health problem and 32.3% ($n = 105$) had two or more significant health problems. The research team wondered about the potential for adverse drug–herb or drug–vitamin interactions with this population of vulnerable older adults, who likely were taking multiple prescription medications and had aging, impaired physiological responses.

Healthcare Choices: Older Rural Women

Additional analyses were conducted on a portion of the data set generated in the first Healthcare Choices study to answer the following research question: What factors predict use of CAM among older rural women (Shreffler-Grant, Hill, Weinert, Nichols, & Ide, 2007)? Men were excluded from this analysis because too few men in the larger data set used CAM, which is consistent with the literature about CAM use. Potential predictors were based on the literature and observations from practice and included education, age, rurality, marital status, income, spirituality, number of chronic illnesses, and health status. Logistic regression analysis was used to examine factors associated with use of CAM by the rural women participants ($n = 156$). A total of 25.6% of the women had used CAM recently and most of the therapies they used were self-prescribed.

Women most likely to use CAM were those who were fairly well educated, not currently married, and in their early older years (60–69 years of age). They had one or more significant chronic illnesses and lower health-related quality of life due to emotional concerns such as depression or stress.

Although this analysis did not yield additional information about health literacy about CAM per se, the results reinforced and expanded the findings of the main study discussed earlier. The women who reported use of CAM in this analysis used primarily self-prescribed CAM, which again raises concern about their level of knowledge about CAM. Women with one or more chronic illnesses were more likely to use CAM than those without chronic illness. Specifically, for each additional chronic illness reported, the odds of CAM use increased by 46%. By identifying characteristics of older rural women who are more or less likely to use CAM, the results can be used to tailor educational interventions to improve health literacy about CAM.

Healthcare Choices: Chronic Illness

The purpose of this study was to provide a better understanding of older rural adults' use of CAM, their perceptions of efficacy of the CAM they used, and the sources of information they used about CAM (Nichols, Sullivan, Ide, Shreffler-Grant, & Weinert, 2005). The study was conducted during 2003 to 2004 and funded by the Center for Research on Chronic Health Conditions (CRCHC) in Rural Dwellers at MSU College of Nursing (NIH/NINR IP20NR07790-01). Ten participants between 60 and 80 years of age who reported using CAM in the original Healthcare Choices study and who had two or more chronic illnesses were interviewed by telephone. Qualitative analysis was used to organize content from the interviews and identify themes. Participants used primarily self-prescribed CAM therapies such as dietary supplements and herbs, taken to compensate for perceived dietary deficiencies. Participants were generally satisfied with the results they attributed to the CAM. With regard to health literacy about CAM, the participants attempted to use reputable sources of information about the CAM products they used, but it was clear that some used the products in an inconsistent manner and did not understand what the products were intended to do for their health. Some individuals reported seeking information about CAM from sources other than their allopathic providers due to a perception that the providers were too busy to answer their questions about CAM.

Healthcare Choices: CAM Providers in Rural Locations

The CAM providers in rural locations study was motivated by the results of the first Healthcare Choices study, in which the older rural adults reported limited use of CAM providers, in contrast to self-prescribed CAM. The study's purpose was to determine the availability of CAM resources in 20 small rural towns in Montana and North Dakota and to explore the contribution of one type of CAM provider, naturopathic physicians, to rural healthcare (Nichols, Weinert, Shreffler-Grant, & Ide, 2006). The study was conducted during 2004 to 2005 and funded by the CRCHC in Rural Dwellers at MSU College of Nursing (NIH/ NINR IP20NR07790-01). CAM resource data were collected from Internet and telephone directory searches and from an online survey of naturopaths in Montana. Seventy-three CAM providers were identified in the 20 towns. Most naturopaths were located in population centers, but some offered outreach clinics to rural communities. Based on the results, the team concluded that local availability is not the critical factor in use of CAM providers by older rural adults. Although there were likely fewer choices of CAM providers in these small rural towns than in larger towns or cities, there were CAM providers available if the rural residents chose to use them. Rural residents are also known to travel outside their local communities to see healthcare providers who are acceptable to them (Shreffler-Grant, 2013).

Healthcare Choices: The MSU CAM Health Literacy Scale

Owing to questions concerning CAM health literacy revealed in the studies discussed earlier, the research team identified the need for an intervention to improve health literacy about CAM among older rural adults, particularly those with chronic health conditions. A measure of health literacy specific to CAM was needed to determine whether the intervention was effective or not. The existing health literacy measures were not suitable for this purpose since they evaluate basic reading and math skills in a conventional healthcare context (IOM, 2004) and not the more complex aspects needed to make reasoned decisions about the use of CAM. Accordingly, the research team designed the next Healthcare Choices project, the purpose of which was to develop a psychometrically sound instrument to measure CAM health literacy. In this project, CAM health literacy was operationally defined as the information about CAM needed to make informed self-management decisions regarding health. The optimal outcome of CAM health literacy is informed self-management of health.

Work to develop and evaluate a new instrument spanned a number of years and was supported by two intramural grants from MSU College of Nursing (2008–2009, 2015–2017) and a federal grant from NIH/NCCAM (1R15T006609-01 2011–2013). The research team utilized DeVellis's (2003) well-established guidelines for scale development to guide the instrument development process and DeVellis served as a consultant as the instrument was developed. A conceptual model of CAM Health Literacy was first developed to clarify concepts to be included in the new instrument (Shreffler-Grant, Nichols, Weinert, & Ide, 2013). A large pool of initial items for the instrument that fit with the empirical indicators in the conceptual model was developed. The draft instrument was reviewed and critiqued by experts and focus groups to assist in evaluating content validity. Following this review, the draft instrument was administered by telephone interview to a sample of 600 randomly selected older adults living in rural areas in the northwestern quadrant of the United States. Psychometric evaluation of the instrument using the data from the telephone interviews was conducted by a lengthy interactive process of examining the effect of individual items on reliability and validity indices. The outcome of this process is the MSU CAM Health Literacy Scale, a 21-item instrument with Cronbach's alpha of 0.753% and 42.27% explained variance (Shreffler-Grant, Weinert, & Nichols, 2014). The scale consists of a list of statements about herbal products, a type of commonly used complementary therapy. Response options range from "agree strongly" to "disagree strongly" based on the respondent's knowledge and understanding of the item content.

The validity of the MSU CAM Health Literacy Scale was further assessed by administering the new scale and two measures of general health literacy to a convenience sample of 110 older rural adults. The general health literacy measures used were the Newest Vital Sign (Weiss et al. 2005) and a single question measure (Chew, Bradley, & Boyko, 2004). The scores on the new scale and general health literacy measures were compared and revealed modest but significant correlations. The research team conducted an additional evaluation of the validity and reliability of the MSU CAM Health Literacy Scale using test–retest procedures. The MSU CAM Health Literacy Scale and two general health literacy measures were administered to a group of rural community–dwelling adults (Time 1) and then again approximately 3 weeks later (Time 2). A total of 188 adults completed both administrations. The results, in brief, supported the validity and reliability of the MSU CAM Health Literacy Scale and the stability of the scale score from Time 1 to Time 2.

Although evaluation of the scale will be an ongoing process, the MSU CAM Health Literacy Scale is now a validated and reliable measure of CAM health literacy. The scale was designed for research purposes to evaluate the effectiveness of an intervention to enhance CAM health literacy. Nurse investigators, however, may find that the scale is useful in other studies in which knowledge about safe use of CAM products or knowledge that supports effective self-care and self-management practices are relevant. The scale may also have important practice applications if used as a screening tool for rural older adults at risk for limitations in health literacy about CAM.

Healthcare Choices: Be Safe and Be Wise

The research team's long-term goal has been to design and implement an intervention to improve health literacy about CAM among older rural adults, particularly those with chronic health conditions. With this goal in mind, the team designed and implemented a project to examine the feasibility of a skill-building intervention to enhance CAM health literacy among older rural adults (Shreffler-Grant, Nichols, & Weinert, 2017). The project was entitled "Healthcare Choices: Be Safe" and was conducted with funding from the National Institutes of Health, National Library of Medicine (HHS-N-276-2011-00008-C 2014–2015) and a MSU intramural grant (2014–2015).

Skill-building modules were developed for the program that focused on concepts and skills important for CAM health literacy, communication with providers, and seeking and evaluating health information. The content of the modules does not encourage or discourage the use of CAM; instead the focus is on encouraging "informed" use. The modules were presented face to face and by webinar with older adults at a senior center in one small rural community in Montana. Participants completed a survey packet including the MSU CAM Health Literacy Scale and measures of general health literacy before and after the intervention. The team determined that conducting the intervention with older adults in a small rural community was feasible, although there were challenges to overcome such as gaining entry to the rural community, recruitment and retention limitations, the cost of an on-site intervention, and limitations of local resources. The feasibly study was not intended to test the effectiveness of the intervention on CAM health literacy; however, the level of CAM health literacy among the participants increased modestly. The team utilized the lessons learned in this feasibility study in the design of a more comprehensive skill-building intervention.

The "Healthcare Choices: Be Wise" research study was initiated in 2016 with support from the National Institutes of Health, NCCIH (1R15AT009097-01 2016–2018). The aims of the study are to implement the skill-building intervention with older rural adults, refine and evaluate the skill-building modules and intervention protocol, and evaluate the impact of the intervention on CAM health literacy and general health literacy. The intervention is designed to enhance CAM health literacy and thus promote more informed health management decisions.

The intervention includes four skill-building modules, three of which were developed for the prior "Healthcare Choices: Be Safe" project. The modules are focused on health literacy and CAM, communication with healthcare professionals, essential CAM knowledge, and health information–seeking skills. The modules have been refined based on the findings of the prior study and will be delivered face to face to older adults living in at least four rural communities. Participants complete survey packets at the first session, following the fourth session, and 6 months after the intervention. The intervention content and protocol will be evaluated using descriptive statistics and qualitative data to determine needed improvements. Statistical analyses will also be used to evaluate the impact of the intervention on CAM health literacy and general health literacy.

At the time of this writing, the intervention has been implemented in two rural communities and is underway in a third community. Although outcomes are not yet known relevant to the issue of health literacy about CAM among rural residents, the anecdotal responses of participants to date demonstrate that they are interested in improving their health literacy about CAM. They are actively engaged in discussions during the sessions, enthusiastic about the skills they are learning, and inquisitive about the material presented. This suggests that the program may lead to more informed self-management decisions about their health, which is the optimal outcome of CAM health literacy.

CONCLUSION

Over the past nearly two decades, this research team conducted the series of studies discussed earlier on the use of CAM among older rural adults. This work has led us to identify a need to enhance the level of health literacy about CAM among this population, particularly those with chronic illnesses. Healthcare consumers in any location, particularly those with chronic illnesses, make numerous decisions about healthcare and use a wide variety of self-care health products and therapies, decisions often made on their own and independent of their regular healthcare providers. This is particularly true of older rural adults, who are known to be more independent, engage in more self-care, and have less access to allopathic care than those living in urban areas (Shreffler-Grant et al., 2007). Those with chronic illnesses are also more likely to use CAM therapies (Astin, 1998; Astin et al., 2000; Barnes et al., 2004; Eisenberg et al., 1998; Shreffler-Grant et al., 2007).

Making informed decisions about the use of CAM requires a sophisticated level of health literacy on the part of the consumer. Without adequate CAM health literacy, older rural consumers may not know of all the appropriate healthcare choices that may benefit them, may fall victim to scams or unscrupulous sales practices, or may ingest potentially harmful substances. Informed use of CAM can increase health and illness management options and support well-reasoned decision making in regard to self-care for older rural adults living with chronic illnesses.

ACKNOWLEDGMENTS

The authors wish to acknowledge Bette Ide, PhD, RN (deceased), professor, University of North Dakota, College of Nursing, a former member of the research team. The research studies were funded in part by the following grants: National Institutes of Health, National Center for Complementary and Alternative Health/National Center for Complementary and Integrative Health (1R15AT095-01 2000–2003, 1R15T006609-01 2011–2013, and 1R15AT009097-01 2016–2018); National Institutes of Health, National Library of Medicine (Contract No. HHS-N-276-2011-00008-C with University of Washington 2014–2015); the Center for Research on Chronic Health Conditions at MSU College of Nursing (NIH/NINR IP20NR07790-01 2003-2005); two intramural grants

(2008–2009, 2015–2017) from MSU College of Nursing, and one Intramural Faculty Excellence Grant from MSU 2014–1015.

REFERENCES

Arcury, T. A., Preisser, J. S., Gesler, W. M., & Sherman, J. E. (2004). Complementary and alternative medicine use among rural residents in western North Carolina. *Complementary Health Practice Review, 9*(2), 93–102. doi:10.1177/1076167503253433

Astin, J. (1998). Why patients use alternative medicine: Results of a national study. *Journal of the American Medical Association, 279*(19), 1548–1553. doi:10.1001/jama.279.19.1548

Astin, J., Pelletier, K., Marie, A., & Haskell, W. (2000). Complementary and alternative medicine use among elderly persons: One-year analysis of a Blue Shield Medicare supplement. *Journal of Gerontology, 55A*(1), M4–M9.

Barnes, P. M., Bloom, B., & Nahin, R. L. (2008). *Complementary and alternative medicine use among adults and children: United States, 2007. National health statistics reports*, No. 12. Hyattsville, MD: National Center for Health Statistics.

Barnes, P. M., Pewell-Griner, E., McFann, K., & Nahin, R. L. (2004). *Complementary and alternative medicine use among adults: United States, 2002. National health statistics reports*, No. 343. Hyattsville, MD: National Center for Health Statistics.

Cherniack, E. P., Senzel, R. S., & Pan, C. X. (2001). Correlates of use of alternative medicine by the elderly in an urban population. *Journal of Alternative and Complementary Medicine, 7*, 277–280. doi:10.1089/107555301300328160

Chew, L. D., Bradley, K. A., & Boyko, E. J. (2004). Brief questions to identify patients with inadequate health literacy. *Family Medicine, 36*(8), 588–594.

DeVellis, R. (2003). *Scale development: Theory and applications* (2nd ed.). Thousand Oaks, CA: Sage.

Eisenberg, D., Davis, R., Ettner, S., Appel, S., Wilkey, S., Van Rompay, M., & Kessler R. C. (1998). Trends in alternative medicine use in the United States, 1990–1997: Results of a follow-up national survey. *Journal of the American Medical Association, 280*(18), 1569–1575. doi:10.1001/jama.280.18.1569

Eisenberg, D., Kessler, R., Foster, C., Norlock, F., Calkins, D., & Delbanco, T. (1993). Unconventional medicine in the United States. *The New England Journal of Medicine, 328*, 246–252. doi:10.1056/NEJM199301283280406

Harron, M., & Glasser, M. (2003). Use of and attitudes toward complementary and alternative medicine among family practice patients in small rural Illinois communities. *The Journal of Rural Health, 19*(3), 279–284. doi:10.1111/j.1748-0361.2003.tb00574.x

Institute of Medicine. (2004). *Health literacy: A prescription to end confusion*. Washington, DC: National Academies Press.

Institute of Medicine. (2005). *Complementary and alternative medicine in the United States*. Washington, DC: National Academies Press.

Johnson, J. (1999). Older rural women and the use of complementary therapies. *Journal of Community Health Nursing, 16*(4), 223–232. doi:10.1207/S15327655JCHN1604_2

King, M. O., & Pettigrew, A. C. (2004). Complementary and alternative therapy use by older adults in three ethnically diverse populations: A pilot study. *Geriatric Nursing, 25*(1), 30–37. doi:10.1016/j.gerinurse.2003.11.013

Lee, H. J., & McDonagh, M. K. (2013). Updating the rural nursing base. In C. A. Winters (Ed.). *Rural nursing: Concepts, theory, and practice* (4th ed., pp. 15–33). New York, NY: Springer Publishing.

Long, K. A., & Weinert, C. (1989). Rural nursing: Developing the theory base. *Scholarly Inquiry for Nursing Practice: An International Journal, 3*, 113–127.

McFarland, B., Bigelow, D., Zani, B., Newsom, J., & Kaplan, M. (2002). Complementary and alternative medicine use in Canada and the United States. *American Journal of Public Health, 92*, 1616–1618. doi:10.2105/AJPH.92.10.1616

Montbraind, M., & Laing, G. (1991). Alternative health care as a control strategy. *Journal of Advanced Nursing, 16*, 325–332. doi:10.1111/j.1365-2648.1991.tb01656.x

National Center for Complementary and Integrative Health. (2017). Complementary, alternative, or integrative health: What's in a name?. Retrieved from https://nccih.nih.gov/health/integrative-health

Nichols, E., Sullivan, T., Ide, B., Shreffler-Grant, J., & Weinert, C. (2005). Health care choices: Complementary therapy, chronic illness, and older rural dwellers. *Journal of Holistic Nursing, 23*(4), 381–394. doi:10.1177/0898010105281088

Nichols, E., Weinert, C., Shreffler-Grant, J., & Ide, B. (2006). Complementary and alternative providers in rural locations. *Online Journal of Rural Nursing and Health Care, 6*(2). Retrieved from http://rnojournal.binghamton.edu/index.php/RNO/article/view/154

Rao, J., Mihaliak, K., Kroenke, K., Bradley, J., Tierney, W., & Weinberger, M. (1999). Use of complementary therapies for arthritis among patients of rheumatologists. *Annals of Internal Medicine, 131*, 409–416. doi:10.7326/0003-4819-131-6-199909210-00003

Shreffler-Grant, J. (2013). Acceptability: One component in choice of health care provider. In C. A. Winters (Ed.), *Rural nursing: Concepts, theory, and practice* (4th ed., pp. 215–224). New York, NY: Springer Publishing.

Shreffler-Grant, J., Hill, W., Weinert, C., Nichols, E., & Ide, B. (2007). Complementary therapy and older rural women: Who uses and who does not? *Nursing Research, 56*(1), 28–33. doi:10.1097/00006199-200701000-00004

Shreffler-Grant, J., Nichols, E., & Weinert, C. (2017). Bee SAFE, A skill-building intervention to enhance CAM health literacy: Lessons learned. *Health Promotion Practice*. doi:10.1177/1524839917700612

Shreffler-Grant, J., Nichols, E., Weinert, C., & Ide, B. (2013). Montana State University conceptual model of complementary and alternative medicine (CAM) health literacy. *Journal of Health Communication: International Perspectives, 18*(10), 1193–1200. doi:10.1080/10810730.3013.778385

Shreffler-Grant, J., Weinert, C., & Nichols, E. (2014). Instrument to measure health literacy about complementary and alternative medicine. *Journal of Nursing Measurement, 22*(3), 489–499. doi:10.1891/1061-3749.22.3.489

Shreffler-Grant, J., Weinert, C., Nichols, E., & Ide, B. (2005). Complementary therapy use among older rural adults. *Public Health Nursing, 22*(4), 323–331. doi:10.1111/j.0737-1209.2005.220407.x

Tanner, L.. (2009, January 13). With economy sour, consumers sweet on herbal medicines. *Associated Press.* Retrieved from http://www.foxnews.com/printer_friendly_wires/2009Jan13/0,4675,MeltdownSupplementSales,00.html

U.S. Department of Health and Human Services. (2000). Healthy people 2010, section 11-2: Health communication objective. Retrieved from https://www.healthypeople.gov

Vallerand, A. H., Fouladbakhsh, J. M., & Templin, T. (2003). The use of complementary/alternative medicine for self-treatment of pain among residents of urban, suburban, and rural communities. *American Journal of Public Health, 93,* 923–925. doi:10.2105/AJPH.93.6.923

Vincent, C., & Furnham, A. (1996). Why do patients turn to complementary medicine? An empirical study. *British Journal of Clinical Psychology, 35,* 37–48. doi:10.1111/j.2044-8260.1996.tb01160.x

Weiss, B. D., Mays, M. Z., Martz, W., Castro, K. M., DeWalt, D. A., Pignone, M. P., . . . Halt, F. (2005). Quick assessment of literacy in primary care: The newest vital sign. *Annals of Family Medicine, 3*(6), 514–522. doi:10.1370/afm.405

Nursing Education

In Chapter 24, four nursing educators sensed a need for a tool to assess the knowledge of rural nursing practice for students and nurses. The educators developed items based on the rural nursing theory (RNT) concepts and common themes found in rural literature. The 27-item Rural Knowledge Scale was structured, successfully psychometrically evaluated, and is available for further testing. In Chapter 25, three of the earlier educators share their strategies, benefits, and challenges in placing nursing students in rural hospital clinical placements.

Using the RNT theoretical statements, Chapter 26 authors summarize the present-day implications for rural education, practice, and policy. Authors of the last chapter in this section/part share ways in which rural healthcare agencies and rural organizations can collaborate to recruit and retain highly qualified nurses through nursing student rural experiences, financial support, and nurse residency programs.

CHAPTER 24

Development and Psychometric Evaluation of the Rural Knowledge Scale

Heidi A. Mennenga, Laurie J. Johansen,
Becka Foerster, and Lori Hendrickx

DISCUSSION QUESTIONS

- What are the strengths and limitations of the Rural Knowledge Scale?
- How does the development of the Rural Knowledge Scale contribute to the science of nursing?
- What are some potential applications for the Rural Knowledge Scale?

According to the 2013 Workforce Analysis Report, only 16% of registered nurses (RNs) working in the United States are currently employed in rural settings (Health Resources and Services Administration [HRSA], 2013). Beurhaus, Staiger, and Auerbach (2009) found that nursing is the largest profession within the healthcare industry in the United States; therefore, it is imperative to have enough of those nurses caring for people living in rural areas. In 2009, the National Advisory Council on Nurse Education and Practice projected a 36% shortage of RNs by 2020. However, more recent data have provided a more optimistic perspective about availability of future RNs. In 2012, the Bureau of Labor Statistics Employment Projections forecasted a 26% increase in employed RNs between 2010 and 2020. Additionally, HRSA (2013) reported a growth rate in the nursing workforce exceeding the growth rate of the U.S. population.

Although the nursing workforce projections are promising for the country as a whole, findings in the literature continue to reveal challenges faced by rural healthcare facilities as they struggle to recruit and retain RNs and other health-care professionals (Schmitz, Claiborne, & Rouhana, 2012). In particular, it is reported that rural populations consistently deal with a scarcity of healthcare professionals (National Rural Health Association, 2016). Several sources caution against being overly optimistic when it comes to the future nursing workforce. Fahs (2012) suggested careful regard for the future availability of RNs in rural healthcare facilities with historic patterns showing greater shortage of RNs in rural locations when compared to their urban counterparts. Likewise, HRSA (2013) also reported that even with the growth rate in the nursing workforce, urban areas continue to have higher per capita rates of nurses with no specific data available on the number of RNs traveling away from their rural communities to more urban areas for employment. To meet the continued healthcare needs and unique challenges of the rural population, rural healthcare facilities need to have the ability to recruit and retain an adequate number of RNs now and in the future.

In addition to an available workforce, it is also vital for rural healthcare professionals to understand the dynamics of the rural population. People living in rural areas have health disparities that add to the complexity of their healthcare needs. Arias (2014) reported that in the United States between 1999 and 2014, rural areas had higher annual age-adjusted death rates from the five leading causes of death when compared to urban areas. In general, people living in rural areas are more likely to be older and more likely to have poorer health than those living in more urban areas (Bolin, Bellamy, Ferdinand, Kash, & Helduser, 2015; Centers for Disease Control and Prevention, 2017). For example, rural women dwellers self-reported higher rates of obesity and rural adolescent dwellers were found more likely to smoke tobacco (Rural Health Research and Policy Centers, 2014). The reality is that the nursing workforce in the rural areas of the United States cares for a population with a significantly different, and often more complicated, health status compared to their urban counterparts.

Discernment of the employment decisions surrounding RNs working in rural healthcare settings is essential to establish effective future recruitment and retention strategies to meet the workforce needs of rural healthcare settings. Thoughtful consideration is necessary when taking into account nurses' choices to not practice nursing in rural settings because of a lack of familiarity with the unique aspects of rural nursing. The rural nursing theory by Long and Weinert (1989) originally shed light on the vast role diffusion needed for a nurse to successfully practice in a rural healthcare setting. Recent research by Medves, Edge, Bisonette, and Stansfield (2015) continued to support the broad scope of practice of the rural nurse and added that the rural nurses truly practice in a specialty area of their own. Nurses' decisions to seek employment in rural healthcare settings may be impacted by their lack of confidence or decreased comfort levels practicing as nurse generalists. This lack of confidence or decreased comfort level sometimes stems from no previous exposure to the nurse generalist role as well as an unfamiliarity with the unique aspects and true expectations that exist in rural nursing practice. Hunsberger, Baumann, Blythe, and Crea (2009) completed a qualitative study of nurses in rural Canada. They found that nurses practicing in rural settings were stressed by the nurse generalist role and that stress was exacerbated by the narrow base of resources available to them. These study findings indicated the need to prioritize education for nurses practicing, or considering practice, in rural healthcare settings by building intentional rural nursing practice considerations into nursing curricula.

Academic institutions play a key role in preparing nurses for their potential roles in rural locations. Nursing students, whether they intend to seek employment in rural or urban areas, need to acquire knowledge of healthcare resources for rural areas as well as to gain an understanding of sociocultural and lifestyle characteristics of patients living in rural areas. Literature shows the value of providing curricular content on rural healthcare to help prepare students to care for rural dwellers in and out of the rural setting (Rutledge, Haney, Bordelon, Renaud, & Fowler, 2014). Programs educating nurses, especially those programs serving rural areas, have a role in providing education that prepares nurse generalists through both course content and clinical experiences alike. Acquiring knowledge, skills, and attitudes to meet the needs of the rural population are essential for nurses to feel comfortable seeking employment in rural healthcare facilities. Studies have revealed a need to have curricular content specific to rural health while increasing the firsthand experiences nursing students get within rural healthcare settings in order to apply appropriate skills unique to rural nursing practice (Molinari, Jaiswal, & Hollinger-Forrest, 2011; Stasser & Neusy, 2010).

As noted by the American Association of Colleges of Nursing (AACN, 2008), baccalaureate-prepared nurses should graduate having experienced an adequate exposure to the practice of nursing across the life span in a continuum of healthcare venues. The effect of rural clinical experiences was studied by Coyle and Narsavage (2012). They found a positive impact on the future recruitment of nursing students to rural healthcare facilities for those nurses having had a rural clinical experience. Likewise, rural hospital managers were surveyed following nursing student exposure to rural clinical sites. Value in the exposure of students to the mixture of patient situations available in rural healthcare settings along with collaborative opportunities with other disciplines and departments was found instrumental in adding to the opportunities for baccalaureate-prepared nurses to gain an understanding of the role of the rural nurse generalist. Students and rural healthcare facilities alike benefited from this unique clinical immersion experience in the rural healthcare setting (Hendrickx, Mennenga, & Johansen, 2013). Ultimately, the clinical opportunities provided for nursing students impact the future nursing workforce, especially that workforce serving the rural population.

Beyond the benefits of rural clinical experiences for nurses, study findings by Daniels, VanLeit, Skipper, Sanders, and Rhyne (2007) revealed the significance of future rural nurses having had some background or prior experiences in rural settings, leading to a desire for them to return to those communities. The firsthand clinical experiences in rural communities serve as the potential recruitment method. As previously noted, workforce issues continue to be a difficult reality in rural healthcare facilities, and ensuring adequate numbers of qualified RNs prepared to practice in rural areas is a priority. Molinari and Monserud (2008) found that many nurses chose to live in a rural community because of their family ties to that community. While summarizing previous systematic reviews about interventions to retain nurses in rural areas, Mbemba, Gagnon, Paré, and Côté (2013) found that successful strategies frequently recommended the creation of organized interactions between nursing students and healthcare professionals in rural settings. They also found success in recruiting students who had previously lived in the rural community and had some form of connection to practicing in a rural setting. The rural community and the rural healthcare system create a context that is important to the future recruitment and retention of nurses and other healthcare professionals.

NURSING STUDENT KNOWLEDGE OF RURAL NURSING CONCEPTS

The knowledge level of baccalaureate nursing students regarding rural nursing concepts is not known; therefore, addressing gaps in knowledge is difficult. By identifying and addressing gaps in knowledge, nursing faculty members may be able to impact student interest and confidence in rural nursing practice, potentially increasing their desire to practice in rural healthcare settings upon graduation. In a review of the literature, no existing instruments measuring knowledge about rural nursing practice were identified.

Purpose of Research

The purpose of this research was to develop an instrument to assess nursing student knowledge of rural nursing practice and conduct psychometric evaluation of the newly developed Rural Knowledge Scale.

Methodology

The Rural Knowledge Scale was developed in three phases: concept clarification, item development, and psychometric testing.

CONCEPT CLARIFICATION

Since no instruments measuring knowledge about rural nursing practice were found, the authors determined the need to develop an instrument. The rural nursing theory (Long & Weinert, 1989) and common themes found in the literature review were used to develop an initial 24-item Rural Knowledge Scale.

ITEM DEVELOPMENT

Based on a literature review and concepts in the rural nursing theory, the initial 24-item tool was developed and divided into six sections:

- Rural environment (two items)
- Rural health risk/issue (four items)
- Rural healthcare access (two items)
- Rural healthcare technology (two items)
- Rural nursing practice (four items)
- Rural characteristics (10 items)

A panel of five experts on rural nursing, several nationally known, was invited to review the instrument for content validity. The initial 24-item instrument had an acceptable scale content validity index of 0.89. The individual items all had a content validity index of 0.6 or above and were retained in the scale. Based on the comments from the panel of five rural nursing experts, three additional items were added, resulting in a 27-item Rural Knowledge Scale.

PSYCHOMETRIC TESTING SAMPLE

Approval was obtained from the institutional review board to conduct psychometric testing on the Rural Knowledge Scale. Undergraduate baccalaureate students at one Midwestern university were asked to complete the 27-item instrument. Participants were enrolled across the five semesters of the nursing program.

Instrument

The 27 items on the Rural Knowledge Scale are organized into six sections, based on the rural nursing theory: rural environment, rural health risk/issue, rural healthcare access, rural healthcare technology, rural nursing practice, and rural characteristics. The 27-item instrument uses a 5-point Likert scale with possible responses ranging from "not at all knowledgeable" to "very knowledgeable." The use of a 5-point Likert scale includes a neutral point, so participants are allowed to express their true reactions (Polit & Beck, 2011).

Results

Statistical analysis was completed using IBM Statistical Product and Service Solutions (SPSS) Statistics Software version 23 (IBM Corporation, Armonk, New York). Descriptive demographic statistics and total scores on the Rural Knowledge Scale were calculated. Factor analysis using principal axis factoring was conducted on the Rural Knowledge Scale.

According to Tabachnick and Fidell's (2012) recommendation that more than 200 participants should be used for instrument development, an adequate sample size was obtained. The convenience sample ($N = 347$) was predominantly female (87.4%), White (83.8%), and under the age of 25 (66.8%). Possible scores on the Rural Knowledge Scale range from 27 to 135. A score of 81 would indicate neutrality, with a score greater than 81 indicating increased knowledge about rural issues. For this research study, scores on the overall instrument ranged from 27 to 135, with a mean of 90.2 (standard deviation [SD] = 20.89), and indicated students self-reported that they were generally knowledgeable about rural issues.

The Kaiser–Meyer–Olkin Measure of Sampling Adequacy was 0.942 for the scale, indicating that factor analysis could be performed (Tabachnick & Fidell, 2012). Extraction of factors was determined by the examination of the scree plot and consideration of eigenvalues greater than 1. The scree plot for the total scale indicated one factor would be appropriate, signifying that all items were interrelated. All items had loadings of more than 0.40 and were retained (Polit & Beck, 2011; Table 24.1).

Reliability for the total scale was determined by calculating a Cronbach's alpha with a result of 0.96. According to Polit and Beck (2011), a Cronbach's alpha greater than 0.70 is desirable for a new instrument. Based on this guideline, the Rural Knowledge Scale demonstrates excellent internal consistency.

Limitations

This research has limited generalizability since it occurred with a fairly homogeneous student sample. Because this nursing school is located in a predominantly rural state, more nursing students may come from rural backgrounds. Students who participated in this study were more likely to have been exposed to rural healthcare issues either through clinical experience in rural facilities or in simulation activities with a rural focus. The Rural Knowledge Scale should also be validated with other populations, such as practicing RNs.

IMPLICATIONS FOR RURAL HEALTH AND NURSING EDUCATION

Rural healthcare facilities and nursing education programs share responsibility for preparing nursing students to practice in a rural setting. The shortage of nurses in rural areas is well documented in the literature and recent efforts to study recruitment and retention of rural nurses have shown that nursing students from rural areas are more likely to remain in rural areas to practice (Bigbee & Mixon, 2013). Healthcare facilities can target recruitment efforts toward high school students who demonstrate an interest in healthcare careers by offering incentives such as tuition reimbursement and guaranteed placement upon graduation. Rural facilities can also use the Rural Knowledge Scale

TABLE 24.1 Factor Loadings for Rural Knowledge Scale

Item	Factor Loading
Longer distances	0.662
Travel conditions	0.628
Availability of transportation	0.686
Occupational safety	0.780
Weather exposure	0.709
Health literacy	0.772
Underinsurance or lack of insurance	0.727
Availability of healthcare services	0.732
Availability of primary care providers	0.726
Availability of specialists	0.721
Impact of public policy on rural healthcare	0.684
Telehealth availability	0.558
Availability of equipment	0.592
Confidentiality and anonymity	0.601
Availability of professional development	0.681
Expert generalist role	0.686
Recruitment/retention of nurses	0.677
Delays in seeking treatment	0.742
Social support networks	0.719
Strong work ethic	0.717
Determination	0.727
Frugality	0.707
Lack of privacy	0.703
Church affiliation/religious	0.694
Resourcefulness	0.775
Self-reliance	0.748
Insider/outsider differentiation	0.765

as an assessment tool for new hires to measure understanding of rural issues prior to practice in a rural area. Having this background information will allow the facility to shape an orientation program that supports newly hired nurses by building on strengths in knowledge about rural healthcare and reinforcing areas of weakness. Having a good understanding of the issues facing rural healthcare should improve the transition from the nursing education environment to actual nursing practice in a rural community.

Although nursing students from rural areas may have a broader knowledge of rural healthcare issues, nursing education programs should include content on rural healthcare in the curriculum for all students. Nursing students from urban areas are often unaware of the richness of a rural clinical rotation and find that the varied opportunities and generalist nature of rural healthcare provide a well-rounded educational experience (Hendrickx et al., 2013). Using the Rural Knowledge Scale to assess nursing students' knowledge prior to delivery of educational content on rural healthcare can provide valuable information to nursing faculty or clinical instructors about the level of understanding of rural issues prior to course development and implementation.

CONCLUSION

Practicing in rural healthcare can be a complex and varied experience that may result in a difficult transition for a newly hired nurse with no rural healthcare background. Providing an educational experience that prepares a nurse for rural practice can be a vital component of a successful move into rural practice. Successful education can be enhanced through the use of the Rural Knowledge Scale. The final 27-item version of the Rural Knowledge Scale demonstrated acceptable psychometric properties and can be utilized to identify gaps in student knowledge related to rural nursing practice and rural healthcare issues. By identifying and addressing gaps, students' interest and confidence in rural nursing practice may be impacted and result in more nurses who are interested in practicing in rural settings.

REFERENCES

American Association of Colleges of Nursing. (2008). *The essentials of baccalaureate education for professional nursing practice*. Washington, DC: Author.

Arias, E. (2014). United States life tables, 2010. *National Vital Statistics Reports, 63*(7). Retrieved from https://www.cdc.gov/nchs/data/nvsr/nvsr63/nvsr63_07.pdf

Beurhaus, P. I., Staiger, D. O., & Auerbach, D. I. (2009). *The future of the nursing workforce in the United States: Data, trends, and implications*. Sudbury, MA: Jones & Bartlett.

Bigbee, J., & Mixon, D. (2103). Recruitment and retention of rural nursing students: A retrospective study. *Rural and Remote Health, 13*, 1–9. Retrieved from https://www.ncbi.nlm.nih.gov/pubmed/24160687

Bolin, J., Bellamy, G., Ferdinand, A., Kash, B., & Helduser, J. (2015). *Rural healthy people 2020* (Vol. 2). College Station: Texas A&M Health Science Center School of Public Health, Southwest Rural Health Research Center. Retrieved from http://sph.tamhsc.edu/srhrc/docs/rhp2020-volume-2.pdf

Bureau of Labor Statistics. (2012). The 30 occupations with the largest projected employment growth, 2010–20. Retrieved from https://www.bls.gov/news .release/ecopro.t10.htm

Centers for Disease Control and Prevention. (2017). About rural health. Retrieved from https://www.cdc.gov/ruralhealth/about.html

Coyle, S. B., & Narsavage, G. L. (2012). Effects of an interprofessional rural rotation on nursing student interest, perceptions, and intent. *Online Journal of Rural Nursing and Health Care, 12*(1), 40–48. Retrieved from http://rnojournal.binghamton.edu/ index.php/RNO/article/view/42

Daniels, Z., VanLeit, B., Skipper, B., Sanders, M., & Rhyne, R. (2007). Factors in recruiting and retaining health professionals for rural practice. *The Journal of Rural Health, 23*(1), 62–71. doi:10.1111/j.1748-0361.2006.00069.x

Fahs, P. (2012). RN labor supply bubble: What does it mean for rural health care? *Online Journal of Rural Nursing and Health Care, 12*(1), 1–2. Retrieved from http:// rnojournal.binghamton.edu/index.php/RNO/article/view/153

Health Resources and Service Administration. (2013). *The U.S. nursing workforce: Trends in supply and education.* Retrieved from https://bhw.hrsa.gov/sites/default/files/ bhw/nchwa/projections/nursingworkforcetrendsoct2013.pdf

Hendrickx, L., Mennenga, H., & Johansen, L. (2013). The use of rural hospitals for clinical placements in nursing education. In C. A. Winters (Ed.). *Rural nursing: Concepts, theory, and practice* (4th ed., pp. 293–301). New York, NY: Springer Publishing.

Hunsberger, M., Baumann, A., Blythe, J., & Crea, M. (2009). Sustaining the rural workforce: Nursing perspectives on worklife challenges. *The Journal of Rural Health, 25*(1), 17–24. doi:10.1111/j.1748-0361.2009.00194.x

Long, K. A., & Weinert, C. (1989). Rural nursing: Developing the theory base. *Research and Theory for Nursing Practice, 3*(2), 113–127.

Mbemba, G., Gagnon, M., Paré, G., & Côté, J. (2013). Interventions for supporting nurse retention in rural and remote areas: An umbrella review. *Human Resources for Health, 11*(44), 1–9. doi:10.1186/1478-4491-11-44

Medves, J., Edge, D., Bisonette, L., & Stansfield, K. (2015). Supporting rural nurses: Skills and knowledge to practice in Ontario, Canada. *Online Journal of Rural Nursing and Health Care, 15*(1), 7–41. Retrieved from http://rnojournal.binghamton.edu/index .php/RNO/article/viewFile/337/272

Molinari, D. L., Jaiswal, A., & Hollinger-Forrest, T. (2011). Rural nurses: Lifestyle preferences and education perspectives. *Online Journal of Rural Nursing and Health Care, 11*(2), 16–26. Retrieved from rnojournal.binghamton.edu/index.php/RNO/ article/download/27/19

Molinari, D. L., & Monserud, M. (2008). Rural nurse job satisfaction. *Rural and Remote Health, 8*(4), 1–12. Retrieved from https://www.rrh.org.au/journal/article/1055

National Rural Health Association. (2016). About rural health care. Retrieved from https://www.ruralhealthweb.org/about-nrha/about-rural-health-care

Polit, D., & Beck, C. (2011). *Nursing research: Generating and assessing evidence for nursing practice* (9th ed.). New York, NY: Lippincott Williams & Wilkins.

Rural Health Research & Policy Centers. (2014). *Rural Health Reform Policy Research Center: The 2014 update of the rural-urban chartbook.* Retrieved from https://ruralhealth.und .edu/projects/health-reform-policy-research-center/pdf/2014-rural-urban -chartbook-update.pdf

Rutledge, C. M., Haney, T., Bordelon, M., Renaud, M., & Fowler, C. (2014). Telehealth: Preparing advanced practice nurses to address healthcare needs in rural and underserved populations. *International Journal of Nursing Education Scholarship*, *11*(1), 1–9. Retrieved from EBSCO Host.

Schmitz, D., Claiborne, N., & Rouhana, N. (2012). Defining the issues and principles of recruitment and retention. *National Rural Health Association Policy Brief*. Retrieved from http://www.ruralhealthweb.org/go/left/government-affairs/policy-documents-and-statements/official-policy-positions/official-policy-positions

Stasser, R., & Neusy, A. (2010). Context counts: Training health workers in and for rural and remote areas. *Bulletin of the World Health Organization*, *88*(10), 777–782.

Tabachnick, B., & Fidell, L. (2012). *Using multivariate statistics* (6th ed.). New York, NY: Allyn & Bacon.

CHAPTER 25

Clinical Placements in Rural Hospitals: Expanding Nursing Students' Knowledge, Skills, and Attitudes Toward Rural Healthcare

Lori Hendrickx, Heidi A. Mennenga, and Laurie J. Johansen

DISCUSSION QUESTIONS

- What are the opportunities that result from placing nursing students in rural hospitals for clinical experiences?
- What are the challenges related to placing nursing students in rural hospitals for clinical experiences?
- How can rural hospital clinical placement affect recruitment and retention in rural healthcare facilities?
- What are some strategies for increasing nursing student exposure to rural healthcare?

Predictions that the current nursing shortage will continue and most likely intensify as the demand for nurses grows have resulted in a variety of recommendations for strategies to reduce the shortage and meet the demands for additional nurses. In 2017, the U.S. Department of Labor projected a 16% growth rate in the need for registered nurses for 2014 to 2024, compared to an average growth rate of 7% for all occupations (U.S. Department of Labor, 2017). Multiple authors and organizations (American Association of Colleges of Nursing [AACN], 2017) have reported the need for additional nurses. Media exposure regarding the nursing shortage has increased national awareness and has resulted in increased numbers of applicants to nursing education programs. The AACN (2017) has reported that several statewide initiatives are being developed to address the nursing shortage; however, challenges continue.

Despite the growing numbers of nursing school applicants, the number of graduates from nursing programs has not sufficiently increased to meet the demand for registered nurses. In many cases, nursing school applicants are turned away due to a shortage of faculty and inadequate numbers of clinical sites or financial constraints. AACN (2017) reported that a faculty shortage and inadequate numbers of clinical education sites were potential barriers to meeting the demand for healthcare providers. Insufficient numbers of clinical sites are an issue faced by many nursing programs that educate students primarily in more urban hospital settings. These urban institutions often have multiple nursing programs competing for clinical time, resulting in the inability to accept more students or add additional clinical groups to facilities already saturated with students.

OPPORTUNITIES FOR RURAL HOSPITALS

In an effort to respond to the nursing shortage, marketing strategies have resulted in substantial increases in the numbers of entering college freshmen declaring nursing as a major. In the last 15 years, South Dakota State University (SDSU) has responded to the increased demand for nursing graduates by increasing the numbers of students accepted from 48 to 64 per semester on one campus, admitting additional students twice a year rather than once a year on another campus, adding two accelerated program sites with the potential for 80 students per year, and adding an additional standard program campus with 40 students per year. These changes resulted in an increase in the number of students accepted yearly from 128 to 312. Despite the large increase in students accepted, in 2011 only one-third of qualified students applying to the SDSU College of Nursing's main campus were accepted on their first application (Hendrickx, 2011). Additional expansion of the nursing program has not occurred in part due to the lack of additional clinical placement sites.

The majority of nursing students at SDSU have traditionally received their clinical education at larger hospitals in a major city, competing with several other nursing programs for clinical placement. Clinical experiences needed to be expanded to include evenings and weekends and changes in the calendar were made so that some groups could do clinical in the summer or early in January before other programs were in session. While these adjustments did result in increased availability of clinical experiences for students, another possible solution was to explore clinical opportunities in smaller, more rural healthcare facilities.

Implementation

SDSU has five semesters in the nursing program with clinical in all the semesters. The first semester clinical experience is in a general medical–surgical setting with emphasis on basic nursing care and physical assessment skills. Several years ago, the first semester coordinator met with nursing directors in two rural hospitals to explore the possibility of placing these beginning students in their facilities for clinical. At the time, there were no other nursing programs doing clinical in these hospitals. Agreements were reached with the two rural facilities and a pilot program for 1 year was completed.

Current nursing instructors from SDSU accompanied the students as clinical faculty for the expansion into the rural hospitals. Clinical group size was limited to eight students for one clinical instructor. After successful implementation of the pilot program, the use of rural hospitals was expanded as the nursing program increased in size.

There were a number of considerations in selection of appropriate rural clinical sites. The proximity to campus was considered with all sites being within an hour's drive. The main campus of SDSU is located near the Minnesota border so hospitals in both South Dakota and Minnesota were considered. Transportation was provided for the faculty member and the students through the campus motor pool fleet.

The size of the facility and average daily census needed to be adequate to accommodate eight students. This did not necessarily mean that there needed to be eight patients in the inpatient setting, just that there were learning opportunities for eight students. Students were usually assigned patients in the inpatient area first and then other learning opportunities were identified. All of the hospitals had active outpatient departments where students could help admit a patient for an outpatient procedure, follow the patient through the procedure, and then provide postprocedural care. Students also rotated through dialysis units, cardiac rehabilitation, and accompanied nurses on home health visits. Some of the hospitals had long-term care facilities attached so students were rotated through the long-term care setting as well as the hospital setting.

As the number of clinical groups increased, the need for additional clinical instructors increased as well. Clinical instructors were selected from the existing faculty first. Administrators in the rural hospitals were concerned that the instructor be familiar with their facility so initially faculty members were approached who had previously worked in one of the rural hospitals. As additional instructors were needed, further discussion revealed that two area rural hospitals had staff nurses in the educator track of SDSU's graduate program. These graduate students were then added as clinical instructors in the hospitals where they had worked as staff nurses. One additional method for recruitment of clinical instructors was having faculty members serve as preceptors for graduate students in the educator track. The graduate student spent one semester in the rural hospital setting doing clinical with a current faculty member. After graduation, these students were more comfortable doing clinical in one of the rural sites. Several of the rural hospitals being used for clinical experiences had instructors who were previously employed by the hospital or assisted with clinical in a rural hospital during graduate school, which resulted in increased trust between the college faculty and the hospital personnel and eased the transition for the clinical instructor and the nursing staff. Since two states were being used, having clinical instructors who had practiced in the hospitals resulted in instructors already holding licensure in their respective states.

Ongoing communication between the hospital and college staffs was maintained through two primary methods. The clinical instructor remained the primary resource for the hospital staff regarding changes in the curriculum, learning needs of the students and responsibilities of the nursing staff in the education of the students. The semester coordinator made periodic site visits to each site to stay in touch with the clinical instructors and the administrators at the clinical site. The semester coordinator addressed any needs of the hospital staff that arose in addition to serving as a mentor for the clinical instructors. The onsite interaction was identified as crucial by the nursing administrators at the clinical sites.

An additional consideration was the day of the week to hold clinical. Since rural hospitals often have surgeons or specialists who are on site only on certain days of the week, it was found to be beneficial to hold clinical experiences on those days as much as possible. For example, patient census was often found to be higher on the day the surgeon had procedures scheduled but typically by Friday some hospitals had discharged most of their patients.

Evaluation

Evaluation of the clinical experiences was done informally each semester and formally through interviews with the nurse managers. Clinical instructors met with the semester coordinator to provide feedback into the type of learning experiences available and appropriate adjustments were made. Face-to-face interviews were done with the nursing managers from the clinical sites. The managers were asked to identify the benefits and challenges associated with having nursing students in their rural healthcare facility.

BENEFITS

The use of rural facilities for clinical experiences results in many benefits not only for students, but also for clinical instructors, patients, staff, and administrators. The managers reported that since rural facilities often have all patients located on a single floor regardless of diagnosis, students have easy access to patients of all ages with many different health problems. A variety of experiences and exposure to other departments also await the student in a rural facility. In a single clinical day, students could observe dialysis, participate in outpatient procedures, and assist in other departments in addition to caring for their primary patient. Additionally, since rural facilities do not typically have intravenous (IV) teams or lift teams, students were often able to perform these types of tasks and participate more in direct patient care.

Respondents indicated that the variety of diagnoses and experiences in one area also presented the clinical instructor with more diverse teaching opportunities. For example, if one student was caring for a patient with pneumonia who had crackles in his or her lungs, the instructor may have all the students listen to the patient's lung sounds, whereas another student may have a surgical patient where wound care could be completed. The clinical instructor could also choose to review the pathophysiology of the different diagnoses to which students were exposed during a single clinical day while at a clinical postconference. The variety of experiences offered by a rural facility allowed the clinical instructor to review a range of diagnoses and improve student understanding of various illnesses. Nurse managers indicated that students also benefited from an increased understanding of the role of the nurse generalist and the level of autonomy that is prevalent in rural hospitals.

Students and clinical instructors are not the only benefactors of the use of rural facilities for nursing education. Respondents indicated that patients also benefited from having students in the rural facility. Since rural facilities are often underused for nursing education, patients often comment on how much they enjoy the one-on-one attention they gain from having a student care for them.

The nurse managers stated that nursing staff were also given the opportunity to mentor students, provide leadership, and share experiences. The presence of students in the clinical setting may also prompt nurses to increase their standard of care as they strive to model evidence-based practices. One nurse manager commented that her nurses "really have to be on their toes and think about what they are doing" when working with students. She commented further that nurses in a rural facility do not get as much exposure to nursing students and faculty and that this is an excellent learning opportunity for the staff as well as the students.

Additionally, results indicated that administrators can use the students' exposure to rural facilities as a recruitment tool. Students often do not consider employment after graduation in a smaller facility, especially if they have never been exposed to the rural environment throughout their education. However, once exposed to the challenges and variety offered by a rural setting, students may seek employment opportunities after graduation. One administrator stated that their last three nurses hired had all been students at that rural facility during a clinical experience.

CHALLENGES

With all the benefits that correspond to the use of rural hospitals for clinical sites, there are also challenges to overcome. As noted by Newhouse (2005), smaller patient bases, along with a variety of acuity levels, are usually experienced in rural hospital clinical sites. This can result in the rise and fall of patient census. Our interviews with nurse mangers paralleled this challenge of a fluctuating census. Patient census was reported to vary from negligible to maximum census while accommodating nursing students. Utilization of a variety of nursing departments does allow facilities the capability of accommodating nursing students while experiencing a fluctuating census, in order to meet student and patient needs.

Constraints with space also presented nurse managers with accommodation barriers for nursing students. Conference rooms, as well as locker rooms, can be modestly available, with the demand for usage extending beyond the capacity of the rural hospitals, even without considering the addition of the nursing students. A desire to provide an environment conducive to learning in a postconference setting can take ingenuity. This ingenuity led to postconferences being held in break rooms and unused patient rooms if conference rooms were not available.

Nurse managers noted the challenge of maintaining communication between SDSU College of Nursing faculty and rural hospital staff. Visits by the semester coordinator helped display the commitment of the College of Nursing to collaborate with rural facilities. In addition, a predominant concern noted was the familiarity of the nurse faculty member with the rural hospital. It was evident that administrators needed to feel comfortable with the level of faculty knowledge about the rural hospital. Respondents reported that utilizing instructors from the facility increased comfort levels by assuring knowledge of the mission and vision of the facility, current policies and procedures, patient types, and staffing patterns.

Implications for Education and Research

The use of rural hospitals for clinical placement in nursing education is an effective way to provide quality clinical educational experiences to beginning nursing students, while relieving some of the clinical congestion from saturated urban settings. At SDSU, the use of rural hospitals has been expanded into the second semester for medical–surgical experience and has resulted in 8 to 10 fewer clinical groups in the larger urban setting each semester. Expanding clinical experiences into rural hospitals has enabled the nursing program to provide additional clinical placement sites as the nursing program increases its enrollment.

Providing clinical experiences in the rural setting enables nursing students to see the importance of the generalist role of the rural nurse and appreciate greater role diffusion. Nursing students are often surprised at the variety of learning opportunities and patient-care situations afforded them in the rural hospitals. This variety of experiences allows the nursing student to appreciate the role of the rural nurse and the flexibility required to care for such a broad range of patients. Nursing practice in a rural hospital requires a specific skill set and range of knowledge that has been described as broader and involving a higher level of responsibility in comparison to urban settings (Strasser & Neusy, 2010). Several of our students who begin their clinical experiences in a rural hospital request to return to a rural setting in their final semester for their preceptorship experience, citing the variety of experiences as the predominant reason for the request.

Increased awareness of the possibilities in rural health can also be promoted through other means. For example, in order to encourage educators to expand clinical education into rural areas, an "Academic Bush Camp" was designed and participants learned about rural health opportunities through experiential learning and workshops. Results indicated that the camp increased awareness of opportunities and has led to increased willingness to place students in a rural clinical experience (Page et al., 2016).

Implications for Practice

Involving nursing students in rural hospital clinical experiences provides an opportunity for rural hospitals to promote their facilities. Rural hospitals have historically struggled to recruit and retain caregivers, with rural nurse vacancy rates significantly higher than urban areas (Cramer, Nienaber, Helget, & Agrawal, 2006; Skillman, Hager, & Frogner, 2015). While many recruitment strategies have been tried, much of the research in this area suggests that exposure to rural hospitals for clinical placements is a major factor in recruitment of healthcare personnel to rural settings and that students often respond positively to their rural healthcare experiences. Research indicates that there are three primary factors associated with students choosing to practice in rural settings: having a rural background, positive clinical experiences in a rural setting, and targeted training for rural practice (Bigbee & Nixon, 2013; Skillman et al., 2015; Strasser & Neusy, 2010; Walters et al., 2016).

Providing rural clinical experiences for undergraduate nursing students has been promoted as a recruitment strategy for rural hospitals. Neill and Taylor (2002) reported that qualitative evaluation of rural clinical placement indicated a positive student response with increased interest in rural nursing following graduation. Other studies have resulted in recommendations for providing rural training and including rural content in the curriculum to improve recruitment and retention (Daniels, VanLiet, Skipper, Sanders, & Rhyne, 2007; Devine, 2006; Orda, Orda, Gupta, & Knight, 2017).

Thrall (2007) identified best practices for recruiting nurses into rural practice that include establishing links with area colleges to provide clinical education and possibly providing funding assistance for employees to attend nursing school in exchange for working at the hospital for a period of time following graduation. Rural hospitals can also develop nurse residency or internship programs for nursing students. These internship opportunities provide additional experiences in rural hospitals that are competing with urban centers that may have similar programs. In South Dakota, several rural administrators have approached the first semester coordinator at South Dakota Rural Health Association meetings to indicate their interest in providing clinical experiences for SDSU nursing students. While some of these rural facilities are located a significant distance from the main campus, it may be possible to consider an overnight or extended experience where students could be housed locally and minimize travel time.

Orda et al. (2017) established a rural internship accreditation program for medical interns. Training in remote geographical locations resulted in an improvement in rural staffing, which led to a decrease in the reliance on locum staffing. The rural training program was recognized as essential for successful recruitment and retention of providers interested in practice in remote areas.

The rural hospitals used for clinical experiences at SDSU have all reported a positive experience with nursing students completing clinical in their facilities. Clinical instructors have had similar positive experiences. While anecdotal data and clinical evaluations from students indicate a positive response to rural clinical placement, additional research is warranted to describe their perceptions of rural clinical experiences and the preparation these experiences provide for subsequent clinical rotations and eventual nursing practice.

CONCLUSION

Rural hospitals have traditionally not been selected as clinical placement sites for nursing education and are an untapped resource for nursing programs needing additional clinical resources. These facilities can provide a wide variety of opportunities for patient care and expose the nursing student to the wealth of experiences that rural healthcare provides. Results from the experiences at SDSU have been positive and should encourage the exploration of rural healthcare facilities for nursing clinical experiences.

REFERENCES

American Association of College of Nursing (2017). Fact sheet: Nursing shortage. Retrieved from http://www.aacnnursing.org/Portals/42/News/Factsheets/Nursing-Shortage-Factsheet-2017.pdf?ver=2017-10-18-144118-163

Bigbee, J., & Mixon, D. (2013). Recruitment and retention of rural nursing students: A retrospective study. *Remote and Rural Health, 13,* 2486. Retrieved from http://www.rrh.org.au/journal/article/2486

Cramer, M., Nienaber, J., Helget, P., & Agrawal, S. (2006). Comparative analysis of urban and rural nursing workforce shortages in Nebraska hospitals. *Policy, Politics, & Nursing Practice, 7*(4), 248–260. doi:10.1177/1527154406296481

Daniels, Z. M., VanLiet, B. J., Skipper, B. J., Sanders, M. L., & Rhyne, R. L. (2007). Factors in recruiting and retaining health professionals for rural practice. *Journal of Rural Health, 23*(1), 62–71. doi:10.1111/j.1748-0361.2006.00069.x

Devine, S. (2006). Perceptions of occupational therapists practicing in rural Australia: A graduate perspective. *Australian Occupational Health Journal, 53*(3), 205–210. doi:10.1111/j.1440-1630.2006.00561.x

Hendrickx, L. (2011, May). *Facing a shortage of clinical sites? Rural hospitals can meet your needs.* Paper presented at the Midwest Healthcare Educators' Academy, Grand Forks, ND.

Neill, J., & Taylor, K. (2002). Undergraduate nursing students' clinical experiences in rural and remote areas: Recruitment and retention. *Australian Journal of Rural Health, 10*(5), 239–243.

Newhouse, R. P. (2005). Exploring nursing issues in rural hospitals. *The Journal of Nursing Administration, 35*(7/8), 350–358.

Orda, U., Orda, S., Gupta, T., & Knight, S. (2017). Building a sustainable workforce in a rural and remote health service: A comprehensive and innovative rural generalist training approach. *Australian Journal of Rural Health, 25*, 116–119. doi:10.1111/ajr.12306

Page, A., Hamilton, S., Hall, M., Fitzgerald, K., Warner, W., Nattabi, B., & Thompson, S. (2016). Gaining a proper sense of what happens out there: An Academic Bush Camp to promote rural placements for students. *Australian Journal of Rural Health, 24*(1), 41–47. doi:10.1111/ajr.12199

Skillman, S., Hager, L., & Frogner, B. (2015, November). *Incentives for nurse practitioners and registered nurses to work in rural and safety net settings.* Retrieved from http://depts.washington.edu/fammed/chws/wp-content/uploads/sites/5/2016/03/CHWS_RTB159_Skillman.pdf

Strasser, R., & Neusy, A. (2010). Context counts: Training health workers in and for rural and remote areas. *Bulletin of the World Health Organization, 88*(10), 777–782. doi:10.2471./BLT.09.072462

Thrall, H. (2007). Best practices for recruiting rural nurses. *Hospitals & Health Networks, 81*(12), 47–50.

U.S. Department of Labor. (2017). Job outlook for registered nurses. Retrieved from http://www.bls.gov/ooh/healthcare/registered-nurses.htm

Walters, L., Seal, A., McGirr, J., Stewart, R., DeWitt, D., & Playford, D. (2016). Effect of medical student preference on rural clinical school experience and rural career intentions. *Rural and Remote Health, 16*, 3698. Retrieved from http://www.rrh.org.au/journal/article/3698

Chapter 26

Implications for Education, Practice, and Policy

Jean Shreffler-Grant and Marlene Reimer[1]

DISCUSSION QUESTIONS

- Discuss opportunities and experiences in nursing education programs that can best prepare graduates for rural practice.
- What are several current societal or secular trends that may affect rural health, rural nursing practice, and rural nursing theory?
- How can national, regional, or local health policies affect rural healthcare in a positive and less positive manner?

As an applied discipline, nursing has traditionally measured the relevance of theory by the extent to which it can inform practice, education, and healthcare policy. Our purpose in this chapter is to make more explicit the relevance of key elements of the rural theory base. We discuss selected educational, practice, and healthcare policy implications of the key concepts and theoretical statements as reported by Long and Weinert (1989) and Lee and McDonagh (2013). We explore how these implications may need to change as rural nursing theory is revised and extended. We also present exemplars from the United States, Canada, and Australia to illustrate how the key concepts and theoretical statements can inform education, practice, and healthcare policy that address rural populations and their health across international borders.

IMPLICATIONS OF THE FIRST THEORETICAL STATEMENT

How a group of citizens perceive health, manage their health, and seek healthcare has broad implications for education, practice, and policy that transcend national borders. The first theoretical statement is "Rural dwellers define health

---

[1] Deceased

primarily as the ability to work, to be productive, to do usual tasks" (Long & Weinert, 1989, p. 120). The interrelated concepts associated with this statement are work beliefs and health beliefs; health is defined in relation to work, and health needs are secondary to work needs.

Education

On the basis of the original rural nursing theory work, the first theoretical statement suggests that nursing programs should include the concept of role performance as health in curricula so that nurses include actual or potential effects of a health problem on the ability to work and to do usual tasks in their assessments and plans of care. Nursing educators should also offer opportunities for students to learn how clients' definitions of health influence their health and illness management behaviors.

Practice

In the practice arena, the first theoretical statement suggests that rural health services should be oriented, structured, and timed to fit with the rhythm of work and role performance. In addition, the benefits of preventive care may be better communicated by framing them according to what will assist rural dwellers to continue to work and do their usual tasks. Data from both Canada and the United States demonstrate the need to find new ways to approach preventive care among rural dwellers, based on trends in rural health indicators such as obesity, hypertension, smoking, lack of regular healthcare visits, and growing rates of suicide and substance use disorders (Medline Plus, 2017; Pong, Desmeules, & Lagace, 2009; Rural Health Information Hub, 2017).

Policy

Policy implications of the original work include establishing funding mechanisms whereby health services can be offered near where people work that are scheduled around the cycle of rural work. Rural residents may not seek timely health services if work must be delayed or disrupted to seek care (Sellers, Poduska, Propp, & White, 1999).

The original theory development work on definitions of health, as well as beliefs about work and health, was conducted in the United States. Research participants were principally Caucasian rural dwellers, the majority population in the Rocky Mountain and High Plains area in which this work was conducted (89.2% of the current Montana population is Caucasian; U.S. Census Bureau, 2017). The original work was not intended to characterize these concepts for American Indians, the primary minority population in the same rural areas (6.6% of the Montana population, U.S. Census Bureau, 2017). Canadian research on health beliefs of rural dwellers, as reported by Winters et al. (2013), was also drawn primarily from Caucasians living in the western part of the country. Further research is warranted to explore how Native American and Aboriginal people living in rural areas define health and how their conception of health is the same as or different from the dominant population. In any case, it is unlikely that one definition of health or one set of health beliefs would emerge that would characterize health beliefs among different Aboriginal communities or tribes, any more than it is likely that one definition would be true for Caucasian groups of different cultures.

As discussed by Lee and McDonagh (2013), rural dwellers' views of health may now be more diverse across different geographical areas, age and ethnic groups, and occupations than when the original theory development work began; so it may require a reconceptualization of definitions of health, work beliefs, and health beliefs. Of particular note are the subpopulations among rural dwellers.

Discussion

Martin (1997) pointed out that farming and ranching are now experienced more as a lifestyle than as an occupation, thus calling for different approaches to affect behavioral change beyond simply appealing to individuals' motivations to continue working. Blank (1999) also referred to traditional farming and ranching as a current lifestyle choice. Since many other forms of rural living are available to Americans besides farming and ranching, and also since most food and commodity crops are now produced on large industrial farms, Blank postulated that the American family farm is a lifestyle that many Americans can no longer afford. Another example of a potential need to reframe rural dwellers' definitions of health can be found within rural subpopulations where unemployment has now persisted for multiple generations. Defining health based on the ability to work may not be relevant for those who have never had regular work (Long, 1993). Some rural areas are now more racially and ethnically diverse than in the past. Culturally based beliefs about what it means to be healthy are likely to result in different definitions of health among racial and ethnic groups. Migration of urban residents to rural areas has resulted in a subpopulation of exurban rural dwellers who bring their urban values and expectations about health and healthcare with them (Troughton, 1999). The "graying" of rural areas is well documented in the literature, as people age in place and younger people migrate out for employment and other opportunities (McLaughlin & Jensen, 1998; Ricketts, Johnson-Webb, & Randolph, 1999). With improved healthcare and healthier lifestyles, people are living many more years postretirement than they once did. How health is defined among this rural population may well have nothing to do with what we traditionally think of as work, but instead may be more consistent with the concept of health as role performance or ability to do usual tasks. Healthy elders may define health as the ability to actively participate in leisure, voluntary activities, and travel. Elders in poor health may define health as nothing more than the ability to complete their activities of daily living. Further research and exploration is warranted to refine the definitions of health for these multiple rural subpopulations.

IMPLICATIONS OF THE SECOND THEORETICAL STATEMENT

The second theoretical statement is "Rural dwellers are self-reliant and resist accepting help or services from those seen as 'outsiders' or from agencies seen as national or regional 'welfare' programs" (Long & Weinert, 1989, p. 120). Related key concepts are self-reliance, outsider, insider, old-timer, and newcomer.

Education

The second theoretical statement underlines the importance of a participative, community development approach in which rural dwellers identify and design health initiatives to fit with their own needs and resources. This approach is consistent with the second theoretical statement as originally conceptualized, as well as with the proposed newer subtheme of symptom–action–timeline (SATL) and the new concept involving choices discussed by Lee and McDonagh (2013). The importance of working in partnership with rural dwellers and communities is an essential content for nursing curricula so that graduates can and will apply the principles of community development and participatory action in rural practice. Skills essential for partnership development and maintenance should also be included in nursing curricula. As a middle-range theory of rural health-seeking behavior evolves, students and scholars should derive and validate the theory in partnership with rural residents themselves so that it is consistent with their local needs and beliefs.

Practice

Goeppinger (1993) advocated partnership as a core intervention strategy in health promotion with rural populations at both individual and aggregate levels. Considering the rural tendency to "make do" and what Weissert, Knott, and Stieber (1994) referred to as the "asymmetry of information between citizens and health professionals . . . about what constitutes good care" (p. 366) in traditional care models, empirical testing of the partnership model in promoting the health of rural residents is needed. A Canadian example of a tool to support participative community development for rural citizens is a workbook that was tested in Manitoba, Canada (Ryan-Nicholls, 2004). The workbook was designed to help rural citizens assess the health of their communities and identify goals and strategies to improve the sustainability of rural communities. In the United States, Findholt (2004) studied how rurality influenced community participation in health promotion initiatives. She found that having a structured process for the initiative appeared to compensate for some of the resource and experiential limitations in rural communities. Communities, for example, that had limited experience and success with previous planning efforts, were not hindered in their current efforts because they had structured support and resources from a state-level office of rural health.

Policy

The question of what healthcare resources are necessary and sufficient in rural and remote areas, given the distance to other sources of care, continues as a focus of debate and policy shifts for which evidence for decision making is scarce. The major constraint is the lack of sufficient population to justify a full mix of acute care, long-term care, and supported residential and home care services (Keyzer, 1995). In a study of home care resources for rural families with cancer, Buehler and Lee (1992) found that the more rural the family, the more limited and inadequate the formal resources available to assist them. These investigators also found that the longer the dying trajectory and the greater the deterioration of the person's health, the more resources became inadequate and the greater became the burden to the caregiver. These findings illustrate one of many policy questions that have emerged: the relationship between length of illness and sustainability of resources through the trajectory of illness in rural versus urban environments. It would seem that a mix of formal and informal resources and the resiliency of each to prolonged illness vary, but few studies have systematically addressed this phenomenon.

The Australian Rural Health Strategy adopted in 1994 (Keyzer, 1995) called for "relocation of resources away from services based on existing facilities towards services based on expressed demand" (p. 28). The strategy included changes that would shift power bases from traditional rural primary and hospital care delivery to a system that relied much more on nurse practitioners and interdisciplinary collaboration. More than two decades later, however, tension still exists in Australia and elsewhere between the economic arguments for downsizing and closure of rural facilities versus advocacy for aging in place, new life-saving treatments that require pretransfer interventions at local healthcare facilities, and other new technologies such as telehealth that minimize the need for travel to urban locations for healthcare (Bolin, et al., 2015; Mueller, 2001; National Rural Health Association, 2017a; Ricketts, 2000).

In the United States, the critical access hospital (CAH) has gained broad support as an alternative to closure of local rural hospitals and has been implemented in rural areas across the nation. CAHs must be located in remote areas and are limited to short-stay lower-intensity services in exchange for more flexibility in staffing and other licensure requirements and more favorable Medicare reimbursement as compared with traditional rural hospitals. The underlying goal is to shift the facility's emphasis from inpatient and surgical services to emergency, outpatient, primary, and long-term care, which are services that may be more sustainable in remote rural areas because they better match the needs of area residents (Shreffler, Capalbo, Flaherty, & Heggem, 1999). One of the prototypes for this national model of care was a grassroots effort initiated by a partnership of rural citizens and legislators in a remote rural area in Montana. There are currently 48 CAHs in Montana and 1,339 CAHs nationwide (Flex Monitoring Team, 2017).

Reform of national health policy in the United States and elsewhere greatly affects the health-seeking behaviors of rural dwellers. In the United States, the Patient Protection and Affordable Care Act (ACA), also referred to as "Obamacare," was passed into law in 2010 and remained highly controversial. Congressional efforts are currently underway to repeal and replace it. How rural dwellers will fare when the federal replacement legislation is finalized is unknown at this time. Despite the contentious features of the ACA, many leaders agreed that its provisions benefited or had the potential to benefit rural consumers and the rural healthcare system (Avery, Finegold, & Xiao, 2016; Hofer, Abraham, & Moscovice, 2011; Newkirk & Damico, 2014). American rural dwellers are much more likely to be uninsured or underinsured than urban dwellers, which limits their access to health insurance and healthcare services. The intent of the ACA was to require insurance coverage for all and to reduce the cost of insurance through purchasing networks, which was seen as advantageous for self-employed or underemployed individuals. The ACA guaranteed renewability of coverage and prohibited preexisting condition exclusions. There were also provisions that addressed the workforce shortage crisis in rural areas and eliminated some payment inequities for rural providers. As national efforts to replace the ACA proceed, rural advocates are voicing their opinions about aspects of the substitute legislation that would disadvantage rural dwellers (Greenwood-Erickson & Abir, 2017; National Rural Health Association, 2017b; Roubein, 2017).

IMPLICATIONS OF THE THIRD THEORETICAL STATEMENT

Finally, the third theoretical statement is "Health care providers in rural areas must deal with a lack of anonymity and much greater role diffusion than providers in urban or suburban settings" (Long & Weinert, 1989, p. 120). A related theme mentioned by Long and Weinert that characterizes rural nursing is "a sense of isolation from professional peers" (p. 120).

Education

Implicit in the third theoretical statement is that students planning or potentially interested in rural practice should be given opportunities to develop skills to function in a generalist role or what McLeod, Browne, and Leipert

(1998) referred to as a multispecialist role that is characteristic of rural nursing practice. Offering undergraduate students a rural elective experience is one such strategy, particularly when it not only involves placement in a rural site but also seminars on rural health and practice issues. Students with an interest in rural practice should have opportunities to develop strategies to cope with or overcome practice isolation, such as skill development in the use of mentors, consultants, and telehealth applications. Through full engagement with their communities, nurses who are newcomers in rural areas may begin to appreciate the familiarity of life in a rural community and gradually may be seen as insiders rather than outsiders, which may mitigate the negative aspects of lack of anonymity and practice isolation. Some nurses, of course, are already insiders, having come from the particular community. The sense of practice isolation may be less acute for them, but the practical issues of limited access to educational opportunities and ready consultation are nevertheless present to varying degrees.

Practice and Policy

Lack of anonymity, role diffusion, and practice isolation may contribute to recruitment difficulties and high turnover of rural healthcare professionals and result in shortages of providers in rural practice settings. Here too, policymakers can look to innovative approaches and exchange of best practices. For example, the Rural Physician Action Plan in Alberta recognized that (a) medical students from rural areas were more likely to go into rural practice, but (b) rural applicants were often disadvantaged in the interview and the selection processes for medical school because of lack of sophistication in interviewing and preparation of materials (Health Workforce for Alberta, 2017; I. Pfeiffer, personal communication, March 4, 2004). An experienced recruiter was hired to help rural applicants prepare for admission interviews. Thus, they went to a root cause with what appear to be positive results.

Stewart et al. (2011) conducted a study to identify factors that predicted intent to leave practice positions among RNs in rural and remote settings in Canada. The investigators found that some predictors were amenable to interventions that may prevent turnover among rural nurses. Workplace and community predictors relevant to the third relational statement are lower local community satisfaction, higher perceived workplace stress, lower satisfaction with autonomy in the workplace, lower satisfaction with workplace scheduling, and a desire to seek further education. Also, being a "newcomer" to the rural practice setting and community was a significant predictor of intent to leave.

An innovative strategy for addressing shortages of nurses and other healthcare providers in rural areas can be seen in the growth of educational outreach efforts via distance-learning technology to rural areas. Rural residents or insiders who are more likely to select rural practice upon graduation can access all or part of educational programs without leaving their rural communities for significant periods of time. Another successful approach for recruitment of health professionals in rural areas has been educational scholarships for rural residents or "grow your own" programs (Hagopian, Johnson, Fordyce, Blades, & Hart, 2003).

CONCLUSION

The radical changes necessary to shift education, practice, and policy for rural health require a strong theory base and depth of understanding of rural health and practice that can emanate only through experience and research. Those who focus on rural health are used to thinking in terms of local contextual factors and the unique nature of a single rural area, region, or nation. Through engagement in cross-border collaborative research and scholarly work on rural nursing theory, we and our respective teams have deepened our understanding of the extent to which larger issues of healthcare reform are also shifting. At the end of the day, the relevance of rural nursing theory and concepts as described in this book will likely be measured by its ability to evolve and change as new knowledge shapes it and its ability to positively influence education, practice, and healthcare policy—and thereby improve the health of rural citizens on both sides of the border.

REFERENCES

Avery, K., Finegold, K., & Xiao, X. (2016). *ASPE issue brief: Impact of the Affordable Care Act coverage expansion on rural and urban populations.* Washington, DC: Department of Health and Human Services. Retrieved from https://aspe.hhs.gov/system/files/pdf/204986/ACARuralbrief.pdf

Blank, S. C. (1999). The end of the American farm. *The Futurist*, 33(4), 22. Retrieved from https://www.questia.com/magazine/1G1-54349265/the-end-of-the-american-farm

Bolin, J. N., Bellamy, G. R., Ferdinand, A. O., Vuong, A. M., Kash, B. A., Schulze, A., & Helduser, J. W. (2015). Rural Healthy People 2020: New decade, same challenges. *The Journal of Rural Health*, 31(3), 326–333. doi:10.1111/jrh.12116

Buehler, J. A., & Lee, H. J. (1992). Exploration of home care resources for rural families with cancer. *Cancer Nursing*, 15, 299–308. doi:10.1097/00002820-199215040-00008

Findholt, N. (2004). *The influence of rurality on community participation in a community health development initiative* (Unpublished doctoral dissertation). Oregon Health & Science University, Portland.

Flex Monitoring Team. (2017). Critical access hospital locations. Retrieved from http://www.flexmonitoring.org/data/critical-access-hospital-locations

Goeppinger, J. (1993). Health promotion for rural populations: Partnership interventions. *Family and Community Health*, 16(1), 1–10. doi:10.1097/00003727-199304000-00004

Greenwood-Erickson, M., & Abir, M. (2017, January 22). Rural America could be hardest hit by repeal of Obamacare. *Newsweek*. Retrieved from http://www.newsweek.com/rural-america-hardest-hit-repeal-obamacare-544813

Hagopian, A., Johnson, K., Fordyce, M., Blades, S., & Hart, L. G. (2003). Health workforce recruitment and retention in critical access hospitals. *CAH/FLEX National Tracking Project*, 3(5). Retrieved from http://www.unmc.edu/ruprihealth/programs/results/vol3num5.pdf

Health Workforce for Alberta. (2017). About health workforce for Alberta. Retrieved from http://www.rpap.ab.ca

Hofer, A. N., Abraham, J. M., & Moscovice, I. (2011). Expansion of coverage under the Patient Protection and Affordable Care Act and primary care utilization. *Milbank Quarterly*, 89(1), 69–89. doi:10.1111/j.1468-0009.2011.00620.x

Keyzer, D. M. (1995). Health policy and rural nurses: A time for reflection. *Collegian*, 2(1), 28–35.

Lee, H. J., & McDonagh, M. K. (2013). Updating the rural nursing base. In C. A. Winters (Ed.), *Rural nursing: Concepts, theory, and practice* (4th ed., pp. 15–33). New York, NY: Springer Publishing.

Long, K. A. (1993). The concept of health: Rural perspectives. *Nursing Clinics of North America*, 28(1), 123–130.

Long, K. A., & Weinert, C. (1989). Rural nursing: Developing the theory base. *Scholarly Inquiry for Nursing Practice: An International Journal*, 3, 113–127.

Martin, S. R. (1997). Agricultural safety and health: Principles and possibilities for nursing education. *Journal of Nursing Education*, 36(2), 74–78.

McLaughlin, D. K., & Jensen, L. (1998). The rural elderly: A demographic portrait. In R. T. Coward & J. A. Krout (Eds.), *Aging in rural settings: Life circumstances & distinctive features* (pp. 15–43). New York, NY: Springer Publishing.

McLeod, M., Browne, A. J., & Leipert, B. (1998). Issues for nurses in rural and remote Canada. *Australian Journal of Rural Health*, 6, 72–78. doi:10.1111/j.1440-1584.1998.tb00287.x

Medline Plus. (2017). Rural health concerns. Retrieved from https://medlineplus.gov/ruralhealthconcerns.html

Mueller, K. J. (2001). Rural health policy: Past as prelude to the future. In S. Loue & B. E. Quill (Eds.), *Handbook of rural health* (pp. 1–23). New York, NY: Kluwer Academic/Plenum.

National Rural Health Association. (2017a). About rural health care. Retrieved from https://www.ruralhealthweb.org/about-nrha/about-rural-health-care

National Rural Health Association. (2017b). *Vote NO to the American Health Care Act*. Retrieved from https://www.ruralhealthweb.org/NRHA/media/Emerge_NRHA/GA/2017-Vote-No-American-Health-Care-Act.pdf

Newkirk, V., & Damico, A. (2014). The Affordable Care Act and insurance coverage in rural areas. *Kaiser Family Foundation*. Retrieved from http://kff.org/uninsured/issue-brief/the-affordable-care-act-and-insurance-coverage-in-rural-areas

Pong, R. W., Desmeules, M., & Lagace, C. (2009). Rural–urban disparities in health: How does Canada fare and how does Canada compare to Australia? *Australian Journal of Rural Health*, 17(1), 58–64. doi:10.1111/j.1440-1584.2008.01039.x

Ricketts, T. C. (2000). The changing nature of rural health care. *Annual Review of Public Health*, 21, 639–657. doi:10.1146/annurev.publhealth.21.1.639

Ricketts, T. C., Johnson-Webb, K. D., & Randolph, R. K. (1999). Populations and places in rural America. In T. C. Ricketts (Ed.), *Rural health in the United States* (pp. 7–24). New York, NY: Oxford University Press.

Roubein, R. (2017, April 18). Groups warn of rural health "crisis" under Obamacare repeal. *The Hill Extra.* Retrieved from http://thehill.com/policy/healthcare/329546-groups-warn-of-rural-health-crisis-under-obamacare-repeal

Rural Health Information Hub. (2017). Rural health disparities. Retrieved from https://www.ruralhealthinfo.org/topics/rural-health-disparities

Ryan-Nicholls, K. (2004). Rural Canadian community health and quality of life: Testing of a workbook to determine priorities and move to action (Preliminary Report). *Rural and Remote Health,* 4(278), 1–10. Retrieved from http://www.rrh.org.au/articles/subviewnew.asp?ArticleID=278

Sellers, S. C., Poduska, M. D., Propp, L. H., & White, S. I. (1999). The health care meanings, values, and practices of Anglo-American males in the rural Midwest. *Journal of Transcultural Nursing,* 10, 320–330. doi:10.1177/104365969901000410

Shreffler, M. J., Capalbo, S. M., Flaherty, R. J., & Heggem, C. (1999). Community decision-making about Critical Access Hospitals: Lessons learned from Montana's Medical Assistance Facility program. *The Journal of Rural Health,* 15(2), 180–188. doi:10.1111/j.1748-0361.1999.tb00738.x

Stewart, N. J., D'Arcy, C., Kosteniuk, J., Andrews, M. E., Morgan, D., Forbes, D., . . . Pitblado, J. R. (2011). Moving on? Predictors of intent to leave among rural and remote RNs in Canada. *The Journal of Rural Health,* 27(1), 103–113. doi:10.1111/j.1748-0361.2010.00308.x

Troughton, M. J. (1999). Redefining "rural" for the twenty-first century. In W. Rampy, J. Kulig, I. Townshend, & V. McGowan (Eds.), *Health in rural settings: Contexts for action* (pp. 21–38). Lethbridge, AB, Canada: University of Lethbridge.

U.S. Census Bureau. (2017). Welcome to quick facts Montana. Retrieved from https://www.census.gov/quickfacts/map/INC110213/30/accessible

Weissert, C. S., Knott, J. H., & Stieber, B. E. (1994). Education and the health professions: Explaining policy choices among the states. *Journal of Health Politics, Policy and Law,* 19, 361–392. doi:10.1215/03616878-19-2-361

Winters, C. A., Thomlinson, E. H., O'Lynn, C., Lee, H. J., McDonagh, M. M., Edge, D., Reimer, M. (2013). Exploring rural nursing theory across borders. In C. Winters (Ed.). *Rural nursing: Concepts, theory, and practice* (4th ed., pp. 35–47). New York, NY: Springer Publishing.

CHAPTER 27

Developing and Sustaining the Rural Nursing Workforce Through Collaborative Educational Models

Polly Petersen, Dayle Boynton Sharp, and Judith M. Paré

DISCUSSION TOPICS

- The main character presented in Case Study 1 is Susan. Susan is torn between the challenges and opportunities of rural nursing practice. Describe at least three strategies that Susan's nurse manager could implement to support her desire for broader clinical experiences while continuing employment in a rural healthcare setting.
- Case Study 2 summarizes the story of Mary, a nurse who had an opportunity to attend a specialty education program in an urban healthcare setting. Discuss the role of nursing administrators in rural and urban settings to advocate and fund these types of residency programs. Do they have a professional obligation to support these programs? What are the benefits and potential challenges? Utilize evidence from the literature to support your views.
- Case Study 4 highlights one federal program that provides funding for nurses who are motivated to enroll in an advanced nursing education program. Select a federal or state program that offers resources for nurses in your area to earn an advanced degree while continuing to practice in a rural healthcare setting. Describe the benefits and limitations of the program in detail.

Rural nursing varies greatly based upon geography and cultural values; however, the attitudes and attributes of rural nurses remain constant. Many registered nurses (RNs) have grown up in the area with family ties that result in their decision to stay and work in rural areas. However, there is a shortage of RNs in these healthcare settings. In the United States, the number of RNs per capita has remained lower in rural areas compared to urban areas from 1980 to present (Skillman, Palazzo, Hart, & Butterfield, 2007; Spring Arbor University, 2017). This distributional imbalance of RNs extends past the United States to throughout the world, with one-half the world's population living in rural settings and only 38% of the total nursing workforce working in rural areas (Dolea, Stormont, & Braichet, 2010). This imbalance is not expected to improve. As baby boomers age, it is estimated that 40% of the current workforce will retire, resulting in the nursing shortage to increase to 1 million RNs by 2020 (Juraschek, Zhang, Ranganathan, & Lin, 2010).

Reasons for shortages in rural settings include lack of educational opportunities and resources, lack of diversity, social support and cultural congruency, policies that are inconsistent to support rural healthcare, and feelings of isolation. Collaborative initiatives in education and institutional support can enhance the professional characteristics of rural nurses. This chapter utilizes case studies to illustrate strategies to build capacity while offering ideas for collaborative educational models that address recruitment, retention, and workforce development of rural nursing.

CASE STUDIES

CASE 1

Susan wanted to be a nurse since she could remember. Growing up on a large cattle ranch in eastern Idaho, she had learned at an early age to care for orphaned lambs, and how to "pull a calf." Susan excelled in science courses in school and was accepted for early admission to the associate degree of nursing program at her local community college, which had the only nursing program within a 150-mile radius. Susan's mother wished that her daughter could have enrolled in the nursing program at the state university but the cost of the program and the distance from the ranch was too great. Susan is very close to her family and she is very proud of her contributions to the family ranch that has been the primary source of income for generations.

Susan just completed her second year as an RN in the critical access hospital (CAH) in her community and she is beginning to wonder about job opportunities that have been posted in the medical center 155 miles away. Her ultimate goal of attaining certification as an emergency department (ED) nurse has yet to be realized. She had registered for a certification conference twice but due to weather and cuts to the educational budget, she was unable to attend either

(continued)

(continued)

conference event. She is frustrated by the lack of a professional career ladder and support for nurses who want to participate in continuing education and pursue advanced degrees but simply do not have the time or funding resources. Susan is grateful for all her parents have done to support her education and her nursing practice but she is torn between a desire to expand her clinical experiences and her obligations to her family and their ranch.

Susan is particularly interested in broadening her experiences with advanced technology to support the needs of trauma patients. She worries about her limited experience working with patients who have multisystem needs and she is frustrated by the lack of resources the CAH has to offer. Susan commented to her mother one evening after an unplanned 16-hour shift, "Nursing is a part of who I am but, I am beginning to wonder if who I am is all that I can be?"

Case 2

Mary grew up in a small town in central Nebraska. She had an opportunity in the middle school to participate in a program that allowed her to volunteer at the local CAH one evening each week. As she spent time feeding Mr. Jones, a patient recovering from a stroke in the long-term care unit, she had a chance to watch the nurses and doctors at the main care station. They were smart and compassionate and she knew she wanted to do exactly what they did.

She finished an associate's degree program at a community college, passed her NCLEX, and returned to her hometown to marry her high-school sweetheart. Working the night shift in the CAH that included a 20-bed long-term care unit and a 2-bed ED, she spent most of her time assisting the aides in turning patients, assisting others to the bathroom, and passing medications. Although she enjoyed the camaraderie of the team of aides with whom she worked, she also felt overwhelmed to think that if there was an emergency, she alone would be responsible for the life of that patient until support came in to assist. This feeling of doom weighed on her, knowing she did not have the experience or education to handle such a situation. Mary chose to attend a 6-week critical care course offered in a large hospital 200 miles away. Mary loved the course; she worked with patients utilizing the knowledge she gained in the classroom setting and felt supported by the staff. She saw patients who were critically ill get better and return to a full life after discharge. She knew she could never go back to the rural CAH setting

(continued)

(continued)

again; she could never transition the care she gave the patients in the critical care course without the team she had come to rely on for that care. Mary left the CAH after returning from the critical care course to work in a big city ICU.

CASE 3

Lucia lives in a rural area of Texas where her family migrated from Mexico so that her parents could work in the cotton fields. Her father had planned to move the family back to Mexico; however, he wanted to offer his children opportunities that were not available in their native country. Lucia has always had an interest in taking care of others. This came naturally to her, as she has been caring for family members since she was a child. She is the oldest and the first in her family to advance her education past the sixth grade. Because of her interest in caring for others, her school guidance counselor suggested that she participate in the Health Occupation Students of America (HOSA) program at her high school. In the HOSA program, she has been able to learn about nursing both in class and at a local clinic. She is excited about being in the HOSA program because when she graduates from high school, she will be a certified nursing assistant.

She is excited about working as a nursing assistant but wants to continue her education to become a nurse. She wants to talk to her parents about attending nursing school but does not know how they will pay the tuition or how she will travel to the university. Before she is able to talk with her parents, she receives an acceptance letter from the community college 45 miles from her home. She had applied to the nursing program with the encouragement of her school counselor. Lucia also applied for multiple scholarships and was excited to receive a scholarship due to her enrollment in HOSA. With this scholarship, Lucia will be able to start her dream of attending college and someday attaining her bachelor's degree in nursing.

CASE 4

Glenn has been an RN for over 20 years, working in the ED in a small CAH in rural New Hampshire (NH). He has become disheartened with the limited healthcare access to his community. He has been caring for individuals who have advanced stages of chronic disease due to lack of follow-up care. Thus, Glenn has begun to investigate options for advancing his education to become a nurse practitioner so that he can

(continued)

(*continued*)

become a primary care provider for his rural neighbors. The nearest graduate program is over 100 miles away. However, he is excited to learn that it is an online program, allowing him to attend graduate school with limited trips to campus.

He contacted his local Area Health Education Center (AHEC), which assists placing students in rural practicums. He learned that they have a current program that will assist him in finding preceptors near his home and find scholarship to help him pay for his tuition. The program is Live, Learn, and Play in Northern NH (North Country Health Consortium, 2017).

CASE 5

Margie is the most senior member of the rural nursing staff in the CAH in northern California. Margie is old enough to retire but financially unable to do so. Four years ago, Margie's husband died suddenly after suffering a major stroke on the ranch where he had worked for more than 40 years. Margie's daughter lives in the same community but her single-parent income often is not enough to pay monthly bills. Margie's salary is now her only income. She often works additional shifts to support the needs of her daughter and grandchildren.

She just celebrated her 43rd anniversary in nursing practice and is proud she has spent her entire career in a CAH but she worries about who will be there to take over her position. She had not met any new nurses in this "new generation" of nurses who have the same attitudes and values that she had that supported a career such as hers.

RURAL NURSING WORKFORCE

Rural and frontier settings have unique characteristics. There are long distances from town to town and from farm to farm. Members of the population have lived there for many generations and know their neighbor's lineage as well as they know their own. In fact, it may often be a shared lineage. When one of them becomes ill, they generally seek care at the local CAH. However, CAHs are in a precarious situation with potential decreases in funding related to healthcare reforms in reimbursement (Balasubramanian & Jones, 2016), fiscal instability, as well as RN and other healthcare provider shortages to care for patients. Reasons for this shortage include the aging RN population and the inability to recruit new graduates. Ninety-one percent of CEOs from one midwestern state reported a critical RN shortage (Cramer, Jones, & Hertzog, 2011) as well as indications that 74% of rural CEOs reported a 73% shortage of RNs

(MacDowell, Glasser, Fitts, Nielsen, & Hunsaker, 2010). The rural RN shortage has skyrocketed compared to urban areas with 52% of frontier counties in the United States reporting a critical shortage compared to 30% of nonfrontier counties (Frontier Education Center, 2004). When geographical regions experience RN shortages, hospitals often decrease RN staffing patterns utilizing licensed practical nurses (LPNs) or temporary RN employees who are not familiar with the area, resulting in a simultaneous drop in patient satisfaction (Cramer, Jones, & Hertzog, 2011).

The average age for practicing RNs in the United States in 2013 was 50 years with 53% of the workforce over the age of 50 years (American Nurses Association, 2014). In 2010, the average age of practicing nurses was close to 55 years; 30% of rural RNs were over the age of 55 years (Gale, 2010). Many of these nurses have been clinically engaged in their profession for more than three decades, demonstrating resiliency and adaptation to enormous changes in healthcare delivery. The total years of experience that these retiring RNs will take with them is estimated to be 1.7 million years (Buerhaus, Auerbach, & Staiger, 2017). This loss of expert, older nurses can potentially compromise quality of care and the assurance of a safe patient and staff environment.

Chief nursing officers (CNOs) from rural hospitals have expressed alarm at the growing trend for nurses to travel from their rural homes to work in metropolitan hospitals, also contributing to the RN shortage in CAHs. These urban facilities offer higher salaries and tuition benefits, the option to be trained in various specialty areas, and promotions that are congruent with levels of education (Havens, Warshawsky, & Vasey, 2012). CNOs in rural settings must create practice environments that support the recruitment and retention of highly qualified RNs resulting in a qualified healthcare workforce that contributes to high patient satisfaction scores.

IMPLICATIONS

These case studies bring to the forefront areas that should be addressed related to educational support from CAHs and other rural healthcare facilities. Programs that provide RNs with knowledge to deliver current, evidence-based care, and tuition support for increasing degree levels such as a BSN as well as advanced education and degrees to move into a primary care provider role are needed. Opportunities for team-based healthcare development, including interprofessional education (IPE) in rural settings, and financial and professional support for diverse populations who are willing to remain in rural facilities to care for family and friends of their own community are also important options for consideration.

For there to be a sufficient number of nurses to care for the rural population, recruitment and retention issues must be addressed. Kulig, Kilpatrick, Moffitt, and Zimmer (2010), in a recent review, identified three categories that address recruitment and retention of the RN workforce for rural and frontier settings: educational opportunities, financial incentives, and enhanced infrastructure.

Educational Opportunities

The literature indicated that one potential solution to address the inability to recruit new RNs to the rural setting is to provide a rural clinical experience within nursing education programs. This model could be supported through a collaboration between state universities and community colleges in rural areas and beyond. These types of programs allow nursing students to have the opportunity to work with students from other healthcare educational programs including medicine, pharmacy, and physical and occupational therapy in rural situations. Application of the Interprofessional Care Access Network (I-CAN) model has shown great promise in strengthening the ability of healthcare students to practice in a collaborative fashion as well as address the needs of populations with limited access to care (Wros, Mathews, & Voss, 2015).

Another resource for IPE is the utilization of healthcare professionals within the rural settings as instructors and mentors. The positive influence of students learning from providers but also providers learning from students enhances collaborative interactions (Pelham, Skinner, McHugh, & Pullon, 2016). Financial incentives for interprofessional experiences may be offered through some governmental agencies. Examples of agency and program support across the country that provide financial and educational support for potential healthcare professionals and CAH staff, include AHEC, HOSA, and Live, Learn and Play in Northern NH.

AREA HEALTH EDUCATION CENTER

AHEC is committed to expanding healthcare providers in rural and underserved areas. Through the introduction of a wide variety of healthcare possibilities, it guides students toward careers in the healthcare field, assisting them with goal setting, educational planning, and critical thinking skills. AHEC works with schools, colleges, and community partners in such programs as "Grow Their Own," to offer culturally appropriate clinical experiences to underrepresented minority students in kindergarten through 12th grade. Working with over 1,000 community health centers, students are exposed to shadowing experiences, mentoring, recruitment, resources, and continuing education (National Area Health Education Center Organization, 2015).

AHEC continues supporting nurses once they are in practice. AHEC works with local hospitals and supports nurses, offering continuing education classes online and in classroom settings. Online courses allow the rural RN to obtain necessary training without having to travel long distances (National Area Health Education Center Organization, 2015). Many courses are offered including Advanced Cardiac Life Support (ACLS), Basic Life Support (BLS), and Pediatric Advanced Life Support (PALS). Face-to-face training can be done at the CAH, other community locations, or a training stimulation van traveling to the nurses.

HEALTH OCCUPATION STUDENTS OF AMERICA

The HOSA program is a student organization recognized by the U.S. Department of Education (HOSA, Inc., 2017). The goal of HOSA is to enhance the delivery of compassionate, quality healthcare by providing opportunities to health science education to students. With the support of health occupation educators as advisors, students develop the knowledge, skills, and leadership to meet the needs of their healthcare community. Since its development, there are over 4,000 HOSA chapters and nearly 180,000 students have participated in HOSA. Along with new skills and experiences, HOSA members are also eligible for additional scholarship opportunities.

LIVE, LEARN, AND PLAY IN NORTHERN NH

Like many rural settings, the North Country of NH is medically underserved. Northern NH has relatively high poverty due to industrial declines. Residents travel long distances for healthcare, especially challenging for older populations with chronic health issues. To address these issues, the North Country Health Consortium (2017) and Northern NH AHEC developed the Live, Learn, and Play in Northern NH. The Northern NH AHEC/North Country Health Consortium assists students with clinical placements through developed partnerships throughout the region including hospitals and community health centers, giving the students a meaningful experience while working on community service projects. Additionally, students are offered a stipend to assist them with costs during their clinical experience.

These are just a few examples of agency educational and financial support and recruitment initiatives of students into healthcare. Many opportunities are not limited to those interested in careers in nursing, but to all healthcare professions. These opportunities also introduce the concept of IPE and team building early in development.

Financial Incentives

While much emphasis could be placed on the wage differences for rural RNs compared to those practicing in urban settings, our focus for financial incentives is on the commitment of CAHs to the RNs to maintain certifications and other educational obligations. Travel presents additional financial burden for rural healthcare providers to maintain these mandated certifications for continued accreditation as well as opportunities for continued education and degree completion. This financial burden of advancing education can be decreased through the use of online courses or offering courses via video conferencing. Likewise, it is of value for CAH facilities to consider financial support of tuition reimbursement or consistent Internet service as individual reliability of Internet services may be a barrier for many rural residents.

The National Rural Health Association (NRHA) advocates for access to quality healthcare for rural residents and CAHs. NRHA has developed initiatives to stop Medicare cuts to rural hospitals and offer innovative delivery models for rural healthcare (NRHA, 2017). The association supports continued funding for professional training such as Teaching Health Center and Rural Track training programs. In addition, NRHA advocates for continued funding to the National Health Service Corps (NHSC), Community Health Center Fund, and annual healthcare policy and fellowship programs.

Collaborative educational and financial support of those interested in rural healthcare professions also includes federal government agencies. Two federal agencies that remain committed to the development of enhancing rural workforce are Health Resources and Services Administration (HRSA) and the NHSC. HRSA offers scholarships to students accepted and enrolled in all levels of nursing education (HRSA Health Workforce, 2017). Students have the potential to receive funding for tuition, fees, and other educational costs. In exchange, the student must work in a facility with a critical nurse shortage upon graduation.

NHSC is a division of HRSA (HRSA, 2017). NHSC was established in 1972 and offered healthcare to individuals in rural and underserved areas. Today over 10,000 NHSC members provide care to more than 11 million people in underserved areas. NHSC accepts applications from individuals committed to becoming primary care providers and who attend an accredited U.S. school to become APRNs.

Enhanced Infrastructure Through Education

Recruitment to practice in rural healthcare settings is extremely difficult. One reason for this is a lack of infrastructure support (Kulig et al., 2010). New nurses may find a lack of support from older, more experienced nurses. This lack of support may be a result of perceptions of generational differences. Older nurses perceive that younger nurses have different values and beliefs; they are interested in working environments that require specialized skills. However, a new graduate nurse may find the lack of other professional team members to be daunting; the potential anonymity is inconsistent with many educators' guidance to select a place of employment that will support a new nurse's professional growth. If the new nurse has not lived in a rural setting, the lack of social and professional cohorts is limiting, resulting in feelings of isolation. Options to address these issues include development of a nurse residency program (NRP) that may enhance socialization and decrease feelings of isolation.

Nurse Residency Programs

New graduate RNs require organizational support when transitioning to their professional role. To assist the new graduate nurse transition into his or her professional role, NRPs designed to introduce the new graduate to critical thinking skills, confidence building, time management, and socialization can be beneficial (Graetz, 2017). Rural healthcare facilities often lack resources to develop such programs. By using NRPs, decreases can be appreciated in both nurse turnover as well as the cost to hire and train new nursing staff. The cost of such turnover is estimated to be from $36,000 to $48,000 per bedside nursing (Nursing Solutions, Inc., 2013), significantly affecting a CAH's profit margins.

Hospitals that have initiated NRPs have reported decreases in turnover rates and an increase in competence of new graduate nurses (Graetz, 2017). Current orientation programs often do not include the information needed for the new graduate to transition to his or her new role. Due to lack of this supportive transition, the agency can accrue the cost of training additional nurses or the use of outside agency nurses, overtime, and increased recruitment processes. In 2012, one rural community hospital estimated the cost of training to be $1,474,000 for salaries of new graduate nurses that left before their first 12 months of employment (Jones, 2013). In addition to turnover, there are concerns of competency. Berman et al. (2014) reported a gap between the actual practice of nursing and what nurses are taught in their formal education. Gaps included lack of critical thinking, communication skills, time management, assessment skills, and the ability to work as a team member. Although nursing curriculums attempt to address these gaps, limitations of time and clinical situations prepare students only in a generalist role.

The use of older nurses as mentors and preceptors for an NRP has the potential to bridge the generational gap. It provides opportunities for older nurses to share their vast knowledge of rural healthcare and begin to understand new graduates' values. Older nurse mentors can minimize the isolation felt by nurses new to the rural community and support growth in competency.

Socialization and Isolation

Rural nurses experience profession isolation: geographical, social, or ideological (Williams, 2012). Geographical isolation results from being a significant distance from places of interest, conferences, or educational opportunities. Social isolation is the lack of contact with family and friends. Ideological isolation is feeling like an outcast, and represented in the rural literature as the "insider outsider" concept (Winters et. al., 2013). Some rural settings have developed support material for individuals working in rural and remote areas. These resources focus on social isolation, pointing out one can feel isolated when moving into a new community and not knowing anyone. Resources offer suggestions that community members can serve as mentors and other ways to care for "self" when relocating.

Retention is affected when nurses feel isolated and unsupported with limited opportunities to advance in their current role. If they do not feel appreciated, RNs may chose to leave for a different opportunity. It is important for rural healthcare providers to consider specific methods to reduce professional isolation. Utilization of information and communication technology can potentially reduce this type of isolation. Nursing research opportunities can also be established, support groups developed, and electronic communications can decrease the feeling of being isolated (Williams, 2012).

CONCLUSION

There is a gap in the literature related to global issues that influence the recruitment and retention of rural and frontier nurses. Educational programs, healthcare facilities, and professional organizations have a responsibility to address this gap. Professional organizations include nursing groups, hospital and state health educational cooperatives, and government agencies. Nursing leaders in rural healthcare settings would benefit from utilizing opportunities to support nurses in education, whether for advanced degrees or continuing education, to maintain skills and knowledge, or for certification reviews. Educators and leaders in rural healthcare settings should consider support of those who are familiar with rural living and all of its implications, including lack of anonymity, isolation, socialization, and work beliefs, and providing care to their community. Areas appropriate to consider include enhanced infrastructure that supports nurses' transition to the rural nursing culture, along with safety and welfare in the workplace setting and education, both for continuing evidence-based knowledge development and advanced degree opportunities.

Rural nurses often feel disenfranchised from their urban colleagues. They are often placed in practice situations where there is no collective support to guide them in defining their role and the boundary of that role. The educational background of rural nurses entering practice must have a foundation in rural theory, leadership, and evidence-based practice information (Long & Weinert, 2013). Rural nurses must demonstrate a competence in assessment and prioritization of care needs within their scope of practice. Although they may not have immediate access to evidence-based information and research, they must know how and where to access that information. CAHs, nursing education programs, and state and federal agencies can all provide those linkages and resources for rural nurses.

REFERENCES

American Nurses Association. (2014). *The nursing workforce 2014: Growth, salaries, education, demographics & trends*. Retrieved from http://www.nursingworld.org/MainMenuCategories/ThePracticeofProfessionalNursing/workforce/Fast-Facts-2014-Nursing-Workforce.pdf

Balasubramanian, S. S., & Jones, E. C. (2016). Hospital closures and the current healthcare climate: The future of rural hospitals in the USA. *Rural and Remote Health, 16*, 3935. Retrieved from https://www.rrh.org.au/journal/article/3935

Berman, A., Beazley, B., Karshmer, J., Prion, S., Van, P., Wallace, J., & West, N. (2014). Competence gaps among unemployed new nursing graduates entering a community-based transition-to-practice program. *Nurse Educator, 39*(2), 56–61. doi:10.1097/NNE.0000000000000018

Buerhaus, P., Auerbach, D., & Staiger, D. (2017). How should we prepare for the wave of retiring baby boomer nurses? *Health Affairs Blog*. Retrieved from http://healthaffairs.org/blog/2017/05/03/how-should-weprepare-for-the-wave-of-retiring-babyboomer-nurse?

Cramer, M. E., Jones, K. J., & Hertzog, M. (2011). Nurse staffing in critical access hospitals: Structural factors linked to quality care. *Journal of Nursing Care Quality, 26*(4), 335–343.

Dolea, C., Stormont, L., & Braichet, J. (2010). Evaluated strategies to increase attraction and retention of health workers in remote and rural areas. *Bull World Health Organization, 88*, 379–387. doi:10.2471/BLT.09.070607

Frontier Education Center. (2004). *Addressing the nursing shortage impacts and innovations in frontier America*. Ojo Sarco, NM: Frontier Education Center National Clearing.

Gale, J. (2010). Rural America: A look beyond the images. Health Progress. *Journal of the Catholic Health Association of the United States, 91*(5), 8–13.

Graetz, J. J. (2017). A nurse residency model for rural and community hospitals: Making a difference in graduate nurse turnover rates. Retrieved from http://hdl.handle.net/10755/595655

Havens, D. S., Warshawsky, N., & Vasey, J. (2012). The nursing practice environment in rural hospitals. *Journal of Nursing Administration, 42*(11), 519–525.

Health Occupation Students of America. (2017). HOSA future health professionals. Retrieved from http://www.hosa.org

Health Resources and Services Administration. (2017.) National Health Service Corps. Retrieved from https://www.nhsc.hrsa.gov

Health Resources and Services Administration Health Workforce. (2017). Nurse corps scholarship program. Retrieved from https://bhw.hrsa.gov/loansscholarships/nursecorps/scholarship

Jones, K. (2013). *RN monthly turnover rate comparison 2011, 2012, & 2013* (Unpublished raw data).

Juraschek, S. P., Zhang, X., Ranganathan, V. K., & Lin, V. (2010). United States registered nurse workforce report card and shortage forecast. *Public Health Resources*. Paper 149.

Kulig, J. C., Kilpatrick, K., Moffitt, P., & Zimmer, L. (2010). Recruitment and retention in rural nursing: It's still an issue! *Nursing Research, 28*(2), 40–50.

Long, K. A., & Weinert, C. (2013). Rural nursing: Developing the theory base. In C. A. Winters (Ed.), *Rural nursing: Concepts, theory, and practice* (4th ed., pp. 1–14). New York, NY: Springer Publishing.

MacDowell, M., Glasser, M., Fitts, M., Nielsen, K., & Hunsaker, M. (2010). A national view of rural health workforce issues in the USA. *Rural and Remote Health, 10*(3), 1531. Retrieved from https://www.rrh.org.au/journal/article/1531

National Area Health Education Center Organization. (2015). *Health Careers Promotion and Preparation*. Retrieved from https://www.nationalahec.org/programs/HealthCareersRecruitmentandPreparation.html

National Rural Health Association. (2017). NRHA fighting for rural. Retrieved from https://www.ruralhealthweb.org/advocate

North Country Health Consortium. (2017). Live, learn, and play in northern New Hampshire. Retrieved from http://livelearnplaynh.org/

Nursing Solutions. (2013). 2013 National healthcare & RN retention report. Retrieved from http://www.nsinursingsolutions.com

Pelham, K., Skinner, M. A., McHugh, P., & Pullon, S. (2016). Interprofessional education in a rural community: The perspectives of the clinical workplace providers. *Journal of Primary Health Care, 8*(3), 210–219. doi:10.1071/HC16010

Skillman, S. M., Palazzo, L., Hart, L. G., & Butterfield, P. (2007). *Changes in the rural registered nurse workforce since 1980*. Seattle, WA: WWAMI Rural Health Research Center.

Spring Arbor University. (2017). What do I need to know about the nursing shortage? Retrieved from https://online.arbor.edu/blog/nursing-shortage-2017/

Williams, M. A. (2012). Rural professional isolation: An integrative review. *Journal of Rural Nursing and Health Care, 12*(2), 3–10. Retrieved from http://rnojournal.binghamton.edu/index.php/RNO/article/view/51/211

Winters, C. A., Thomlinson, E. H., O'Lynn, C., Lee, H. J., McDonagh, M. K., Edge, D. S., & Reimer, M. A. (2013). Exploring rural nursing theory across borders. In C. A. Winters (Ed.), *Rural nursing: Concepts, theory, and practice* (4th ed., pp. 35–47). New York, NY: Springer Publishing.

Wros, P., Mathews, L. R., & Voss, H. (2015). An academic-practice model to improve the health of underserved neighborhoods. *Family Community Health, 38*(2), 195–203. doi:10.1097/FCH.0000000000000065

Rural Public Health

The last section contains three chapters that address important challenges facing rural healthcare providers, educators, and researchers. Chapter 28 provides readers with a basic overview of local public health systems and structures in the United States with special emphasis on the rural public health system. The roles of nurses in rural settings and systems, and implications of the changing structures on the future of public health nursing are examined. The focus of Chapter 29 is substance abuse and use in rural communities. Service availability for substance users and abusers in rural areas, evidence practices, and implications for practice by public health systems are reviewed. The final chapter focuses on engaging rural residents in research. Partnerships between community members and academic investigators are integral to the success of human studies in rural communities. In Chapter 30, we report on the Rural Participatory Research Model *(RPRM). The RPRM may be useful to researchers conducting community-based research with rural partners.*

CHAPTER 28

Rural Public Health Structure and Practice and the Role of the Public Health Nurse

Jo Ann Walsh Dotson and Jane Smilie

DISCUSSION TOPICS

- Select a rural or frontier county of interest to you. Contact the local public health nurse and interview him/her regarding a typical day. Ask about challenges and opportunities of meeting the roles and responsibilities of a public health nurse in that county.
- Identify specific strategies to address lack of resources to support needed public health services identified by the public health nurse with whom you spoke in the selected county.
- Share your conversation and strategies with your classmates.

The public health system in the United States is a complex network of services and programs, consisting of national, state, tribal, county, and other substate health units. In addition to governmental organizations, public health systems include all organizations that contribute to the health and well-being of a community, including " . . . all public, private, and voluntary entities that contribute to the delivery of essential public health services within a jurisdiction" (Centers for Disease Control and Prevention [CDC], 2013). The system has been visualized as a web-like network (Figure 28.1) that varies from region to region and area to area depending upon the available resources.

For the purposes of this chapter, a brief summary of the national and subunit governmental public health structures is presented, providing some context for the structure of rural health systems in the United States. The process and impact of accreditation on the public health system including rural communities is addressed, as well as the funding of rural health systems.

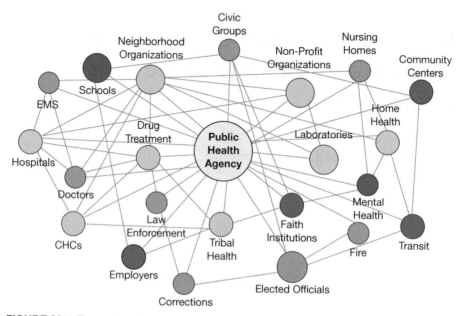

FIGURE 28.1. The public health system.
Source: Centers for Disease Control and Prevention. (2013). *United States Public Health 101. National Public Health performance standards.* Retrieved from https://www.cdc.gov/nphpsp/essentialservices.html
CHCs, community health centers; EMS, emergency medical services

The role of the nurse in public health systems in rural settings is explored, with implications for the future of nurses in rural public health systems briefly addressed.

THE U.S. NATIONAL PUBLIC HEALTH SYSTEM

The public health system in the United States dates back to 1798 with the creation of the U.S. Marine Hospital Service, which was created to provide healthcare to seaman. The role and responsibilities of the service expanded over the next century to provide care to seamen and their families as well as to assume responsibilities for quarantining incoming travelers with a goal of protecting the public from communicable diseases entering the country. The complexity of coordinating quarantine and other public health challenges in the rapidly expanding United States resulted in the expansion of the service, which was renamed the Public Health and Marine Hospital Service in 1902. In 1912, the title of the service was again changed to the Public Health Service (PHS), and over the next century, the roles assumed expanded to include the provision of healthcare to underserved groups and to the public following natural disasters, controlling food and drug supplies, and conducting biomedical research. In 1944, the Public Health Service Act was passed, clarifying and codifying public health rules and regulations, expanding the scope of the PHS, and establishing major administrative units of the service, including the Office of the Surgeon General, the National Institutes of Health, the Bureau of State Services, and the Bureau of Medical Services (Description of Public Health Service Act, 1944). According to Bufford and Lee, the federal government addresses population health through mechanisms that may be categorized under the three core functions of public health: (a) assessment (collecting and disseminating information), (b) policymaking, and (c) assurance, which includes development of the capacity of the public health system and workforce (Bufford & Lee, 2001). Federal agencies are supported by powers granted to them by the U.S. Supreme Court to protect the public's health and safety, and courts have generally upheld governmental efforts to protect the public's health as with mandatory vaccinations, or by supporting minimum ages for purchasing alcohol and tobacco (Gostin, 2000).

THE STATE-LEVEL PUBLIC HEALTH SYSTEM

The 10th amendment to the U.S. Constitution, ratified in 1791, is the last amendment in the Bill of Rights. The 10th amendment assures that states retain powers that are not specifically assigned to Congress (Rutkow & Vernick, 2011), including public health responsibilities such as keeping people safe and the environment clean. Early state-level efforts included child labor laws that protected children's health and safety, and laws that protected water and crops from contamination. More recent examples of public health emergencies that required multistate or regional action included the 9/11 attacks on New York City, Hurricane Katrina in 2005, the H1N1 epidemic in 2011, and notably the present opioid epidemic being addressed at all levels of government by city, state, tribal, and national agencies (CDC, 2013).

State agencies address the health of the public in many ways, including developing and maintaining surveillance systems that monitor health indicators, including birth, death, injury, immunization, and disease in order to identify and target interventions to moderate poor outcomes. States are also responsible for individuals and groups with communicable diseases and protecting others from exposure, and assuring that access to high-quality healthcare services is available not only for the privileged but also for the poor and vulnerable. State agencies, in partnership with local and regional agencies, also protect the public by assuring that food sellers and service providers comply with requirements that keep the public and those in group housing or care facilities safe (Institute of Medicine [IOM], 2002). Similarly, tribal departments address the health needs of sovereign nations either in part or whole with the Indian Health Service or as independent agencies per the Indian Self-Determination and Education Act of 1975 (Warne, 2011).

State, tribal, and local agencies are often mired by ambiguous, redundant, and sometimes conflicting laws. Local, state, and tribal agencies also routinely receive funding from federal and other coffers that are inadequate to provide high-quality services for the entire population, with high-risk vulnerable populations frequently suffering the most. States, tribal communities, and other areas with rural settings frequently have less revenue to supplement federal and other programs and services.

THE LOCAL LEVEL PUBLIC HEALTH SYSTEM

The National Association of City and County Health Officers (NACCHO) conducted a survey of local health departments (LHDs) in the United States in 2013. NACCHO defined a LHD as " . . . an administrative or service unit of local or state government, concerned with health, and carrying some responsibility for the health of a jurisdiction smaller than the state" (NACCHO, 2014, p. 2). The survey was sent to 2,532 LHDs in 48 states and the District of Columbia; Hawaii and New Hampshire do not have LHDs, so were not included in the survey. Two thousand or 79% of the LHDs responded, with 15 states having a 100% response rate, 12 states having 90% or better. LHDs serving smaller populations were less likely to respond to the survey, as evidenced by only 72% of the 1,040 health departments serving less than 25,000 people responding compared to 93% of the 137 health departments serving 500,000 or more people responding. About 1,500, or 60% of the responding LHDs, served 50,000 or fewer people, and over 400 served fewer than 10,000 people.

Most health departments (68%) are county governed and 20% are city governed. Almost 40% of LHDs share responsibilities for one or more services with another jurisdiction; emergency preparedness and epidemiology/surveillance are the most commonly shared functions. About 60% of LHDs have a chief health officer who has either a nursing, public health, or medical degree, and half of those are nurses. Sixty percent of LHDs have 25 or fewer employees, and clerical staff and registered nurses (RNs) are the most frequently employed disciplines at LHDs. In very small health departments, serving less than 10,000 people, RNs and clerical staff were typically the only full-time employees, and in all health departments, regardless of size, only clerical staff outnumbered RNs.

Overall, LHD staffing has decreased 12% since the last NACCHO survey in 2008, from 166,000 full-time equivalents (FTEs) overall to 146,000 in 2013. Behavioral health professional positions were the most likely to be eliminated, with 46% of the 7,400 positions lost between 2008 and 2013. RN positions were the second most likely to be eliminated with the number of nurse positions dropping 16% from 32,900 to 27,700.

RURAL PUBLIC HEALTH SYSTEMS

Rural health systems are critically important because of the economic and social disadvantages in rural communities, but are challenged by the lack of healthcare resources that are contingent upon availability of a qualified workforce (Weinhold & Gurtner, 2014). The term "rural" is defined variably in this text and throughout the literature, but for the purposes of this chapter, rural is defined using the U.S. Census Bureau definition that classifies rural as any area *not* urban, including urbanized areas with 50,000 or more people, urban clusters with 2,500 to 50,000 people, or areas with a population density of approximately 200 people per square mile (Weinhold & Gurtner, 2014). The U.S. Census Bureau further applies data regarding total population thresholds, density, land use, and distance, which results in the portion of the United States considered rural to include not only the sparsely populated and remote areas, but also small, yet densely populated, towns and housing subdivisions located on the perimeters of urban areas (Ratcliffe, Burd, Holder, & Fields, 2016).

The limited availability of primary and supportive health services in rural communities in the United States is complicated by the documented reluctance of rural populations to seek healthcare, due in part to cultural and financial constraints, limited public transport, and poor access to Internet and cell phone services (Dotson, Nelson, Young, Buchwald, & Roll, 2017; Douthit, Kiv, Dwolatzky, & Biswas, 2015). The ongoing lack of primary health services results in LHDs often focusing on the assurance role of public health, facilitating access for individuals as well as communities. The accreditation of public health departments is therefore especially important in rural communities, as the process requires the health department and community leadership to focus on the full range of public health responsibilities.

Accreditation of Public Health Agencies

Accreditation is a process adopted by many health organizations to improve organizational capacity, program delivery, and outcomes. The origin of healthcare organization accreditation in the United States began in the early 1900s with the establishment of *Minimum Standards for Hospitals* by the American College of Surgeons (ACS) in 1917. The ACS was joined by the American College of Physicians, the American Hospital Association, the American Medical Association, and the Canadian Medical Association in 1951 to form the Joint Commission for Accreditation of Hospitals. The name was changed with the expansion of focus to the Joint Commission on Accreditation of Health Care Organizations in 1987, and shortened to The Joint Commission in 2007 (The Joint Commission, 2016). The Commission's work over the last century is primarily a voluntary program of accreditation, which uses trained, external reviewers to examine an organization's compliance with and performance on preestablished indicators (Kilsdonk, Siesling, Otter, & Harten, 2015). The process of accreditation has been demonstrated to be associated with improved clinical outcomes of a wide variety of healthcare settings (Alkhenizan & Shaw, 2011).

The purpose and process of public health accreditation has been in development for approximately 20 years, spurred first by the IOM report on the Future of Public Health (IOM, 1988) and then by the Future of the Public's Health in the 21st century in which the IOM encouraged the exploration of a public health accreditation process (IOM, 2003). In the early 2000s, public health accreditation standards were drafted and in 2007, the Public Health Accreditation Board (PHAB) was created to develop the process and explore and educate public health agencies and the public about the benefits of accreditation of public health agencies (Bender, Kronstadt, Wilcox, & Lee, 2014). The accreditation process was launched in 2011, and requires agencies to document compliance with a multitude of standards and measures, including that they have completed a community health assessment, a community health improvement plan, and an agency-wide strategic plan within the last 5 years. The benefits and drivers for pursuing accreditation include the potential to reduce costs and meet customer demands, improving efficiency and productivity, and most importantly, survive in an era of public health and governmental cuts (Hamm, 2007). The PHAB recently reported that 198 million people, or 64% of the U.S. population, reside in areas served by nationally accredited public health agencies. As of 2017, 30 state health departments, one tribal health department, one centralized integrated state/local public health system, and 169 LHDs have achieved PHAB designation (PHAB, 2017).

Despite the evidence supporting accreditation and specifically public health agency accreditation (L. W. Chen et al., 2015), rural health departments continue to lag behind in the accreditation process. In 2013, the NACCHO conducted a survey of LHDs. Of the 490 participating departments, about 40% were located in a rural community, another 40% in an urban community, and about 20% in a "micropolition community," which using the U.S. Census definition would be considered urban. LHDs in rural communities were significantly less likely to be actively working on accreditation ($p < .001$). Respondents reported that the time and efforts required to both seek and obtain accreditation were the biggest barriers. Beatty, Erwin, Brownson, Meit, and Fey (2017) noted that additional financial and technical support would be needed if rural LHDs were to more actively purse accreditation and that even then, the benefits of accreditation will need to be more clearly described to both LHD staff and to county commissioners and/or boards of health that oversee the departments.

Recognizing barriers and capacity issues faced by smaller public health departments in achieving accreditation, the PHAB has assembled an advisory group comprising representatives from these departments. The group is assisting PHAB as it develops a strategy to better support small health departments to achieve accreditation, rather than lessening the rigor of the PHAB accreditation standards and measures. Through the work of this group, PHAB has defined "small" health departments as those that serve populations of fewer than 50,000 people and/or have fewer than 10 nonclinical FTE staff members; therefore, some are rural and some urban. As of July 2017, there are 17 small health departments (using this definition) that have achieved accreditation. The smallest accredited health department serves a population of 17,000 with seven FTEs.

To identify lessons learned, PHAB and the advisory group have also examined how the small health departments that are accredited were successful. One option for consideration by small health departments is to use the PHAB's multijurisdictional application category. With this category, two or more health departments that work together and share documentation can jointly apply and submit their documentation. Although this application category is not limited to small health departments, it may be an appropriate means for these agencies to achieve accreditation. To date, two multijurisdictional applications have been received by PHAB (R. Wilcox, personal communication, July 5, 2017).

Financing of Rural Public Health

Federal expenditures for public health continue to account for a very small percentage (0.08%) of the gross domestic product (GDP) and only 0.5% of total health-related U.S. expenditures (Kinner & Pellegrini, 2009). Funding for PHSs varies both by state and locality and by urban and rural setting. Federal funding of PHSs is distributed based on a variety of factors, including the number or population in the target group for the particular federal funding, risk and resiliency factors affecting the federal funding target, and the availability of state and/or local match required for federal grants. A detailed investigation of state and local public health funding was conducted by the National Opinion Research Center (NORC) at the University of Chicago. Seven states (Alabama, Arkansas, California, Georgia, Massachusetts, North Dakota, and Oregon) were selected, chosen to be representative of multiple states based on governance type, location, and administrative structure. Data were collected from Association of State and Territorial Health Officials (ASTHO) and other databases on the topics of revenue by funding source (including the American Recovery and Reinvestment Act and Affordable Care Act), expenditures by program area, and expenditures by recipient, expenditures for maternal and child health services, and tobacco use prevention expenditures. The report, published in 2013, summarized the ratios, distribution, and per capita expenditures for PHSs (Meit et al., 2013).

The NORC report revealed large variability in annual expenditures per capita, from $113 per capita in Massachusetts to $53 in Oregon. States with centralized departmental structure tended to have higher cost per capita, with the exception of Massachusetts, whose budget includes administration of five public hospitals. Percent of funds attributable to federal and state funding also differs, with Georgia reporting that 75% of its total public health budget comes from the federal government compared to 27% of the budget of Massachusetts.

The U.S. Department of Agriculture (USDA) was the source of over 40% of the federal funding received by all states, followed by Centers for Disease Control and Prevention (CDC) and the Health Resources and Services Administration. The state general fund accounted for over 50% of expenditures in Massachusetts, compared to about 8% of expenditures in Oregon. States also vary by the percentage of state revenue attributable to Medicaid and Medicare services, with almost 30% of Alabama's revenue from those sources, compared to just over 1% of Georgia's billing.

Distribution of federal and state funding to local agencies also differs by state. In North Dakota, about 85% of funding is allocated to and expended at the state level, with the remaining 15% expended by local public health agencies. This differs from California, where about 34% is expended at the state level and 64% at the local level. Local agency per capita expenditures vary even more widely than state level, with Boston, Massachusetts, public health agency spending $254 per capita compared to $40 per capita in Fulton County, Georgia. The small sample of both state and local agencies make generalizability ill advised, but in general, states and local agencies serving higher percentages of rural populations have less funding and spend less per capita than agencies in urban settings. Public health agencies continue to face shrinking budgets and increasing demands. This finding differed from the NACCHO survey, which reported that health departments serving smaller populations had higher expenditures *and* revenues per capita than larger health departments. In that survey, the per capita expenditures varied widely from state to state, with four states spending less than $15 per person and three states more than $100 per person. Expenditures were not examined based on rurality, but it was noted that the per capita expenditures also ranged widely in states with rural and frontier areas. Health departments serving smaller populations were also more likely to provide and bill for clinical services paid for by Medicaid, Medicare, and private insurances than those serving larger populations (NACCHO, 2014).

The NORC study reported that all seven of the health departments included in the NORC study reported decreased budgets, attributable in large part to reductions in the Tobacco Master Settlement, but also to decreases in other state and federal funding. All departments reported some program cuts and layoffs between 2008 and 2011 (Meit et al., 2013).

Nursing Roles

The important role of public health nurses in rural settings cannot be overestimated. Public health nurses utilize nursing knowledge and skills to address and improve the health of populations. Public health nurses in rural settings practice independently and in partnership with health professionals, government officials, social service agencies, and others to assess health needs, plan and implement policies, and assure access to programs and services that influence health. As noted in NACCHO surveys, nurses in rural settings may be the only LHD professionals, with a broad scope of responsibilities. A typical day for a public health nurse in a rural county health department may start with a morning of providing breastfeeding and nutritional education to new or expectant mothers in the women, infants, and children (WIC) program, a noon meeting with county commissioners to present a budget increase proposal, an afternoon teleconference with health departments in neighboring counties to discuss planning for an upcoming emergency preparedness exercise, followed by a visit to an elderly resident in response to a call from a surgeon's office in a neighboring town asking for a welfare check after a missed postoperative visit. The expansive skill set required to prioritize and perform these tasks is both complex and constantly changing.

Kulbok, Thatcher, Park, and Meszaros (2012) report that public health nursing developed as a distinct specialty in order to facilitate coordinated responses to risks to the population's health, including environmental hazards, knowledge deficits, and resource limitations. Present day public health emergencies, including the epidemics of obesity and substance use and abuse, continue to require nursing knowledge and skills, especially in rural settings where the lack of health professionals and other resources make community-specific evidence-based practice critical. Public health nursing visionaries like Lillian Wald and Mary Osborne developed and demonstrated the community-based process of identifying and addressing health issues with service recipients and local leaders (Lundy & Janes, 2016; Stanhope & Lancaster, 2015). The PHS Act recognized the role of nurses by authorizing the commissioning of nurses and other healthcare professionals to the Commissioned Corps in 1949. This restructuring created the position of Chief Nurse Officer (CNO) in the Office of the Surgeon General. The CNO was charged with advising the surgeon general regarding policy issues and overseeing the largest category in the Commissioned Corps (Debisette, Martinelli, Couig, & Braun, 2010; Nurse Professional Advisory Committee [NPAC], 2016).

PHS Corp nurse responsibilities include provision of clinical services, responding to public health emergencies, development and implementation of health policies, development of training and educational programs, and development of clinical practice guidelines and evidence-based practices through the development or facilitation of research (Debisette et al., 2010). Public health nurses at state and local agencies, including those in rural settings, assume these same responsibilities.

Public health nurses address and support the assertion by Douthit et al. (2015) that "Rural residents have the same right to quality health care as their urban counterparts" (p. 612). The rural public health nurse faces challenges, however, including limited access to services and health information. The expansion of information technology, which was anticipated to greatly improve care and access for rural residents through telemedicine, has actually had limited impact on health outcomes in rural areas to date. The "digital divide" is manifested by place-specific and or time-variable limited access to the Internet and to readily accessible computers, with 39% of the population in rural areas *not* having access to broadband access, with that percent much higher in some states like Alaska (67%), Nevada (65%), and Arizona and Wyoming (63%; "Access to telecommunications technology: Bridging the digital divide in the United States," 2013; Dotson et al., 2017; Kruger & Gilroy, 2016).

Other challenges faced by public health nurses in rural settings include food deserts (areas with limited access to affordable and nutritious food), limited access to health education and health promotion classes and programs for tobacco and other addictions, unavailable or underfunded mental health services including suicide prevention and very limited home care services for those requiring posthospitalization or chronic condition–related services (Brooks, McBee, Pack, & Alamian, 2017; Searles, Valley, Hedegaard, & Betz, 2014; Whitley, 2013). Lower average incomes and lack of public transportation may contribute to fewer healthcare provider visits by rural residents as compared to urban counterparts, but there is also some evidence that rural dwellers may choose to manage their own healthcare, including mental health needs (Ziller, Anderson, & Coburn, 2010). The rural public health nurse is challenged to both be aware of these tendencies, and to work with health and social service professionals to incorporate anticipatory guidance into care protocols and engage the community to recognize and refer appropriately. Public health nurses also often help individuals function more independently by assuring that community members are aware of resources like transport services and telemedicine options.

Implications for the Future of Public Health Nursing

Derose, Gresenz, and Ringel (2011) conceptualized the role that public health can and does have on the health system and individual factors impacting the health of the public. Their work demonstrates the impact of public health core services moderated by health systems and individual factors on health outcomes. Conscious efforts by academics to include content on population health and the role of the public health nurse in undergraduate and graduate health professional programs, such as the one presently in process in Washington state, can improve the readiness of nurses to practice in public health environments. Development and dissemination of certificate programs in leadership, which include rural health system structure and strategy, could also be developed and marketed to health departments and nurses in rural areas.

Strategies to support nurses to practice and lead health services in rural areas have been developed and documented by Hauenstein et al. (2014). Hauenstein documented a practice/academic partnership designed to prepare nurse leaders, with specific expertise in rural healthcare, who were prepared to guide policy and practice to address preventable health problems for disadvantaged rural dwellers in their communities, including those with chronic conditions (p. 467). Partnerships with academia, as well as with entities like the PHS CNO, and organizations like the National Rural Health Association, and the Rural Nurse Organization, can help, strengthen, and disseminate these efforts and strengthen the support of rural health nursing.

Continued efforts to increase the number of public health agencies that are accredited would also improve the capacity of local public health agencies to effectively address the core functions of public health. Partnership with academia could enhance the ability of rural health departments to develop the required assessments, health improvement, and strategic plans, to increase nursing student and faculty exposure to rural health structure and function, and to increase the potential for dissemination of findings and processes through publication. These partnerships could also increase the volume of research by and with rural public health nurses that could examine the characteristics of rural health departments that are located in communities with better-than-average health outcomes, providing other rural agencies with realistic targets to improve outcomes (Douthit et al., 2015).

CONCLUSION

Nurses, and their partners in healthcare, have the ability and potential to improve the health of rural populations. According to the World Health Organization, "Universal access to skilled, motivated and supported health workers, especially in remote and rural communities, is a necessary condition for realizing the human right to health, a matter of social justice" (L. C. Chen, 2010, p. 1). It is critical that nurses be informed about and active in efforts to understand, improve, and lead healthcare in rural communities.

REFERENCES

Access to telecommunications technology: Bridging the digital divide in the United States. (2013). *Congressional Digest, 92*(4), 2–5.

Alkhenizan, A., & Shaw, C. (2011). Impact of accreditation on the quality of healthcare services: A systematic review of the literature. *Annals of Saudi Medicine, 31*(4), 407–416.

Beatty, K. E., Erwin, P. C., Brownson, R. C., Meit, M., & Fey, J. (2017). Public health agency accreditation among rural local health departments: Influencers and barriers. *Journal of Public Health Management and Practice, 24*(1), 49–56. doi:10.1097/PHH.0000000000000509

Bender, K., Kronstadt, J., Wilcox, R., & Lee, T. P. (2014). Overview of the Public Health Accreditation Board. *Journal of Public Health Management and Practice, 20*(1), 4–6. doi:10.1097/PHH.0b013e3182a778a0

Boufford, J. I., & Lee, P. R. (2001). *Health policies for the 21st century: Challenges and recomendations for the U.S. Department of Health and Human Services.* New York,

NY: Milbank Memorial Fund. Retrieved from https://www.milbank.org/wp-content/uploads/2016/06/Health-Policies-for-the-21st-Century-Challenges-and-Recommendations-for-the-U.S.-Department-of-Health-and-Human-Services.pdf

Brooks, B., McBee, M., Pack, R., & Alamian, A. (2017). The effects of rurality on substance use disorder diagnosis: A multiple-groups latent class analysis. *Addictive Behaviors, 68*, 24–29. doi:10.1016/j.addbeh.2017.01.019

Centers for Disease Control and Prevention. (2013, April 27). National Public Health Performance Standards. Retrieved from https://www.cdc.gov/nphpsp/essentialservices.html

Chen, L. C. (2010). Striking the right balance: Health workforce retention in remote and rural areas. *Bulletin of the World Health Organization, 88*(5), 323–323. doi:10.2471/BLT.10.078477

Chen, L.-W., Nguyen, A., Jacobson, J. J., Gupta, N., Bekmuratova, S., & Palm, D. (2015). Relationship between quality improvement implementation and accreditation seeking in local health departments. *American Journal of Public Health, 105*(S2), S295–S302. doi:10.2105/AJPH.2014.302278

Debisette, A. T., Martinelli, A. M., Couig, M. P., & Braun, M. (2010). US public health service commissioned corps nurses: Responding in times of national need. *Nursing Clinics of North America, 45*(2), 123–135. doi:10.1016/j.cnur.2010.02.003

Derose, K. P., Gresenz, C. R., & Ringel, J. S. (2011). Understanding disparities in health care access—and reducing them—through a focus on public health. *Health Affairs, 30*(10), 1844–1851. doi:10.1377/hlthaff.2011.0644

Dotson, J. A. W., Nelson, L. A., Young, S. L., Buchwald, D., & Roll, J. (2017). Use of cell phones and computers for health promotion and tobacco cessation by American Indian college students in Montana. *Rural & Remote Health, 17*, 1–11. Retrieved from https://www.rrh.org.au/journal/article/4014

Douthit, N., Kiv, S., Dwolatzky, T., & Biswas, S. (2015). Exposing some important barriers to health care access in the rural USA. *Public Health (Elsevier), 129*(6), 611–620. doi:10.1016/j.puhe.2015.04.001

Gostin, L. O. (2000). Public health law in a new century: Part I: Law as a tool to advance the community's health. *Journal of the American Medical Association, 283*(21), 2837–2841.

Hamm, M. (2007). Quality improvement initiatives in accreditation: Private sector examples and key lessons for public health. Retrieved from http://www.phaboard.org/wp-content/uploads/QIInitiativesinAccreditation.pdf

Hauenstein, E. J., Glick, D. F., Kane, C., Kulbok, P., Barbero, E., & Cox, K. (2014). A model to develop nurse leaders for rural practice. *Journal of Professional Nursing, 30*(6), 463–473. doi:10.1016/j.profnurs.2014.04.001

Institute of Medicine. (1988). *The future of public health.* Washington, DC: National Academies Press. Retrieved from https://www.nap.edu/read/1091/chapter/1

Institute of Medicine. (2002). *The future of the public's health in the 21st century* (p. 510). Washington, DC: National Academies Press (US).

Institute of Medicine. (2003). *The future of the public's health in the 21st century.* Washington, DC: National Academies Press. Retrieved from https://www.ncbi.nlm.nih.gov/books/NBK221239

The Joint Commission. (2016). *The Joint Commission: Over a century of quality and safety.* Retrieved from https://www.jointcommission.org/assets/1/6/TJC-history-timeline_through_20161.PDF

Kilsdonk, M., Siesling, S., Otter, R., & Harten, W. V. (2015). Evaluating the impact of accreditation and external peer review. *International Journal of Health Care Quality Assurance, 28*(8), 757–777. doi:10.1108/IJHCQA-05-2014-0055

Kinner, K., & Pellegrini, C. (2009). Expenditures for public health: Assessing historical and prospective trends. *American Journal of Public Health, 99*(10), 1780–1791.

Kruger, L., & Gilroy, A. (2016). *Broadband Internet access and the digital divide: Federal assistance programs.* Washington, DC: Congressional Research Service. Retrieved from https://fas.org/sgp/crs/misc/RL30719.pdf

Kulbok, P. A., Thatcher, E., Park, E., & Meszaros, P. S. (2012). Evolving public health nursing roles: Focus on community participatory health promotion and prevention. *Online Journal of Issues in Nursing, 17*(2), 1. doi:10.3912/OJIN.Vol17No02Man01

Lundy, K. S., & Janes, S. (2016). *Community health nursing: Caring for the public's health* (3rd ed.). Burlington, MA: Jones & Bartlett.

Meit, M., Knudson, A., Dickman, I., Brown, A., Hernandez, N., & Kronstadt, J. (2013). *An examination of public health financing in the United States.* Washington, DC: Office of the Assistant Secretary for Planning and Evaluation. Retrieved from http://www.norc.org/PDFs/PH%20Financing%20Report%20-%20Final.pdf

National Association of City and County Health Officers. (2014). *2013 National profile of local health departments.* Washington, DC: Author. Retrieved from http://archived.naccho.org/topics/infrastructure/profile/upload/2013-National-Profile-of-Local-Health-Departments-report.pdf

Nurse Professional Advisory Committee. (2016). History of nursing in the USPHS. *Nurse Resource Manual.* Retrieved from https://dcp.psc.gov/OSG/Nurse/nurse-resource-manual.aspx

Public Health Accreditation Board. (2017). Public health accreditation board's rigorous national standards now benefiting 178 million U.S. residents [Press release]. Retrieved from http://www.phaboard.org/wp-content/uploads/PressReleaseFinal032117.pdf

Public Health Service Act, 1944. Public Health Reports, 59(28), p. 468. Retrieved from https://www.ncbi.nlm.nih.gov/pmc/articles/PMC1403520/pdf/pubhealthrep00059-0006.pdf

Ratcliffe, M., Burd, C., Holder, K., & Fields, A. (2016). *Defining rural at the U.S. Census Bureau.* (ACSGEO-1). Washington, DC: U.S. Census Bureau. Retrieved from https://www2.census.gov/geo/pdfs/reference/ua/Defining_Rural.pdf

Rutkow, L., & Vernick, J. S. (2011). The U.S. Constitution's Commerce Clause, the Supreme Court, and public health. *Public Health Reports (Washington, D.C.: 1974), 126*(5), 750–753.

Searles, V. B., Valley, M. A., Hedegaard, H., & Betz, M. E. (2014). Suicides in urban and rural counties in the United States, 2006–2008. *Crisis: The Journal of Crisis Intervention & Suicide Prevension, 35*(1), 18–26. doi:10.1027/0227-5910/a000224

Stanhope, M., & Lancaster, J. (2015). *Public health nursing: Population-centered health care in the community* (9th ed.). St Louis, MO: Elsevier.

Warne, D. (2011). Policy issues in American Indian health governance. *Journal of Law, Medicine & Ethics, 39,* 42–45. doi:10.1111/j.1748-720X.2011.00564.x

Weinhold, I., & Gurtner, S. (2014). Understanding shortages of sufficient health care in rural areas. *Health Policy, 118*(2), 201–214. doi:10.1016/j.healthpol.2014.07.018

Whitley, S. (2013). Changing times in rural America: Food assistance and food insecurity in food deserts. *Journal of Family Social Work, 16*(1), 36–52. doi:10.1080/10522158.2012.736080

Ziller, E. C., Anderson, N. J., & Coburn, A. F. (2010). Access to rural mental health services: Service use and out-of-pocket costs. *Journal of Rural Health, 26*(3), 214–224.

CHAPTER 29

Substance Use and Abuse in Rural Communities

Jo Ann Walsh Dotson, Ekaterina Burduli,
and Sterling McPherson

DISCUSSION TOPICS

- Rural communities often lack services targeting substance abuse, or facilities that provide evidence-based treatments for substance use disorders. Consider one to two innovative and culturally tailored evidence-based substance abuse treatment strategies that you could implement within your rural community to address substance abuse within the rural youth population.
- Identify key stakeholders in a rural community needed to develop and implement a collaborative nurse-led project (nurse-led clinic, community-based action project, etc.) to address a specific substance use issue. Outline the process you would use to make the project come to life.

Substances are consumed for a variety of personal and social reasons. However, substance use turns into a disorder when people either use illegal drugs or use legal drugs improperly. The most recent edition of the *Diagnostic and Statistical Manual of Mental Disorders (DSM-5)* merged the two previously existing classifications of substance abuse and substance dependence into a single classification: substance use disorder.

DEFINITION AND PREVALENCE

Definition

The *DSM-5* currently defines a *substance use disorder* as a recurrent use of alcohol and/or drugs that causes clinically and functionally significant impairment, including impaired control, social impairment, risky use, and pharmacological criteria (i.e., tolerance and withdrawal; American Psychiatric Association, 2013). Substance use disorders can be classified as either mild, moderate, or severe, depending on the number of diagnostic criteria met by a person. This is intended to capture the continuous nature of such disorders and how best to implement various treatments.

A related term is drug *addiction*. While the *DSM-5* does not classify drug *addiction* as a diagnosis, this term is still commonly used by the National Institute on Drug Abuse (NIDA) and a variety of other reputable research and treatment centers and institutes. Drug addiction is considered a complex and often chronic disease affecting the body and brain functioning. Recently, there have been increasing calls to treat substance use as a chronic, relapsing condition not unlike diabetes or hypertension.

The defining characteristic of drug addiction is the inability to control one's impulses to use drugs despite adverse, sometimes severe, consequences (NIDA, 2016). Other addiction symptoms include loss of control, obsession with using the drug, failed efforts to quit, and tolerance and withdrawal. Other indirect effects often involve the individual's family, medical treatment for other diagnoses, employment, legal entanglements, and psychiatric health. Substance use disorder and drug addiction roughly overlap as central to both definitions is impairment in functioning and adverse physical, mental, and social consequences (NIDA, 2016).

Prevalence

According to the Substance Abuse and Mental Health Services Administration's (SAMHSA) 2014 National Survey on Drug Use and Health (NSDUH), approximately 21.5 million (8.1%) adults (ages ≥12) in the United States met the criteria for a substance use disorder in the previous year. Of those, 2.6 million abused both alcohol and drugs, 4.5 million abused drugs but not alcohol, and 14.4 million abused alcohol only (SAMHSA, 2015). The most common substance use disorders in the United States in order of prevalence are alcohol use disorders, tobacco use disorders, cannabis use disorders, stimulant use disorders, hallucinogen use disorders, and opioid use disorders (SAMHSA, 2015). Substance abuse disorders in general are a major public health concern in the United States as alcohol and illicit and prescription drugs are linked to approximately 90,000 American deaths yearly, whereas tobacco use alone is linked to an estimated 480,000 deaths yearly (U.S. Department of Health & Human Services [USDHHS], 2014). Substance use disorders also have a negative economic impact as they cost Americans over $700 billion a year in greater healthcare costs, crime, and loss of work productivity (Rehm et al., 2009). Finally, both alcohol and smoking are two of the top three leading causes of preventable deaths in the United States (Schroeder, 2007). Thus, alcohol and drug use are clearly key areas to focus on when discussing any aspect of important public health domains in need of improvement.

THE RURAL LANDSCAPE

Rural Substance Abuse Prevalence

A common misconception about substance use is that it is urban in nature. Although in general rural and urban areas have similar rates of substance use and abuse, surprisingly, rural Americans are at a higher risk than their urban counterparts for abuse of some substances, especially when considering they often have worse access to evidence-based treatment programs (Dotson et al., 2014; Edmond, Aletraris, & Roman, 2015; SAMHSA, 2012, 2015). Substance abuse is growing at an alarming rate in rural areas that have a shortage of means and infrastructure to offer access to necessary education, support, and health services to persons struggling with substance use disorders. This is especially true for the use of alcohol, smoking, and in the West, methamphetamine use (Grant et al., 2007). Furthermore, most medically underserved areas of the United States lie in rural counties; thus considerable substance abuse mortality is concentrated in rural areas (Health Resources & Services Administration [HRSA], 2016). Therefore, the most vulnerable rural communities have the least resources to help its citizens with substance use disorders.

Rural Versus Urban Youth

Rural adolescents are more likely to use alcohol than their peers in urban areas and use is highest among adolescents living in remote rural areas (Lasser, Schmidt, Diep, & Huebel, 2010). Studies find that alcohol use and binge drinking, and drinking and driving under the influence (DUI), are more common among rural youth than among urban youth (Lasser et al., 2010), suggesting that adolescents who begin drinking alcohol at an early age may engage in problem drinking as they get older (Lambert, Gale, & Hartley, 2008). A 2011 study by Rhew and colleagues found that alcohol, smokeless tobacco, inhalant, and other illicit drug use were more prevalent among high school–aged youths living on farms than among those living in towns (Rhew, David, Hawkins, & Oesterle, 2011). In addition, farm-dwelling students were exposed to increased drug use risk factors when compared with urban-dwelling students. Rural youth are also significantly more likely to smoke tobacco (Meit et al., 2014), and abuse prescription drugs (Havens et al., 2011; Havens, Oser, & Leukefeld, 2011; Havens, Young, & Havens, 2011) when compared with youth living in urban areas. According to one 2011 study, rural youth also reported greater lifetime prevalence (13% vs. 10%) of nonmedical prescription drug use than urban adolescents (Havens et al., 2011). Although there have been several hypothesized reasons for this, the scant literature does not yet have a clearly articulated cause of this phenomenon.

Rural Illicit Drug Use

Illicit drugs fall into one of two categories: (a) illegal drugs or (b) prescription, and or over-the-counter drugs that are used inappropriately. The *2014 Update of the Rural-Urban Chartbook* reports that alcohol, followed by marijuana, stimulants, opiates, and cocaine were the primary substances for substance abuse treatment admissions in rural settings (Meit et al., 2014). In 2004, the rate of methamphetamine use by young rural adults was double the rate of young urban adults ages 18 to 25 (2.9% vs. 1.5%). Although methamphetamine use by teens across the nation has declined by approximately 70% since 1999, the pattern of higher use in rural areas continues to be of concern (Substance Abuse Among Rural Youth: A Little Meth and a Lot of Booze, 2007). This rate continues to grow, especially among disadvantaged populations including American Indians (AI) and people with low socioeconomic status.

Although heroin has historically been more common in urban areas, an increasing percentage of rural heroin users is reported, with opioids being especially prevalent among rural dwellers. A 2015 article published in the *International Journal of Drug Policy* investigating rural/urban use of opioids found that 4.9% of rural adults (vs. 5.9% of urban adults) reported nonmedical use of prescription opioids in the past year (Rigg & Monnat, 2015). Research also suggests that death and injury from opioids are more prevalent in states with significant rural populations (Paulozzi, 2011).

A 2012 Treatment Episode Data Set (TEDS) report comparing rural and urban substance abuse treatment admissions found that rural admissions were younger than urban admissions and were more likely to report primary abuse of alcohol (49.5% vs. 36.1%) or nonheroin opiates (10.6% vs. 4.0%). Urban admissions were in turn significantly more likely than rural admissions to report primary abuse of heroin (21.8% vs. 3.1%) or cocaine (11.9% vs. 5.6%; SAMHSA, 2012). However, rural admissions were more likely than urban admissions to be referred by the criminal justice system (51.6% vs. 28.4%) and less likely to be self- or individually referred (22.8% vs. 38.7%; SAMHSA, 2012).

Examples of Health Disparities in Rural Settings

In terms of access to healthcare, rurality is a disparity unto itself and when layered onto another disparate population, such as racial and ethnic minorities, or pregnant women, it exacerbates existing disparities already at work. Racial and ethnic minorities carry an elevated burden of some substance use disorders. For example, AI and Alaska Natives (AN) are at a higher risk for alcohol, tobacco, and opioid abuse. Scientific research coupled with the Indian Health

Service (IHS) along with SAMHSA, and the U.S. Department of Justice, have established that substance use disproportionately affects Native populations in the United States. An estimated 5% of AIs and ANs, compared to 2.9% of the general U.S. population, had a substance use disorder in the past year. Among the most prevalent problems on many reservations today are alcohol dependence and prescription opiate misuse (SAMHSA, 2015). Alcohol is the most frequently abused substance, with a use rate of 10.7% for Native people and 7.6% for the general population (Feldstein, Venner, & May, 2006; SAMHSA, 2015). Alcohol-associated deaths account for 11.7% of all AI/AN deaths, and the age-adjusted death rate is approximately twice that of the U.S. general population (CDC, 2008). Relative to other ethnic groups, AIs have a 2.5 times higher rate of accidental deaths by poisoning (Murphy et al., 2014). In addition, among alcohol drinkers of all races, AI/ANs are the most likely (11.7%) to concurrently use an illicit drug (SAMHSA, 2015). Among ANs receiving inpatient treatment for alcohol dependence, 11% to 15% suffered from opiate dependence at some time during their lives.

Another disparate group is pregnant women or women of reproductive age. The Centers for Disease Control and Prevention (CDC) reports that roughly 6% to 9% of women of reproductive age use one or more substances (CDC, 2009). A reported 5.9% use illicit drugs, 8.5% use alcohol, and 2.7% binge drink (SAMHSA, 2014). A 2015 study by Shaw and colleagues implementing an intervention for substance-abusing mothers found that rural mothers were more likely to use alcohol and binge drink at the start of the intervention and at the end of the 3-year intervention program. Rural women were also less likely to complete outpatient substance abuse treatment and used less mental health services compared to urban participants throughout the 3-year period (Shaw et al., 2015).

Service Availability in Rural Communities

Availability of resources for individuals and communities experiencing high rates of substance use and abuse and associated mental health needs are often woefully inadequate in rural settings. A study conducted by Edmond et al. (2015) examined differences between rural and urban substance and mental health treatment centers. Facilities participating in the U.S. National Treatment Center Study (National Treatment Center Study, 2016) were included as potential study sites, and using a stratified sampling, 591 geographically representative centers were selected from a pool of 636 centers. About 68% or 432 responded to the survey, which was conducted using face-to-face interviews of clinical and administrative directors. Data elements included agency staffing patterns and characteristics, funding, assessment strategies, and treatment methods used, including pharmacotherapy, and availability of "specialized treatment tracks" like those for adolescent substance users. As hypothesized, the authors reported that rural centers had a lower percentage of providers with advanced degrees (masters or higher), but unexpectedly, rural treatment centers were *more* likely to employ a nurse than urban centers. Analysis also supported the hypothesis that rural centers were more likely to be publicly funded, which the authors attributed to the facts that smaller populations and higher poverty levels in rural areas likely made for-profit or privately funded centers less sustainable. They also reported that, as hypothesized, rural centers offered fewer services, such as including buprenorphine. It was noted that while rural centers were less likely to offer programs or "tracks" for certain populations, a higher percentage of centers in rural areas offered specialized treatment for adolescents than their urban counterparts. The authors noted that this service availability was "encouraging" in light of the higher incidence of binge drinking and methamphetamine use among rural youth (Lambert et al., 2008; Rhew et al., 2011).

Rural substance abuse can have deleterious effects on individuals, their families, and the community. Substance abuse can lead to increased rates of unemployment, homelessness, risky sexual behavior, infectious diseases, crime, fetal alcohol syndrome, and injuries and accidents. These negative consequences are amplified by distinctive challenges that rural communities face including long distance travel required for patients seeking services, rural medical staff with little experience in providing care to a drug overdose patient, no readily available substance abuse treatment services, sparingly spread law enforcement, and treatment-hesitant patients due to privacy concerns associated with small rural areas.

Obstacles specific to treatment may include lack of employment and educational attainment, substandard living conditions, racial discrimination, geographical isolation, and acculturation stress. Clinicians in rural areas who try to address substance misuse also face complex barriers such as far-flung service areas, limited financial resources, few addiction treatment professionals, and few medical providers who are able to prescribe medication targeting substance abuse, or facilities that provide evidence-based treatments for substance use disorders. Although many innovative and culturally tailored evidence-based substance abuse treatments are being implemented with rural populations recently, challenges remain in the service delivery of evidence-based substance abuse treatments in rural settings.

NURSING ROLES

Public health nurses (PHNs) possess skills that can help identify risk and resiliency factors in individual and community clients, and knowledge of resources that can be mobilized to address those risks and maximize resiliency (Dudgeon & Evanson, 2014; Strass & Billay, 2008). The Public Health Nurse

Core Competencies, as outlined by the Quad Council Public Health Nursing Organization, describe an array of skills and abilities that guide nursing activities at many levels. For example, generalist PHNs implement the most basic or Tier 1 competencies as they perform their day-to-day activities as part of state and local public health organizations. These skills include delivery of individual and population-based services by nurses not in management positions. Tier 2 competencies extend to program planning, management, and implementation that may include supervision of nurses and other health professionals and support staff in the delivery of individual- and population-based programs. Tier 3 competencies are those demonstrated by executive or senior level nurses in leadership positions in public health organizations. At this level, PHNs are responsible for guiding and developing the mission and vision of health organizations and for assuring that activities and programming support the overall intent and continuously improve the health of the public. These competencies are further described in terms of eight "domains" which address, by tier, expectations for PHN practices in the areas of (a) analytic and assessment, (b) policy development/program planning, (c) communication, (d) cultural competence, (e) community practice, (f) public health science, (g) financial planning and management, and (h) leadership and systems thinking (Council, 2011). These competencies identify the skills and knowledge PHNs have that allow them to link need with resources in ways that practitioners in clinical settings and/or neighboring communities may not be aware of (Barrett, Terry, Lê, & Hoang, 2016). Nurse run programs, like the community-based participatory action studies conducted by Nyamathi and colleagues in California and by Kulbok and associates in Virginia, have demonstrated a positive impact on tobacco and other substance use in targeted populations, including those in rural communities (Kulbok, Thatcher, Park, & Meszaros, 2012; Nyamathi et al., 2012).

Implications for the Future of Public Health Nursing

As described in the Institute of Medicine's (IOM's) Future of Nursing Report, it is critical that all nurses, including PHNs and those in rural settings, practice to the full extent of their education and training (IOM, 2011). It is the responsibility of the profession to partner with academia to assure that nurses can seamlessly progress through degree options and achieve higher levels of education, allowing more nurses to operate at Tier 2 and Tier 3 levels as described by the Quad Council. It is also critical that nurses continue to advocate for and lead in community-based participatory research that partners with communities to assure that the health of the public is a paramount consideration when planning and implementing studies (Kulbok et al., 2012). Nursing organizations must also consistently assess and update research priorities to assure that the changing needs of the public are incorporated, and that the profession strives for ever-increasing rigor in the planning and implementation of community-based research.

REFERENCES

American Psychiatric Association. (2013). *Diagnostic and statistical manual of mental disorders* (5th ed.). Arlington, VA: American Psychiatric Publishing.

Barrett, A., Terry, D. R., Lê, Q., & Hoang, H. (2016). Factors influencing community nursing roles and health service provision in rural areas: A review of literature. *Contemporary Nurse: A Journal for the Australian Nursing Profession, 52*(1), 119–135. doi:10.1080/10376178.2016.1198234

Centers for Disease Control and Prevention. (2008). Alcohol-attributable deaths and years of potential life lost among American Indians and Alaska Natives—United States, 2001–2005. *Morbidity & Mortality Weekly Report, 57*(34), 938–941. Retrieved from https://www.cdc.gov/mmwr/preview/mmwrhtml/mm5734a3.htm

Centers for Disease Control and Prevention. (2009). Alcohol use among pregnant and nonpregnant women of childbearing age—United States, 1991–2005. *Morbidity and Mortality Weekly Report, 58*(19), 529–532. Retrieved from https://www.cdc.gov/mmwr/preview/mmwrhtml/mm5819a4.htm

Council, Q. (Producer). (2011, March 19). Quad Council competencies for public health nurses. Retrieved from http://www.achne.org/files/Quad%20Council/QuadCouncilCompetenciesforPublicHealthNurses.pdf

Dotson, J. A., Roll, J. M., Packer, R. R., Lewis, J. M., McPherson, S., & Howell, D. (2014). Urban and rural utilization of evidence-based practices for substance use and mental health disorders. *The Journal of Rural Health, 30*(3), 292–299. doi:10.1111/jrh.12068

Dudgeon, A., & Evanson, T. A. (2014). Intimate partner violence in rural U.S. areas: What every nurse should know. *American Journal of Nursing, 114*(5), 26–36. doi:10.1097/01.NAJ.0000446771.02202.35

Edmond, M. B., Aletraris, L., & Roman, P. M. (2015). Rural substance use treatment centers in the United States: An assessment of treatment quality by location. *American Journal of Drug & Alcohol Abuse, 41*(5), 449–457. doi:10.3109/00952990.2015.1059842

Feldstein, S. W., Venner, K. L., & May, P. A. (2006). American Indian/Alaska Native alcohol-related incarceration and treatment. *American Indian & Alaska Native Mental Health Research: The Journal of the National Center, 13*(3), 1–22.

Grant, K. M., Kelley, S. S., Agrawal, S., Meza, J. L., Meyer, J. R., Romberger, D. J. (2007). Methamphetamine use in rural midwesterners. *American Journal on Addictions, 16*(2), 79–84. doi:10.1080/10550490601184159

Havens, J. R., Oser, C. B., Knudsen, H. K., Lofwall, M., Stoops, W. W., Walsh, S. L., . . . Kral, A. H. (2011). Individual and network factors associated with non-fatal overdose among rural Appalachian drug users. *Drug Alcohol Depend, 115*(1–2), 107–112. doi:10.1016/j.drugalcdep.2010.11.003

Havens, J. R., Oser, C. B., & Leukefeld, C. G. (2011). Injection risk behaviors among rural drug users: Implications for HIV prevention. *AIDS Care, 23*(5), 638–645. doi:10.1080/09540121.2010.516346

Havens, J. R., Young, A. M., & Havens, C. E. (2011). Nonmedical prescription drug use in a nationally representative sample of adolescents: Evidence of greater use among rural adolescents. *Archives of Pediatrics & Adolescent Medicine, 165*(3), 250–255. doi:10.1001/archpediatrics.2010.217

Health Resources and Services Administration (HRSA). (2016). *Guidelines for medically underserved area and population designation.* Rockville, MD: Author. Retrieved from https://bhw.hrsa.gov/shortage-designation/muap

Institute of Medicine (IOM). (2011). *The future of nursing: Leading change, advancing health.* Washington, DC: National Academies Press.

Kulbok, P. A., Thatcher, E., Park, E., & Meszaros, P. S. (2012). Evolving public health nursing roles: Focus on community participatory health promotion and prevention. *Online Journal of Issues in Nursing, 17*(2), 1. doi:10.3912/OJIN.Vol17No02Man01

Lambert, D., Gale, J. A., & Hartley, D. (2008). Substance abuse by youth and young adults in rural America. *The Journal of Rural Health, 24*(3), 221–228. doi:10.1111/j.1748-0361.2008.00162.x

Lasser, J., Schmidt, E., Diep, J., & Huebel, A. (2010). Underage rural drinking: Survey data and implications for educators. *Rural Educator, 31*(3), 38–46.

Meit, M., Knudson, A., Gilbert, T., Tzy-Chyi Yu, A., Tanenbaum, E., Ormson, E., . . . Popat, S. (2014). *The 2014 update of the rural-urban chartbook.* Grand Forks, ND: Center for Rural Health. Retrieved from https://ruralhealth.und.edu/projects/health-reform-policy-research-center/pdf/2014-rural-urban-chartbook-update.pdf

Murphy, T., Pokhrel, P., Worthington, A., Billie, H., Sewell, M., & Bill, N. (2014). Unintentional injury mortality among American Indians and Alaska Natives in the United States, 1990–2009. *American Journal of Public Health, 104*(Suppl. 3), S470–S480. doi:10.2105/AJPH.2013.301854

National Institute on Drug Abuse. (2016). *Media guide.* Retrieved from https://www.drugabuse.gov/publications/media-guide/dear-journalist

National Treatment Center Study. (2016). *Behavioral healthcare services: Organization, delivery, and quality.* Retrieved from http://ntcs.uga.edu

Nyamathi, A., Branson, C., Kennedy, B., Salem, B., Khalilifard, F., Marfisee, M., . . . Leake, B. (2012). Impact of nursing intervention on decreasing substances among homeless youth. *American Journal on Addictions, 21*(6), 558–565. doi:10.1111/j.1521-0391.2012.00288.x

Paulozzi, L. J. (2011). Drug-induced deaths—United States, 2003–2007. *MMWR Supplements, 60*(1), 60–61. Retrieved from https://www.cdc.gov/mmwr/preview/mmwrhtml/su6001a12.htm

Rehm, J., Mathers, C., Popova, S., Thavorncharoensap, M., Teerawattananon, Y., & Patra, J. (2009). Global burden of disease and injury and economic cost attributable to alcohol use and alcohol-use disorders. *The Lancet, 373*(9682), 2223–2233. doi:10.1016/S0140-6736(09)60746-7

Rhew, I. C., David Hawkins, J., & Oesterle, S. (2011). Drug use and risk among youth in different rural contexts. *Health & Place, 17*(3), 775–783. doi:10.1016/j.healthplace.2011.02.003

Rigg, K. K., & Monnat, S. M. (2015). Urban vs. rural differences in prescription opioid misuse among adults in the United States: Informing region specific drug policies and interventions. *International Journal on Drug Policy, 26*(5), 484–491. doi:10.1016/j.drugpo.2014.10.001

Schroeder, S. A. (2007). Shattuck Lecture: We can do better: Improving the health of the American people. *The New England Journal of Medicine, 357*(12), 1221–1228. doi:10.1056/NEJMsa073350

Shaw, M. R., Grant, T., Barbosa-Leiker, C., Fleming, S. E., Henley, S., & Graham, J. C. (2015). Intervention with substance-abusing mothers: Are there rural-urban differences? *American Journal on Addictions/American Academy of Psychiatrists in Alcoholism and Addictions, 24*(2), 144–152. doi:10.1111/ajad.12155

Strass, P., & Billay, E. (2008). A public health nursing initiative to promote antenatal health. *The Canadian Nurse, 104*(2), 29–33.

Substance abuse among rural youth: A little meth and a lot of booze. (2007). Retrieved from http://muskie.usm.maine.edu/Publications/rural/pb35a.pdf

Substance Abuse and Mental Health Services Administration. (2012). *The TEDS report: A comparison of rural and urban substance abuse treatment admissions.* Rockville, MD: Author. Retrieved from https://www.samhsa.gov/sites/default/files/teds-short-report043-urban-rural-admissions-2012.pdf

Substance Abuse and Mental Health Services Administration. (2014). *Results from the 2013 National Survey on Drug Use and Health: Summary of National Findings* (NSDUH Series H-48, HHS Publication No. (SMA) 14-4863). Rockville, MD: Author. Retrieved from https://www.samhsa.gov/data/sites/default/files/NSDUHresultsPDFWHTML2013/Web/NSDUHresults2013.pdf

Substance Abuse and Mental Health Services Administration. (2015). *Behavioral health trends in the United States: Results from the 2014 National Survey on Drug Use and Health* (HHS Publication No. SMA 15-4927, NSDUH Series H-50). Rockville, MD: Author. Retrieved from https://www.samhsa.gov/data/sites/default/files/NSDUH-FRR1-2014/NSDUH-FRR1-2014.pdf

U.S. Department of Health and Human Services. (2014). *The health consequences of smoking: 50 years of progress. A report of the surgeon general.* Atlanta, GA: Author. Printed with corrections, January 2014. Retrieved from https://www.surgeongeneral.gov/library/reports/50-years-of-progress/full-report.pdf

Engagement of Rural Residents in Research: The Rural Participatory Research Model

Sandra W. Kuntz, Tanis Hernandez, and Charlene A. Winters

DISCUSSION TOPICS

- You are a researcher at a distinguished university. Discuss how you would apply the Rural Participatory Research Model (RPRM) for a study you will lead in a distant rural community.
- Describe strategies to engage rural community members in research.
- Explain the notion of "erosion of trust" that can occur following a technological disaster.

Partnerships between community members and academic investigators are integral to the success of human studies in rural communities. Research to explore the holistic impact of a rural, slow-motion, technological environmental disaster relies on questions raised and probed by community members living with the direct or indirect social, emotional, physical, or economic effects of exposure. In October 2005, clinicians from the Center for Asbestos Related Disease (CARD) contacted Montana State University (MSU) nurse researchers and queried the possibility of collaborating with MSU on a specific project. The CARD clinic's search for a research partner emanated from their mission as a "non-profit specialty asbestos clinic devoted to healthcare, research, and outreach to benefit all people impacted by exposure to Libby amphibole asbestos" (CARD, 2017). The CARD clinicians were looking for a partner to help analyze a data set that included results from the St. George's Respiratory Questionnaire (SGRQ) survey linked to clinical data from 1,200 CARD clients. The SGRQ is "an index deigned to measure and quantify health-related health status in patients with chronic airflow limitation . . . [the SGRQ] has been shown to correlate well with established measures of symptom level, disease activity and disability" (Jones, Quirk, Baveystock, & Littlejohns, 1992, p. 1321).

The initial partnership resulted in the joint submission of a grant to the Health Resources and Services Administration (HRSA) Office of Rural Health Policy [R04RH07544]. The funding supported Study 1, a comprehensive understanding of the biopsychosocial health status of persons exposed to Libby amphibole asbestos (LAA) and the human response to chronic illness resulting from asbestos exposure. The study utilized a community-based participatory research (CBPR) approach and analysis of the CARD clinic existing client data. Results of this study are reported in the *International Scholarly Research Network* (Weinert et al., 2011), *Journal of Environmental and Public Health* (Winters et al., 2011), and *BMJ Open* (Winters et al., 2012).

Next, the CARD/MSU team developed Study 2 in response to the National Institutes of Health (NIH) Public Trust Initiative to explore ways to improve the communication and interaction between researchers and the public. The funded proposal, *Exploring Research Communication and Engagement in a Rural Community: The Libby Partnership Initiative* included the following three aims and specifically called for the development of a rural CBPR model as a part of the grant deliverables.

- Determine the research milieu in Libby, Montana, by conducting a focused community assessment to include:
  - History of research in the community
  - Infrastructure (services and resources) available to support the communication and translation of research in the community
  - Libby residents' awareness, knowledge, and acceptance of research
  - Libby residents' preferred method of communication about research
- Design, implement, and evaluate strategies for communicating research opportunities and results to Libby residents to
  - Be used by researchers to facilitate research communication in Libby, Montana
  - Increase community residents' awareness, knowledge, and acceptance of research
- Enhance the existing local research infrastructure for communication of research to community members. Develop the foundation for a rural CBPR model that fosters community involvement in research and guides researchers working in rural communities.

Finally, Study 3 contributed further insight toward the development of the model described in the third aim of Study 2. An MSU master's in nursing student and Libby community member, Natasha Nicole Blata-Pennock, worked with the CARD/MSU team to conduct a study entitled *Communication and Information Exchange in Libby, Montana: A Secondary Data Analysis of Community Advisory Group Meeting Summaries.* This retrospective, qualitative study was launched based on the following problem statement:

Effective communication is an essential component to the success of community-based activities. Although the Libby Community Advisory

Group (CAG) was developed [by the Environmental Protection Agency (EPA)] as a forum for two way communication and information exchange between the community and agencies involved in the (Libby) clean-up efforts, little is known about preferred modes of communication and the community's acceptance and resistance to biomedical and behavioral research. (Blata-Pennock, 2010, p. 10)

The study of existing documents identified "concerns, perceptions, and preferences of rural Libby residents related to research communication and other issues critical to the population's health and well-being" (p. 10). The qualitative analysis of themes utilized rural nursing theory (Long & Weinert, 1989; Winters & Lee, 2010) and Covello's risk communication model (Covello & Allen, 1988) and increased awareness of communication preferences related to research in a rural community.

The purpose of this chapter is to report on the development of the community-generated Rural Participatory Research Model (RPRM) that emerged from results of the three studies conducted in Libby, Montana between 2006 and 2010. The RPRM (Figure 30.1) was developed to help guide researchers working with rural communities experiencing the ongoing effects of an environmental disaster.

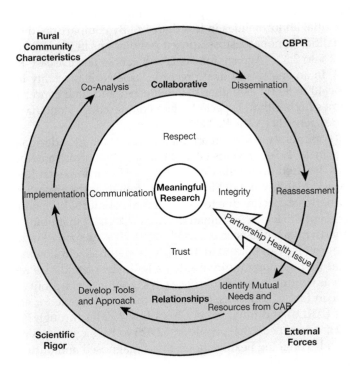

FIGURE 30.1 Rural Participatory Research Model (RPRM).

BACKGROUND

According to the 2010 census, Libby, Montana is designated rural (population 2,628) as well as the surrounding county frontier (population 19,687; 5.4 people/square mile; U.S. Census Bureau, 2010). From the 1920s until 1990, vermiculite ore contaminated with amphibole asbestos was mined, processed, and distributed from Libby to more than 200 processing facilities across the United States accounting for 80% of the world's supply (U.S. EPA, 2017). Vermiculite is a natural-occurring fibrous mineral widely used in industry and construction (U.S. Environmental Protection Agency, 2003). Contaminated vermiculite was also widely disbursed in south Lincoln County as it was available by the truck load, free of charge. Therefore, it was used as a soil conditioner in gardens, insulation for homes and business, and as foundations for school running tracks and driveways.

In 1999, a media exposé revealed possible community-wide amphibole asbestos exposure. Amphibole asbestos is a toxic mineral associated with lung cancer, mesothelioma, and nonmalignant lung and pleural disorders, including asbestosis, pleural plaques, pleural thickening, and pleural effusions (Amandus, Althouse, Morgan, Sargent, & Jones, 1987; Amandus, Wheeler, Jankovic, & Tucker, 1987). In 2000 and 2001, medical screening of more than 6,668 current and former Libby residents revealed pleural abnormalities in 18% of participants and interstitial abnormalities in less than 1%. By comparison, the rate of pleural abnormalities in nonasbestos-exposed populations in the United States ranged from 0.2% to 2.3% (Agency for Toxic substances and Disease Registry [ATSDR], 2003). In an analysis of death records, asbestosis mortality in Libby was found to be 40 to 80 times higher than expected and lung cancer mortality 1.2 to 1.3 times higher than expected when compared to Montana and the United States, respectively (ATSDR, 2002).

The extent of community-wide contamination warranted EPA designation as a Superfund site in 2002. Seven years later, the first public health emergency in U.S. history was declared under the Comprehensive Environmental Response, Compensation, and Liability Act (CERCLA), also known as the Superfund Law for the Libby asbestos exposure due to the high rates of morbidity and mortality (U.S. Department of Health & Human Services, 2009). At that point in time, generations of individuals had been exposed over a 70-year span of time. Since respiratory compromise can take 10 to 40 years to materialize following exposure, it was clear that the community needed a long-term healthcare response as the disaster was continuing to unfold. The CARD clinic, a nonprofit community-based clinic in Libby, continues to this day to screen people for asbestos-related diseases (ARDs) and lung cancer. From July 1, 2011 through February 28, 2017, CARD has screened 4,500 people and 2,025 were diagnosed with ARD. CARD also provides ongoing healthcare for those diagnosed and outreach and education to a regional audience.

METHODS

Development of the RPRM (see Figure 30.1) evolved over time as the CARD/MSU team addressed research questions posed by community members, CARD clinicians, and MSU nurse researchers. Study 1 provided entry to the community and the initial opportunity to work with the CARD clinic personnel. All three studies used a CBPR approach and created an opportunity to work continuously with the CARD clinicians. To assure community engagement and voice, a community-advisory board (CAB) was formed at the beginning of the first study to provide input to the investigators at every stage of the research. The research design and methods used for each study varied based on the project goals and specific aims.

For Study 1, a descriptive cross-sectional study design was used by the team to explore the (a) respiratory health status and respiratory health-related quality of life (HRQOL) of a cohort of persons exposed to LAA (Winters et al., 2012); (b) the psychosocial health status (depression, stress, and acceptance of illness) and differences in psychosocial health based on age, gender, residence, exposure pathway, insurance status, and access to care (Weinert et al., 2011); and (c) the perceived satisfaction with access/financial aspects of care among the CARD clinic's local and distant clients (Winters et al., 2011).

For Study 2, case study research methods (Yin, 2009) were applied to the study aims. The embedded single-case design followed three principles of data collection. First, multiple sources of both quantitative and qualitative evidence included archival records, direct observation, and community member surveys. Data were analyzed to begin building the case during the first year of the project. Second, a case study database was created to organize and document the evidence. The database contributed to outcome reliability, project evaluation, and the final report. Finally, construct validity and an enhanced quality of case design was achieved as the chain of evidence was maintained. Throughout the 2-year investigation, a study protocol guided each phase of the project and provided structure for the evaluation of project inputs (e.g., research and process data), formative outputs (e.g., data analysis), and summative outcomes (e.g., final case study and foundation for the rural research model). The initial case study research protocol developed by the CARD/MSU team was enhanced and revised through community input and feedback from the CAB (Winters, Rowse, Kuntz, & Weinert, 2008).

Study 3 (Blata-Pennock, 2010), a retrospective, descriptive, qualitative study, used content and thematic analysis of existing documents to search for and identify concerns, perceptions, preferences, and research communication themes critical to the population's health and well-being within the Libby community. Four years of meeting summaries (2001, 2003, 2006, and 2008) from the CAG formed by the EPA were selected for analysis. Years chosen for review coincided with seminal events associated with asbestos mitigation in the community.

For instance, year 2001 was the first year of CAG and the year ATSDR released the asbestos medical screening report. Year 2003 represents the year after Libby was placed on the EPA National Priorities List (NPL) as a Superfund site. Year 2006 represents a time of continued cleanup efforts by the EPA, and 2008 is the year leading up to the CAG dissolvement and the period of time shortly before the federal public health emergency was declared in Libby. A total of 53 meeting summaries were analyzed with themes sorted based on five topics: information exchange; communication characteristics; community awareness, concerns, perceptions, preferences, knowledge, acceptance and resistance to healthcare, cleanup, and biomedical and behavioral research; characteristics of rural residents; and evidence of rules of risk communication.

RESULTS: RPRM COMPONENTS

Study 1

Findings related to all three studies contributed to the development of the RPRM; components of the model are *italicized* in this section. In Study 1, the direct contribution to RPRM included identifying the importance of establishing a relationship with the community by responding to specific needs raised by CARD on behalf of community members impacted by exposure to LAA. The research questions were generated from the community and a partnership was established that respected the tenets of CBPR. Study 1 allowed the MSU team entry to the community and *an opportunity to build trust, establish mutual respect, observe and exhibit integrity, and create effective methods of communicating with the CARD clinicians and community members.* For instance, in addition to creating the community advisory board, the MSU/CARD team planned special evening events and participated in community-based research rallies to better inform and connect with community members. At the center of the RPRM, *meaningful research* is surrounded by basic principles of partnership and *collaborative relationships—mutual trust, respect, integrity, and communication.*

For Study 1, the research team first used existing clinical data of 329 clients (chest radiographs, pulmonary function tests, smoking history, demographic characteristics, and SGRQ results) to examine the respiratory health status (55% had pleural abnormalities; 21% had both pleural and interstitial abnormalities; 18% had no documented lung abnormality based on chest x-ray) and HRQOL scores from the SGRQ. The SGRQ results for the Libby cohort indicated significantly lower scores for HRQOL compared to healthy people and "appreciably worse than some persons with chronic obstructive pulmonary disease" (Winters et al., 2012, p. 8).

Next, the team applied three measures (Center for Epidemiological Studies-Depression Scale [CES-D]; Perceived Stress Scale [PSS]; and Acceptance of Illness Scale [AOI]) to determine the psychosocial health status (depression, stress, and acceptance of illness) of 386 CARD clinic clients. Results indicated "participants demonstrated moderate levels of stress and acceptance of illness however more than one-third (34.5%) had depression scores indicating a clinically significant level of psychological distress" (Weinert et al., 2011, p. 9). For the CARD/MSU research team, these findings pointed to the importance of caring for not just the physical/pulmonary health of citizens exposed to LAA but the emotional health needs as well. "Psychological distress identification, prevention, and intervention strategies, including self-management skills, are needed for persons exposed to environmental and workplace contamination such as the LAA disaster." (p. 9)

The final inquiry addressed the perceived satisfaction with access/financial aspects of care among the CARD clinic's local and distant clients. Two of seven subscales of the Medical Outcomes, Patient Satisfaction Questionnaire (PSQ-III) were used. The 12-item Access, Availability, and Convenience subscale measured perception of availability of medical resources, waiting times, and continuity of care. The Financial Aspects of Care subscale assessed perception of difficulty in paying for medical care (Ware & Hays, 1988). The two PSQ-III subscales were administered to 426 CARD clients during regular clinic visits. The research team concluded:

> The presence of the CARD clinic providing .... specialty care services may serve as a stopgap and somewhat of an equalizing factor for the provision of care to ... patients; however, when compared to persons with other chronic illnesses, the Libby cohort was significantly less satisfied with access and financial aspects of care. Among the Libby cohort, younger participants were less satisfied with access and financial aspects of care than older members, while exposure through a family member or household contact (versus other routes of exposure) and having a limited source of insurance .... resulted in the lowest scores on satisfaction with financial aspects of care. (Winters et al., 2011, p. 6)

In addition to a robust biopsychosocial description of a sample of CARD patients exposed to LAA, the three inquiries for Study 1 helped demonstrate the value and capability of the team to apply *scientific rigor* to community questions. At each stage of the research, *(identification of needs and resources, selection of tools and approaches, implementation, co-analysis of the results, dissemination, and reassessment needs for the next project)*, community members on the CAB and clinicians of the CARD clinic provided insight and an explanation of the meaning of the findings to the researchers.

Study 2

Study 1 set the stage for development of RPRM. Study 2 took the model to the next step by exploring "the community's history of asbestos-related research, community-based research infrastructure, and rural residents' views on and willingness to participate in research" (Winters, Kuntz, Weinert, & Black 2014,

p. 214). The case study investigation involved multiple data sources and a complex data management tracking system. The results were summarized based on four study propositions that related directly to issues raised by community members. The case study model was grounded in theory and advanced based on context and proposition development. Data were collected from a variety of archival sources (records, media, and meeting minutes) or generated from interviews and surveys as needed. The result (discovery) led to the case results and confirmation of RPRM key components.

The first proposition addressed community history and the erosion of trust that took place over a period of at least three decades. Early studies uncovered high mortality rates among mine workers and subsequently, family members who received secondary exposure to asbestos. When community environmental hazards are identified, decisions to remove the public from potential exposures often result in closing areas or moving people away from the hazard. However, in Libby, the EPA conducted the cleanup as citizens went about their daily lives. Communication conflicts between the public and scientific/technical experts, business, community, and political leaders and policymakers frequently resulted in skepticism, mistrust, and increased public wariness. The obstacles and stages of risk communication (Covello & Allen, 1988) provide credence to the value of reciprocal listening and consistent messaging since once *trust, respect, integrity/ authenticity, and communication* are lost, all are difficult to reclaim.

The second proposition involved the infrastructure to support communication and translation of research. A critical resource noted by community members is the CARD specialty clinic, which not only provides diagnostic and supportive care to clients but also serves as liaison and gatekeeper between the community and outside researchers. Rural nursing theory proved valuable in understanding the value of CARD as an internal resource to community members. *Characteristics of rural people* include "hardiness, self-sufficiency, independence, work oriented, distrusting of 'outsiders' and 'newcomers' and trustful and respectful of 'old timers' (people who have lived in the community for an extended period of time" (Long & Weinert, 1989; Winters et al., 2011, pp. 215–216). Trusted gatekeepers with insight into community characteristics, beliefs, and values are best suited to support communication and translation of research.

The third proposition identified divergent views related to communication resources including the most common, effective, trusted, and preferred methods for receiving research information (by community members) or transmitting study results (by researchers). Residents identified the local newspaper (72%) and the local radio station (61%) as the most common methods for learning about research. The most effective but least trusted communication source was "word of mouth" (67%, 50%). When researchers were asked this question, they named a different set of communication resources—scientific publications, public forums like CAG, or CARD-sponsored research rallies. This *dissemination* variation depicts an important cultural gap between residents and researchers that should be investigated and resolved with the help of the community liaison.

The fourth proposition highlighted the importance of community engagement factors and confirmed agreement between residents and researchers. Residents indicated they were more likely to participate in research if the research "was worthwhile (52%); helped the community (49%); benefitted their family (48%); or improved their healthcare (40%)" (Winters et al., 2011, p. 222). Researchers believed residents would be more likely to participate "if the research was perceived as having a potential to benefit participant health" (p. 223). A principal components analysis related to propositions three and four (communication and community engagement factors) examined "empirical dimensions of attitudes towards research participation including community engagement at a designated Superfund site" (Winters et al., 2016, p. 7). Principal components showed four dimensions of community members' attitudes toward research engagement: (a) researcher communication and contributions to the community, (b) identity and affiliation of the researchers requesting participation, (c) potential personal barriers, including data confidentiality, painful or invasive procedures, and effects on health insurance, and (d) research benefits for the community, oneself, or family.

Study 3

"The purpose of this study was to use existing documents (CAG meeting summaries) to identify concerns, perceptions, and communication preferences of rural Libby residents related to research and other issues critical to the community's health and well-being" (Blata-Pennock, 2010, p. 48). Qualitative results from analysis of 53 CAG meeting summaries identified critical *external forces* that impacted the community from 2001 to 2008 including political and economic impacts; governmental intervention by the EPA; external research funding; health issues; mine ownership litigation; federal asbestos and healthcare legislation; and public health emergency and Superfund designations. This study identified 11 primary information exchange topics that emerged from participants of CAG and were noted in the meeting summaries. Table 30.1 lists the topics, number of meeting summaries cited, and the associated citation percentages.

TABLE 30.1 Frequency of Primary Information Exchange Topics

Primary Information Exchange Topic	Number of Meeting Summaries Cited	Percentage of Meeting Summaries Cited
CAG purpose and process	24	45
Cleanup activities	51	96
Economy	23	43
Funding and finances	48	91
Government agency involvement	50	94
Health	43	81

(continued)

TABLE 30.1 Frequency of Primary Information Exchange Topics (*continued*)

Primary Information Exchange Topic	Number of Meeting Summaries Cited	Percentage of Meeting Summaries Cited
Litigation and legislation	25	47
Public health emergency designation	19	36
Research	40	75
Schools and children	33	62
Superfund designation	11	21

CAG, Community Advisory Group.

Source: Blata-Pennock, N. (2010). *Communication and information exchange in Libby, Montana: A secondary data analysis of community advisory group meeting summaries* (p. 50; MN thesis). Montana State University, Bozeman, MT.

Examples of *rural community characteristics* including independence/self-reliance, hardiness/resilience, distance/isolation, and insider/outsider perceptions are captured in comments from CAG community members (Blata-Pennock, 2010, pp. 86–88).

- Independence and self-reliance: "We need to continue working hard and persistently with the tools available to us. The heavens are not going to open and rain money on us" (p. 87).
- Hardiness and resilience: "As frustrating as things are, we should recognize how far we have come . . . It is important not to dwell on the negative" (p. 87).
- Distance and isolation: "Community isolation from specialty healthcare services . . . [caused concern] since the only pulmonologist that worked with the community [was retirement age]" (p. 87).
- Outsider/insider: "People in Libby have trust and confidence in the CARD clinic and willing to provide information to it. They may not be as willing to share their information with an outside university" (p. 88).

Study 3 confirmed and reinforced many of the RPRM concepts, especially precepts located in the outer circle of the model: *rural community characteristics, external forces, CBPR, and scientific rigor of research.*

CONCLUSION

The rural community of Libby, Montana was thrust into the national spotlight in the 1990s and, to this day, the population continues to deal with the sequelae and fallout of this technological, environmental disaster. The RPRM was developed to help guide researchers working with rural communities experiencing the ongoing effects of an environmental disaster. Although not specifically designed or patterned after logic-model metrics, the CARD/MSU team recognized the critical nature of inputs (knowledge of community history, patterns, and beliefs); activities and outputs conducted based on community member insights (meaningful research grounded on mutual respect, integrity/ authenticity, trust, and communication); a research plan with short-term and long-term outcomes (publishable scientific data that will lead to new knowledge and improved health outcomes for the population).

The RPRM may be used by research teams when conducting research within and with other rural communities, whether experiencing an environmental disaster or another type of event. Research in rural communities cannot be adequately conducted by the application of research models developed for urban or suburban areas, but requires unique approaches emphasizing the special needs of these communities and populations. Building upon the tenets of rural nursing theory and CBPR, the RPRM is well suited for research conducted in partnership with rural residents.

REFERENCES

Agency for Toxic Substances and Disease Registry. (2002). *Mortality in Libby, Montana (1979–1998)*. Retrieved from https://www.atsdr.cdc.gov/hac/pha/LibbyAsbestosSite/MT_LibbyHCMortalityRev8-8-2002_508.pdf

Agency for Toxic Substances and Disease Registry. (2003). *Public health assessment*. Retrieved from https://www.atsdr.cdc.gov/news/libby-pha.pdf

Amandus, H. E., Althouse, R., Morgan, W. K., Sargent, E. N., & Jones, R. (1987). The morbidity and mortality of vermiculite miners and millers exposed to tremolite-actinolite: Part III. Radiographic findings. *American Journal of Industrial Medicine, 11*(1), 27–37.

Amandus, H. E., Wheeler, R., Jankovic, J., & Tucker, J. (1987). The morbidity and mortality of vermiculite miners and millers exposed to tremolite–actinolite: Part I. Exposure estimates. *American Journal of Industrial Medicine, 11*(1), 1–14.

Blata-Pennock, N. (2010). *Communication and information exchange in Libby, Montana: A secondary data analysis of community advisory group meeting summaries* (MN thesis). Montana State University, Bozeman, MT.

Center for Asbestos Related Disease. (2017). CARD today. Retrieved from http://www.libbyasbestos.org/about-card

Covello, V., & Allen, F. (1988). The EPA's seven cardinal rules of risk communication. Retrieved from http://www.wvdhhr.org/bphtraining/courses/cdcynergy/content/activeinformation/resources/epa_seven_cardinal_rules.pdf

Jones, P. W., Quirk, F. H., Baveystock, C. M., & Littlejohns, P. (1992). A self-complete measure of health status for chronic airflow limitation. The St. George's Respiratory Questionnaire. *American Review Respiratory Disease, 145*(6), 1321–1327. doi:10.1164/ajrccm/145.6.1321

Long, K. A., & Weinert, C. (1989). Rural nursing: Developing the theory base. *Scholarly Inquiry for Nursing Practice, 3*(2), 113–127.

U.S. Census Bureau. (2010). Libby City, Montana. Retrieved from https://factfinder .census.gov/faces/nav/jsf/pages/community_facts.xhtml#

U.S. Department of Health & Human Services. (2009). EPA announces public health emergency in Libby, Montana. Retrieved from https://yosemite.epa.gov/opa/ admpress.nsf/bd4379a92ceceeac8525735900400c27/0d16234d252c98f9852575d800 5e63ac!opendocument

U.S. Environmental Protection Agency. (2003). ABCs of asbestos in schools. Retrieved from https://www.epa.gov/sites/production/files/documents/abcsfinal.pdf

U.S. Environmental Protection Agency. (2017). Libby site background. Retrieved from https://cumulis.epa.gov/supercpad/cursites/csitinfo.cfm?id=0801744

Ware, J. E. Jr., & Hays, R. D. (1988). Methods for measuring patient satisfaction with specific medical encounters. *Medical Care, 26*(4), 393–402.

Weinert, C., Hill, W. G., Winters, C. A., Kuntz, S. W., Rowse, K., Hernandez, T.,... Cudney, S. (2011). Psychosocial health status of persons seeking treatment for exposure to Libby amphibole asbestos. *ISRN Nursing, 2011.* doi:10.5402/2011/735936

Winters, C. A., Hill, W. G., Kuntz, S. W., Weinert, C., Rowse, K., Hernandez, T., & Black, B. (2011). Determining satisfaction with access and financial aspects of care for persons exposed to Libby amphibole asbestos: Rural and national environmental policy implications. *Journal of Environmental and Public Health, 2011,* 789514. doi:10.1155/2011/789514

Winters, C. A., Hill, W. G., Rowse, K., Black, B., Kuntz, S. W., & Weinert, C. (2012). Descriptive analysis of the respiratory health status of persons exposed to Libby amphibole asbestos. *BMJ Open, 2*(6). doi:10.1136/bmjopen-2012-001552

Winters, C. A., Kuntz, S. W., Weinert, C., & Black, B. (2014). A case study exploring research communication and engagement in a rural community experiencing an environmental disaster. *Applied Environmental Education & Communication, 13*(4), 213–226. doi:10.1080/1533015X.2014.970718

Winters, C. A., & Lee, H. S. (Eds.). (2010). *Rural nursing: Concepts, theory and practice* (3rd ed.). New York, NY: Springer Publishing.

Winters, C. A., Moore, C. F., Kuntz, S. W., Weinert, C., Hernandez, T., & Black, B. (2016). Principal components analysis to identify influences on research communication and engagement during an environmental disaster. *BMJ Open, 6*(8), e012106. doi:10.1136/bmjopen-2016-012106

Winters, C. A., Rowse, K., Kuntz, S. W., & Weinert, C. (2008). *The Libby Project.* Health Services and Resources Administration 1P20NR07790-01.

Yin, R. (2009). *Case study research: Design and methods* (4th ed.). Thousand Oaks, CA: Sage.

Index